Voice Disorders and their Management
Third Edition

Voice Disorders and their Management

Third edition

Edited by

MARGARET FREEMAN
DipLCST, MPhil, MRCSLT (Reg)
University of Sheffield

and

MARGARET FAWCUS
DipLCST, MSc, MRCSLT (Reg), FRCSLT
lately City University, London

W
WHURR PUBLISHERS
LONDON AND PHILADELPHIA

© 2000 Whurr Publishers Ltd
19b Compton Terrace, London N1 2UN, England and
325 Chestnut Street, Philadelphia PA 1906, USA

First published by Croom Helm Ltd 1986
Second edition published by Chapman & Hall 1991

British Library Cataloguing in Publication Data
A catalogue record for this book is available from the
British Library.

ISBN: 1 86156 186 5

Printed and bound in the UK by Athenaeum Press Ltd,
Gateshead, Tyne & Wear

Contents

Preface   ix
Preface to the second edition   xi
Acknowledgements   xii
Contributors   xiii

Chapter 1   **1**

The physiology of phonation
Robert Fawcus

Chapter 2   **18**

Voice development and change throughout the life span
Margaret Freeman

Chapter 3   **32**

Surgical management of laryngeal disorders
Andrew Johns

Chapter 4   **47**

The causes and classification of voice disorders
Margaret Fawcus

Chapter 5   **69**

The speech and language therapist's assessment of the dysphonic patient
Paul Carding

Chapter 6   89

Children with voice problems: a perspective on treatment
Moya Andrews

Chapter 7   110

Voice disorders associated with hyperfunction
Jennifer Oates

Chapter 8   137

Psychogenic, psychological and psychosocial issues in
diagnosis and therapy
Margaret Freeman

Chapter 9   156

Voice problems of speakers with dysarthria
Lorraine Ramig

Chapter 10   172

Vocal fold paralysis – paresis – immobility
Janina Casper

Chapter 11   192

Spasmodic dysphonia redefined: diagnosis, assessment and treatment
Renata Whurr

Chapter 12   219

Managing voice with deaf and hearing impaired speakers
Sheila Wirz

Chapter 13   234

Mutational disorders of voice
Robert Fawcus

Chapter 14   245

The voice of the transsexual
Judith Chaloner

Chapter 15   268

Post radiotherapy voice quality
Eva Carlson

Chapter 16   283

Voice care for the professional voice user
Stephanie Martin

Chapter 17   301

Phonosurgery
Marc Bouchayer and Guy Cornut

Chapter 18   319

The multidisciplinary voice clinic
Sara Harris, Tom Harris, Jacob Lieberman and Dinah Harris

References   340
Index   377

Preface to the third edition

Like the previous editions, this book contains contributions from clinicians who have special interest and expertise in voice disorders and their management. Again like the previous editions, the main aim of the book is to consider how current knowledge, research and practice can enable all voice care professionals to meet the needs of people with voice disorders.

In the introduction to the first edition, nearly fifteen years ago, Margaret Fawcus emphasized the need for changes in all aspects of diagnosis and management for voice disorders. At that time, laryngologists, therapists and other voice care workers generally had very little professional contact, and clinical diagnosis and therapy were predominantly based on perceptual judgements. Therapists placed great emphasis on the art of therapy, although, in some cases, the therapy for voice disorders did not match the theory. Margaret made a strong case for more rigorous approaches to diagnosis, better application of theory in practice and greater emphasis on the need to evaluate the efficacy of treatment methods.

The contributions to this new edition show that we are now addressing some of these key issues. Many more specialist voice clinics have been established, and the technology which enables us to evaluate many aspects of vocal dysfunction is available in the clinic, as well as in the research laboratories. There has also been a massive explosion of information about voice and voice disorders; research findings and clinical information on voice disorders can be found in a wide range of journals and books, as well as in the electronic media. Whereas we once had difficulties locating the occasional useful journal article, clinicians and students can now feel overwhelmed by the vast body of information on both diagnosis and treatment. At the same time, we know that many clinicians do not have (and some may be hoping to avoid!) access to the information superhighway or to computer-based equipment. Despite all the changes, it can still be difficult to see how theory and therapy come together for a particular patient in a specific clinical setting.

The aim of this book is to reflect on the developments that have taken place during the past ten years in some of the key areas of voice and voice therapy, and particularly to consider how they affect our work with our clients. Two strong themes are clearly identifiable in each chapter; the first is the recognition that vocal impairments can have significant social and psychosocial consequences. Many of the contributors have also addressed issues such as evidence-based practice, efficacy and the outcomes of intervention.

With each new edition of this book, the chapters have grown larger. Most of the original chapters in this volume have been rewritten or substantially updated, and some new chapters have been contributed by expert practitioners in the UK, the United States and Australia. This welcome sharing of international expertise has also meant that editorial decisions needed to be taken, and a small number of chapters from previous editions have been omitted. We hope, nevertheless, that we have produced a balanced volume which will continue to be a useful reference for all those who are involved in voice care.

Margaret Freeman
October 2000

Preface to the second edition

Since this book was first published, four years ago, there has been a considerable upsurge of interest in the field of both normal and abnormal voice production. Tangible evidence of this lies in the publication of the *Journal of Voice* in the United States, and in the UK, the formation of the British Voice Association. This organization has attracted an increasing membership from professionals involved in all aspects of voice care and use – actors and singers, laryngologists and speech therapists, teachers and phoneticians. The Association holds regular study days, holds an annual two-day symposium, and publishes a Newsletter which attracts entries from this broad spectrum of professionals.

We have also seen an increase in the number of specialist voice clinics, and in the two final chapters in this book a contrast is presented between a specialist setting and the more typical clinic that operates in the majority of general hospitals. The last chapter now contains a breakdown of referrals over an eight-year period, which must represent a unique published study in this country. There still remains, however, little research into the management of voice disorders. There is clearly a need for more efficacy studies into specific treatment methods, and the single case-study designs developed in aphasia would seem to be appropriate here.

Recent studies, notably from Japan and the United States, have continued to shed light on vocal fold structure and movement and the co-ordinated mechanisms of respiration and phonation. We have included a chapter on technical support in the management of dysphonia, reflecting the increasing sophistication of the instrumentation available for presenting objective data on normal and abnormal voice use.

Developments in the field of phonosurgery over the past few years have certainly justified the inclusion of a chapter on this increasingly specialist area of ENT management.

The majority of the original chapters have either been rewritten or updated, and we hope that this volume will continue to be a useful source of reference for all those involved, in one way or another, with voice care.

Margaret Fawcus

Acknowledgements

Many thanks are due to all the people who have helped with the completion of this edition. My warm thanks are especially due to Maggie for her tolerance and empathic support as I attempted to follow in her experienced editorial footsteps.

Each of the authors agreed to contribute to this edition with an enthusiastic readiness to share their knowledge and expertise. I would like to thank all of these people for the time and work that went into writing these thoughtful and informative chapters, despite their many other professional commitments. Thanks are also due to Colin Whurr and his staff for their sterling support in bringing the final product into production.

I also want to thank colleagues in the Department of Human Communication Sciences at the University of Sheffield, who have provided advice, friendship, academic and practical support in lots of ways during the writing and editorial process. Louise Turton deserves a special mention for her tremendous support with secretarial jobs. Finally, I want to say a special thank you to Peter Stubley for his love, encouragement and practical help with everything from computing to coffee, and to Lucy Stubley who has been remarkably tolerant of her mother's vagaries throughout the whole process.

Table 4.4 'Classification: after Verdolini', in the chapter by Margaret Fawcus, has been reproduced by kind permission of Katherine Verdolini and Singular Publishing Group, Inc.

Contributors

Moya Andrews, PhD, CCC-SLP is Professor of Speech and Hearing Services at Indiana University, Bloomington, Indiana, USA.

Marc Bouchayer, MD is Consultant ENT surgeon, Polyclinique des Minguettes, Venissieux, France.

Paul Carding, PhD, MRCSLT is Head of the Speech and Language Therapy Department at the Freeman Hospital and Senior Lecturer at the Medical School, Newcastle University, Newcastle upon Tyne, UK.

Eva Carlson, PhD, MRCSLT is Chief Speech and Language Therapist and Specialist in Voice at St Thomas's Hospital, London, UK.

Janina Casper, PhD, CCC-SLP is Associate Professor of Otology and Communication Sciences at the State University of New York Health Science Centre at Syracuse and has taught at Syracuse University, Syracuse, New York, USA.

Judith Chaloner, BA, MRCSLT was Specialist Speech and Language Therapist at the West Middlesex University College Hospital until her retirement in March, 1999. Judith ran group classes for male-to-female transsexuals at the Gender Identity Clinic, Charing Cross Hospital, London, UK for many years and is still involved in voice training for these clients.

Guy Cornut, MD is a phoniatrician in Lyon, France.

Margaret Fawcus MSc, MRCSLT, FRCSLT was formerly Reader in Clinical Communication Studies at City University, London, UK.

Robert Fawcus, BSc, MRCSLT, FRCSLT was formerly Professor in Clinical Communication Studies at City University, London and is now Consultant Speech and Language Therapist at the Nuffield Hospital in Tunbridge Wells, Kent, UK.

Margaret Freeman, MPhil, MRCSLT is lecturer in speech and language therapy in the Department of Human Communication Science, University of Sheffield, UK.

Dinah Harris, ARCM is a singing teacher and voice coach, part of the Voice Clinic Team at Queen Mary's Hospital, Sidcup, Kent, UK.

Sara Harris, MCSLT is Speech and Language Therapist and co-founder of the Voice Clinic Team at Queen Mary's Hospital, Sidcup, Kent, UK.

Tom Harris, MA, FRCS is Consultant Laryngologist in the Voice Clinic, Queen Mary's Hospital, Sidcup, Kent and at University Hospital, Lewisham, London, UK.

Andrew Johns, MA, FRCS is Consultant ENT Surgeon at the Kent County Ophthalmic and Aural Hospital, Maidstone, Kent, UK.

Jacob Lieberman, DO, MA is an osteopath and dynamic psychotherapist in the Voice Clinic at Queen Mary's Hospital, Sidcup, Kent, UK.

Stephanie Martin, MSc, MRCSLT is a part-time lecturer/clinical tutor at the University of Ulster and also works with student teachers at University of Greenwich, London, UK.

Jenni Oates, PhD, MAASH is Associate Professor in the School of Human Communication Sciences at La Trobe University, Melbourne, Australia.

Lorraine Ramig, PhD, CCC-SLP is Professor in the Department of Speech, Language, Hearing Sciences at the University of Colorado–Boulder, Colorado, USA and a Research Associate at the Wilbur James Gould Voice Research Centre of the Denver Centre for the Performing Arts.

Renata Whurr, PhD, MRCSLT is Senior Clinical Research Fellow in Speech and Language Therapy at the National Hospital of Neurology and Neurosurgery, Queen Square, London, UK.

Sheila Wirz, PhD, MRCSLT is Course Director of the MSc in Community Disability Studies for International Child Health, University College London, UK.

CHAPTER 1

The physiology of phonation

ROBERT FAWCUS

Introduction

The elaboration of phonatory behaviour observable in the processes of human communication demands levels of physiological complexity which generally exceed those encountered in any other species. This represents arguably the most advanced sensorimotor system to be found in the human organism. To divorce phonation from the function of articulation is, however, misleading and highly artificial. It is, in fact, the co-ordination of phonatory and articulatory behaviours which represents the advanced levels of evolutionary performance in perceptuomotor processing.

The basic process of phonation is well established and displays high levels of organization in many mammals and birds (Negus, 1949; Kirchener, 1988). In man, however, these activities have developed into a pattern of movements involving precise co-ordination of reflexive and learned behaviours resulting in accurate, intricate manoeuvres executed with flexibility and speed.

Lenneberg (1967) estimated that the production of a single phoneme could involve up to one hundred muscular contractions and adjustments. The majority of these adjustments form part of respiratory and phonatory activity, and the most subtle are those involving the complex lattice of intrinsic and extrinsic muscles of the larynx. In fluent speech this would represent over five hundred muscular adjustments per second within the speech tract. The control system specifications required to achieve the level of precision evident in even casual speech are quite beyond our imagination.

Respiratory studies

The primary source of power for phonation is derived from egressive respiratory air flow which is brought about by finely controlled contractions of the intercostal musculature. This contrasts markedly with the relatively passive process involved in quiet breathing (Widdicombe and Davies, 1983; Nunn, 1987). During speech the major contribution to the intake of air is achieved by contraction of the diaphragm, which produces a negative pressure in the thoracic cavity.

In shouting, singing or public speaking the intercostal musculature is also employed to provide greater levels of air intake to satisfy the increased rate of flow required to sustain vocal intensity (Bunch, 1982; Sundberg, 1987).

In their seminal study of electromyography of the respiratory system, Draper et al. (1960) showed the different functions of the external and internal intercostals. Figure 1.1 shows an oscillographic record of the repetition of the syllable [ma].

- The first trace provides a time marker in x seconds.
- The second shows a gradual decrease in the electrical activity of the external intercostals as each syllable is uttered.
- The third trace shows the acoustic signal derived from a microphone – a sequence of nine syllables.
- The fourth trace shows the gradual reduction in lung volume in the course of the utterance.
- The final trace indicates increasing activity in the internal intercostals. Electromyography of the respiratory musculature and other muscle systems in the speech tract usually requires the insertion of needle electrodes to detect electrical activity in individual muscles or small muscle groups. Surface electrodes pick up voltages from a range of contiguous muscles and therefore lack the precision afforded by needle electrodes.

Hixon and Weismer (1995) acknowledge the importance of this original study but make a number of severe criticisms of both the technique and the interpretation of the findings. They are concerned that the muscle tissue selected in the earlier study could not provide an adequate or valid representation of muscular function of the rib cage wall nor the abdominal musculature. They believe that the comparison of pleural pressure for speech production to alveolar pressure for relaxation is not meaningful. They contend that errors made in the Edinburgh study can explain the differences found in later studies at Harvard (c.f. Hixon et al., 1976).

Wilder (1983) and Baken (1987) discuss the findings yielded from pneumographic and related physiological studies of the contribution of the respiratory system to phonatory behaviour. Wilder investigated movements of the rib cage and abdominal wall using Whitney gauges and electronic spirometry and found that there were significant differences between the respiratory movements detectable in male and female subjects (Figure 1.2). Her findings supported earlier claims that there is a precisely preprogrammed adjustment of the chest wall immediately prior to phonation onset (Baken and Cavallo, 1981).

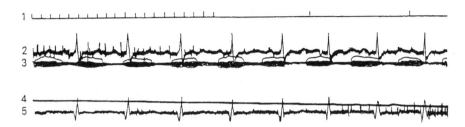

Figure 1.1 The electrical activity of several muscles of the chest during speech. The traces were recorded on an oscilloscope during the repetition of the syllable [ma] (1) time marker, seconds; (2) decreasing electrical activity of the external intercostals; (3) acoustic signal recorded by microphone; (4) volume of air in the lungs gradually decreasing; (5) increasing activity of the internal intercostals. (After Draper et al., 1960).

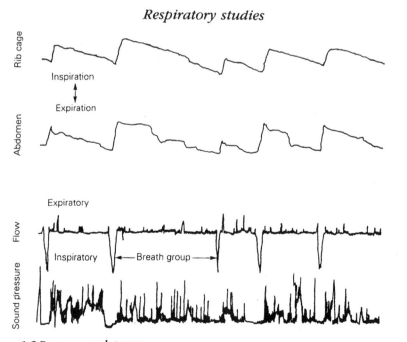

Figure 1.2 Pneumograph traces

A wide variety of pneumograph devices have been constructed in order to detect gross respiratory activity. They all require some form of transducer, usually a strain gauge, which converts the stretching of a belt placed around different levels of the thorax and abdomen into electrical signals that can be displayed and recorded. More accurate data may be obtained from a pneumotachograph, in which air flow is detected and measured during fluent speech or singing. This procedure requires the subject to wear a face mask, however, which increases the artificiality of the assessment.

Winkworth and Davis (1997) employed linearized magnetometers to study the strategies employed by a group of female speakers responding to variations in the intensity of background noise and found no consistent pattern of change in lung volume. McHenry et al. (1996) compared findings derived from tracheal puncture with indirect intra-oral measurements to investigate the accuracy of the latter in the determination of laryngeal airway resistance. Considerable variation was observed which brought into question the value of the less invasive technique.

Baken (1987) presents a meticulous examination of different methods of study of both respiratory and phonatory activities. He outlines the limitations and difficulties of each technique and provides examples of findings from a wide range of studies of both children and adults.

Laryngeal physiology – vegetative function

The primary purpose of the laryngeal mechanism is the protection of the airway to the trachea. The drainage of saliva and mucus from the oropharynx requires periodic reflexive closure to ensure the transfer of accumulated liquid to the oesophagus rather than the trachea, which would result in aspiration, with life-threatening consequences. Effort closure, which occurs during coughing, 'bearing down', and the fixation of the thorax during the lifting of heavy weights can involve a marked degree of muscular tension. Such closure can resist the maximal pressures generated in the thorax which is evident in the severe stutterer during a laryngeal block or the weight-lifter during a final effort. These pressures can reach levels in excess of 90 mmHg (Fink and Demarest, 1978).

Effort closure involves apposition of the cuneiform cartilages and vestibular folds, approximation of the thyroid cartilage and the hyoid bone with infolding of the aryepiglottic folds, and apposition of the median thyrohyoid fold to the lower part of the adducted vestibular folds. The closure which occurs during deglutition involves far less powerful contraction of the extrinsic and intrinsic laryngeal musculature. The co-ordination of laryngeal contractions and high thoracic pressures can result in linear velocities approaching the speed of sound when the pressure is abruptly released during coughing (Nunn, 1987).

Linguistic demands

Birds, cats, dogs, primates and other mammals display complex levels of respiratory and phonatory control to achieve communicative ends, but it is in the movement patterns of the human larynx where one can observe the level of physiological complexity which is characteristic of man's communicative behaviour. The achievement of an acoustic power source by means of driving a respiratory outflow through contracted sphincteric membranes is a basic feature of both mammalian and avian communication. Some birds produce patterns of considerable complexity which can closely resemble human musical utterances, while certain species of whales are noted for extended vocal output. In the human larynx the subtlety of the control available has been exploited in different ways by diverse language groups. The communication of meaning through tonal patterns in some African and Asian languages requires the precise tuning of laryngeal vibration with changes at each syllable boundary. This developmental skill tends to precede the associated articulatory patterns of the language even though the structure of syllables is generally less complex than typical Indo-European languages (Li and Thompson, 1978; Gandour et al., 1989). Similarly the child learning English, Russian or any other Indo-European language will normally learn to imitate the intonation patterns in his or her environment well before achieving accuracy in articulatory skills.

In Indo-European languages the patterns of intonation run in parallel with the structure of a sentence or phrase and are employed to convey emphasis, emotion, and overall meaning of an utterance. Speakers in tonal languages such as Cantonese employ meaningless 'tags', which are inflected to convey signals relating to emphasis and feelings (Ladefoged, 1983; Ladefoged et al., 1988).

In addition to this important demand for control of intonation, the laryngeal mechanism is employed to signal differences in intensity in order to impose patterns of rhythm and emphasis. Stress patterns are closely linked to variations in intonation in English and many other languages and these are brought about by precise adjustments of the internal intercostals.

The achievement of voiced–voiceless contrasts, the timing of aspiration, and voice onset all impose complex demands upon the function of the control system. To these must be added the requirement to produce glottal plosives and fricatives in many languages, and in some, such as

Vietnamese, phonatory quality changes that are used to convey meaning (Ladefoged, 1983; Ladefoged et al., 1988). It must not be overlooked that in the production of fluent speech the system needs to revert to vegetative respiratory function about ten times in every minute.

Phonatory registers

Modal

Three principal types of phonation are claimed to occur during fluent speech. Modal register, described by Hollien (1974), occurs most frequently in normal phonation and consists of a pattern of vocal cord closure in which the mass of the cords is brought together with sufficient stiffness to interrupt the pulmonary air flow briefly. This results in a train of glottal pulses which occur at about 100 Hz in adult males and in the region of 200 Hz in female adults and children.

Daniloff et al. (1980) provide a cogent description of the Bernoulli effect, which plays a vital role in modal phonation. The lower edges of the vocal folds are more compliant than the upper edges. As a result, air pressure rising below the vocal folds first pushes aside the lower edges. As the lower edges move aside, they drag the upper edges with them towards the glottal opening. Once the folds open, air begins to flow through the slit. Due to an aerodynamic coupling effect, as the upper fold edges move apart, the airflow and the Bernoulli drop in air pressure become very large in the region of the lower edges. Because of their greater compliance and the fact that the Bernoulli pressure drop is greatest at the bottom edge of the glottis, the lower vocal fold edges begin to move towards closure once again in advance of the stiffer upper edges that they pull along with them.

Glottal vibration generally does not begin with the vocal folds completely closed. Instead, the folds are brought towards the midline, but not fully closed. As air pressure rises, air flows through the small glottal opening. The Bernoulli drop in pressure causes the folds to move towards the midline. As the folds are pulled towards midline closure, elastic recoil increases and airflow is reduced. The folds recoil outward, airflow rises and the Bernoulli effect increases once again drawing the folds towards the midline. As momentum increases with each successive cycle of vibration, the vocal folds move nearer and nearer until they finally achieve closure.

Wyke (1983a) describes a prephonatory inspiratory phase that occurs prior to each sequence of speech. The vocal cords are rapidly abducted and remain so until completion of an ingressive air flow, which provides the volume of air required for the ensuing utterance. Simultaneously the body of the larynx descends slightly in relation to the extent of the inspiratory tidal volume.

This process, he explains, is accomplished by simultaneous bilateral activation of a large proportion of neurons in the motor neuron pools serving the posterior cricoarytenoid muscles. These pools are located in the nucleus ambiguus in the medulla. At the same time the adductors of the vocal folds relax as a result of coincident inhibition of their motor neurons. The descent of the larynx referred to above results partly from the elastic traction applied from the trachea and in part from reflex augmented motor unit activity in the sternothyroid muscles.

Wyke then outlines the prephonatory expiratory phase which is subsequently initiated. This involves relaxation of the previously contracted diaphragm and inspiratory intercostal muscles, permitting recoil of the stretched elastic tissues of the lungs and chest wall. This process is supplemented by augmented motor unit activity in the abdominal and expiratory intercostal muscles. The cortically evoked motor unit activity in the posterior cricoarytenoid muscles is abruptly (but only briefly) switched off, while corticobulbar activation of the vocal fold adductor motor neurons is switched on. Wyke's description of the neural and muscular events occurring in a few hundred milliseconds at the junction of every breath group does not include the important differences due to the presence or absence of voicing required at the beginning of the ensuing syllable. Neither does it consider the influence of articulatory activities of the larynx in the production of the glottal stop or a variety of glottal fricatives.

Hollien (1983) discusses the contribution of both radiographic studies and electromyographic investigations to our understanding of the mechanisms underlying the control of vocal frequency. He concludes that frequency control is mediated by variation in vocal fold mass and stiffness plus changes in subglottal air pressure. He considers that vocal fold mass and stiffness plus the impedance to respiratory air flow in the glottis appear to vary as a consequence of changes in laryngeal physiology, which include variation in vocal cord length. Such variation, he suggests, results from at least two mechanisms.

The primary system (said to 'stretch' the vocal folds which have previously been shortened for phonation) results from contraction of the cricothyroid muscles. In turn these contractions operate to lengthen the vocal folds by increasing the distance between the thyroid cartilage and the vocal processes of the arytenoids. A second mechanism which functions to elongate the folds is one resulting from anteroposterior movement of the arytenoids – events that are mediated by co-ordinated activity among the interarytenoid and posterior cricoarytenoid muscles.

This secondary process is most often seen to occur for the higher frequencies within the modal register.

Hollien prefers the term stiffness to muscle tension, as he considers the latter is non-specific and rarely properly defined. He also emphasizes that the vocal folds are not in fact 'stretched' during phonation, as they are in fact longest during respiratory activity and are shortened for all types of phonation.

Pulse register

Creak, known in the United States as glottal fry, was termed 'pulse register' by Hollien (1974) in his attempt to clarify terminology. It is a form of phonation that occurs in almost every utterance in some speakers. It can occur to a greater or lesser extent in individuals according to mood, level of fatigue, or even degree of misuse of the laryngeal system. It occurs at lower frequencies than modal voice and is characterized by a relatively random rate of vibration in comparison with the high degree of consistency evident in normal modal phonation. McGlone (1967, 1970) found significantly lower flow rates in speakers using pulse register at a comfortable intensity. The air flow for males producing vowels with pulse register ranged between 10 and 72 ml/s. Females producing similar phonation used from 2 to 63 ml/s. Creaky voice is a mixture of modal and pulse register (Table 1.1.).

Table 1.1 Mean air flow in modal and pulse registers in normal males*

Register	F_o (Hz)		Flow (ml/s)	
	Mean	Range	Mean	Range
Modal	107.9	87–117	142.2	74.9–267.8
Pulse	34.4	18–65	40.4	0.0[†]–145.3

* Nine young adult males † Indicates a flow too small to be measured

Loft Register

The third type of phonation occurring in normal speech, but tending to be rarer than pulse register, is commonly described as falsetto. Fawcus (1991) described the range of human vocal activities in which 'loft register' is typically observed. These include the singing of the counter-tenor or male alto, and many types of popular singing styles from the traditional Irish tenor to the Beach Boys. War cries in many cultures, including the shouting of orders on the military parade ground, frequently include an element of loft register, as do gentler activities such as yodelling, giggling, laughing, and the upper ranges of intonation in many male adults (Van Riper and Irwin, 1958).

McGlone (1970) studied air flow during phonation in eight college-age women who sustained a vowel for 4 s at 10% of their intensity range and also 10% of their pitch range while using loft register. Flow rate was derived by dividing the volume of air used by the duration of phonation (Table 1.2).

Table 1.2 Mean air flow in the loft register: females (ml/s)

Intensity level (percentage intervals)	Pitch level (percentage intervals)									Mean for intensity level
	10	20	30	40	50	60	70	80	90	
10	92.4	96.9	91.7	87.8	100.8	132.8	130.7	121.9	131.8	109.6
20	121.1	120.6	114.4	123.4	133.9	149.2	154.4	151.8	158.6	136.4
30	162.0	158.6	138.0	154.2	144.3	165.6	167.2	159.1	180.2	158.8
40	185.7	187.8	177.3	164.6	148.7	183.3	169.5	173.9	186.1	175.2
50	208.9	200.5	174.2	203.1	179.4	184.1	198.4	182.0	188.5	191.0
60	207.5	217.4	183.9	216.4	188.8	200.5	227.8	190.1	188.8	202.4
70	242.4	232.0	194.3	224.5	205.5	220.6	229.7	215.2	206.2	218.9
80	239.8	240.4	211.5	246.4	202.6	237.8	242.2	223.1	216.4	228.9
90	266.4	249.7	223.9	249.0	198.4	232.9	268.7	213.3	224.0	236.3
Mean for pitch level	191.8	189.8	167.7	185.5	166.9	189.6	198.7	181.2	186.7	

From McGlone (1970). Reprinted by permission

Hirano (1975, 1982) presented electromyographic evidence on the activity of the phonatory musculature during the transition between different registers in singing. In speech the transitions are usually much faster and, although frequent, are rarely deliberately undertaken. The spectrographic and simultaneous laryngographic record (Figure 1.3) shows the shift from loft register through modal into pulse within 300 ms in a single syllable 'you'.

Vilkman et al. (1995) introduced the concept of a 'critical mass' in an attempt to explain register transitions. They employed electroglottography and inverse filtering of the acoustic output from male and female subjects who had different levels of training in singing. All subjects were able to achieve an abrupt register shift from soft falsetto to soft modal phonation. They report that the differences between the male and female subjects on the EGG waveforms were smaller than anticipated.

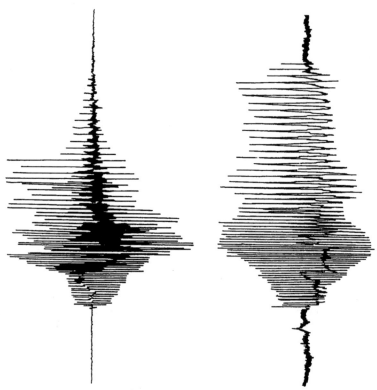

Figure 1.3 Laryngeal control mechanisms

We think that eliciting and sustaining a chest register phonation calls not only for contact between the vocal folds or vocal processes as stated by Titze (1988) but also for a powerful enough collision between the vibrating folds in the vertical and longitudinal dimensions.

They discuss observations of vibrations on the skin in the laryngeal region using holographic interferometry and consider that the mucosal wave on the upper surface of the vocal folds during modal phonation is a further sign of the tissue deformation caused by collision.

Laryngeal reflex mechanisms

Wyke (1983b) provides further information regarding reflexogenic contributions to the control of phonatory behaviour. He describes three sets of low-threshold mechanoreceptors which are embedded in the subglottic mucosa, muscle tissue, and laryngeal joint capsules. Afferent discharges from these receptors are relayed via the laryngeal nerves to the brain stem motor neuron pools serving the laryngeal musculature upon which they exert reciprocally co-ordinated facilitatory and inhibitory influences. He goes on to describe a further three types of extrinsic modulatory reflexogenic system situated in pulmonary tissues, and a final one, the cochleolaryngeal, which, when stimulated, results in facilitation of laryngeal adductor motor neurons.

Histological studies of the structure of the vocal folds

The major contribution of Hirano (1977, 1981) to our understanding of the cellular structure of the vocal folds has introduced a completely new dimension to studies of normal and pathological patterns of phonatory behaviour. Hirano and his colleagues have described a five-layered structure (Figure 1.4, see p. 12):

1. A surface of squamous cell epithelium which has been described as a thin stiff capsule whose purpose is to maintain the shape of the vocal fold.
2. Lying below the epithelium there is a superficial layer of the lamina propria consisting of a matrix of loose fibrous components not unlike a mass of soft gelatin.
3. The intermediate layer of the lamina propria consists chiefly of elastic fibres and has been likened by Hirano to a bundle of soft rubber bands.
4. The deep layer of the lamina propria consists primarily of collagenous fibres and has been compared to a bundle of cotton thread.
5. Finally the body of the vocalis muscle makes up the bulk of the vocal fold and is said to be similar to a bundle of rather stiff rubber bands.

The physiology of phonation

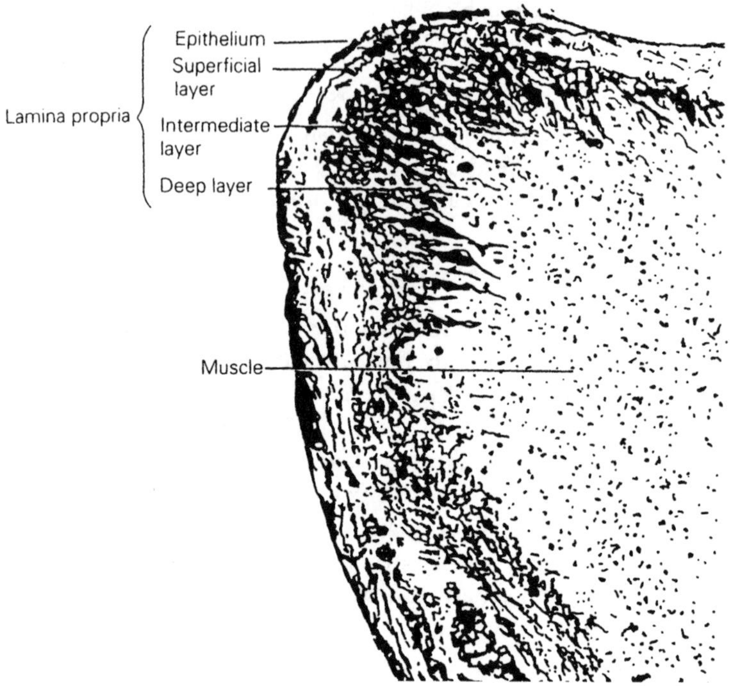

Figure 1.4 Frontal section of a human vocal fold through the middle of the membranous portion (Hirano, 1981).

Hirano has further simplified the concept of the layered folds by referring to a mechanical classification consisting of a cover containing the epithelium and the superficial layer of the lamina propria, the transition consisting of the vocal ligament – the intermediate and deep layer of the lamina propria, and the body constituting the vocalis muscle. Hirano's studies have also involved examination of the different roles of pairs of muscles within the larynx. Table 1.3 summarizes the functions of the muscles in vocal fold adjustments.

Hammond et al. (1997) used electron microscopy to investigate the morphology of the lamina propria because of its vital importance in the production of voice. They were particularly concerned with two of the prime constituents, elastin and hyaluronic acid.

Previous studies had determined that the human lamina propria comprised mainly fibroblasts and matrix substances secreted by these cells including glycosaminoglycans, proteoglycans and fibrous proteins including collagen and elastin. Other constituents included capillaries,

Table 1.3 Functions of muscles in vocal fold adjustments

	CT	VOC	LCA	IA	PCA
Position	Paramed	*Adduct*	*Adduct*	*Adduct*	*Abduct*
Level	Lower	Lower	*Lower*	0	*Elevate*
Length	*Elongate*	*Shorten*	Elongate	(Shorten)	*Elongate*
Thickness	*Thin*	*Thicken*	Thin	(Thicken)	Thin
Edge	*Sharpen*	*Round*	Sharpen	0	Round
Muscle (body)	*Stiffen*	*Stiffen*	Stiffen	(Slacken)	Stiffen
Mucosa (cover and transition)	*Stiffen*	*Slacken*	Stiffen	(Slacken)	Stiffen

0 = no effect; ( ) = slightly; italics = markedly; CT = cricothyroid muscle; VOC = vocalis muscle; LCA = lateral cricoarytenoid muscle; IA = interarytenoid muscle; PCA = posterior cricoarytenoid muscle. From Hirano (1981)

nerves and macrophages. Elastin is found in three distinct forms in the lamina propria and hyaluronic acid is one of the major glycosaminoglycans (GAGs) encountered in biological systems. GAGs are hydrophylic molecules that are relatively inflexible. This gives them their 'space filling' characteristic through gel formation.

The lamina propria was shown to consist of three distinct layers and although the quantities of elastin were not gender specific there was a significant difference between males and females in the proportion of hyaluronic acid. They conclude that the consequent extra hydration of the male vocal fold would make it morphologically distinct. Swelling involved in injury is related to a build-up and secretion of hyaluronic acid and the presence of greater quantities of this substance in the male vocal fold could explain the lower incidence of vocal fold nodules in men.

Laryngeal neuromuscular activity

Faaborg-Anderson (1957) presented the results of his studies of laryngeal myography having inserted needle electrodes in the intrinsic laryngeal musculature via the oral cavity and further transcutaneous electrodes in the cricothyroid muscles via cervical tissues. Hirano (1981) comments that this approach led to difficulties in achieving normal phonation and this restricted its use in clinical examination.

Hirano and Ohala (1967) extended earlier Japanese work (Hiroto et al., 1962) and reported the successful insertion of hooked wire electrodes into the major intrinsic laryngeal musculature. Hirose (1971) modified their technique and inserted needles into the cricothyroid space, through submucous tissue into the vocalis muscle, avoiding the need to pass through the subglottic space. In order to insert electrodes into the posterior cricoarytenoid and interarytenoid muscles, Hirose employed the peroral route.

Theories of vocal fold function

The late 1950s saw the elaboration of a number of theories of vocal fold function, some highly controversial. Husson and his collaborators had worked in Paris for over 20 years and proposed a revolutionary neurochronaxic theory, which suggested that achievement of phonatory frequency was dependent upon direct cortical control rather than being purely the result of the interaction of air flow, the gestures of the vocal folds, and auditory feedback (Husson 1953, 1957, 1962). Van den Berg (1958) strongly rejected this theory and propounded the myoelastic-aerodynamic theory, which has been the most commonly accepted view of laryngeal function for the past quarter of a century. The most graphic form of his attack came in a film he made showing phonatory activity in an excised human larynx. By reversing the sequence of dissection in the film he was able to show a larynx constructed piece by piece from cartilages and muscles and finally able to vibrate in an artificial air stream without any neuromotor input. The muscles were contracted by means of externally applied tension (Van den Berg et al., 1960).

Lecluse (1977), also working in Holland, compared electroglottograms derived from living human subjects with those from a series of excised larynges, and found consistencies between the results when air was pumped through the laryngeal preparations. The vocal cords were mounted between two clamps and a force transducer achieved either slow or rapid extension of the vibrating structures.

Smith (1954, 1957) put forward the membrane-cushion (mucosamuscle) theory to explain the vertical phase difference between the upper and lower borders of the vocal fold margins. He employed high-speed film pioneered by Bell Laboratories, laryngeal stroboscopy, and observation of ingenious rubber models of the vocal cords.

Stevens (1977, 1988) postulated that the phase difference could be explained by a two-mass mechanical model of the vocal folds, and this has been developed by Titze (1981) and Ishizaka (1981) in the form of kinetic descriptions derived from computer simulations. Hirano et al. (1974), Hirano (1982) and Hirano et al. (1988) have elaborated the 'body-cover' structure of the vocal folds and its mechanical contribution to phonatory physiology. Their findings tend to support Smith's membrane-cushion theory and are derived from both histological and physiological evidence. Austin and Titze (1997) and Scherer et al. (1997) have tested these theories by means of physiological experiments and have now extended the studies into potential clinical applications.

Physiological studies in the management of dysphonia

The physiological processes underlying the production of normal voice and singing have received considerable international attention over the past three decades, and our knowledge and understanding are growing rapidly. Scant attention has so far been paid to the physiological study of dysphonia, but important work is in progress in Japan, the United States, and Europe, which is beginning to provide a firm scientific basis for the assessment and management of disorders of voice.

It must be emphasized that these studies cannot be confined to the realm of physiology because this would ignore the important contribution of anatomical, acoustic, clinical, and psychological investigations. To date the overwhelming majority of studies of laryngeal function and dysfunction have taken place in a few specialized laboratories in the United States, Japan and Europe, and there has been a strong tendency for medical interests to dominate the investigations. The task of the voice therapist is to bring together these diverse factors, to establish a working hypothesis, and to devise regimes that will facilitate efficient and effective voice use.

It is noteworthy that the first two major steps in the study of phonation came from a singing teacher in London (Garcia, 1855) and a century later from a biological physicist in Lille (Fabre, 1957). More recently the work of Hirano and associates shifted the focus of laryngeal physiology to Japan and firmly into the medical field. Studies in the US, Australia and Europe are showing increasing collaboration between surgeons, voice scientists and speech and language pathologists.

Three major levels of physiological investigation have a bearing on the clinical management of disorders of phonation. Few clinics have the time, the staff, or the technical resources to attempt most of the investigations reported in current literature, even in the countries where considerable developments have taken place. This does not mean that laboratory-based physiological studies are irrelevant to the everyday problems faced by the therapist working with dysphonic patients, but merely underlines the differences between the levels of resource that are both practical and accessible. The top-flight laboratory capable of employing medical staff, physiologists, specialists in acoustic phonetics, and therapists skilled in the assessment and management of patients with phonatory disorders is likely to be a rare phenomenon in any country. The hardware alone would prove to be a prohibitive requirement, and yet most developed countries have at least one centre that approximates to this model. The most frequent manifestation is, however, a less formal arrangement involving co-operation between different interested departments in a university setting.

The voice clinic (see Harris et al., Chapter 18, this volume) represents an intermediate level of activity. Both accounts, however, describe features which clearly converge with the first level. The more typical voice clinic would rarely offer physiological investigations as a routine, and accompanying acoustic analysis would probably be even less common. Advances in microprocessor-based assessment techniques, particularly non-invasive procedures, should lead to wider availability of measurement, display and analysis of physiological and acoustic phenomena.

In a study at the Royal National Throat, Nose and Ear Hospital, London, it was found that the proliferation of data acquisition devices interfered significantly with the normal running of the clinic and placed greater demands on the patient than could be reasonably justified. The principal mode of investigation was by means of a flexible or rigid fibreoptic endoscope connected to a miniature videocamera. The image of the laryngeal structures could be displayed on a large monitor and was recorded by means of a video cassette recorder. The addition of a microphone enhanced the procedure, but when we started to introduce laryngograph electrodes we were clearly at times stretching patient co-operation to its limits.

While some patients approach the situation with confidence and even enthusiasm, a large number find the technology baffling and even threatening. The laryngograph electrodes are non-invasive but can be the object of considerable suspicion and concern for a patient who is already finding the endoscopy something of an ordeal. Our original intention was to employ both the laryngograph and air-flow monitoring transducers, but there is no satisfactory means available at the present time that would allow air-flow measurement to occur simultaneously with the insertion of a nasoendoscope.

For the voice therapist working in a hospital clinic the detection of laryngeal vibration by means of a laryngograph, with the possible addition of air-flow measurement and acoustic analysis, can greatly enhance the initial assessment of the patient. The possibilities for recording and analysing progress as well as providing appropriate feedback are now well established. Because of limited resources in the field such facilities continue to be rare in the United Kingdom.

The Laryngograph (Abberton and Fourcin, 1984; Abberton et al., 1989) and the IBM Phonetic Workstation (Trudgeon et al., 1988) provide a tangible means to achieve more objective and effective monitoring of dysphonic patients, as both provide for simultaneous recording of a range of acoustic and physiological parameters. The inclusion of techniques for analysis of the recorded data means that for the first time a voice therapist has the opportunity to base therapy on hard evidence rather than subjective impressions.

McGlashan and colleagues have investigated the development of a stereoscopic laryngostroboscope connected to a powerful computer which was capable of providing modelling of the vocal folds and precise measurements of both structures and lesions (Bootle et al., 1998). The timing of the strobe was derived from a PCLX. The system offers considerable possibilities for the study of both normal function and the analysis of phonatory disorders.

Crary et al. (1996) report on their use of dynamic Magnetic Resonance Imaging to investigate the configuration of the vocal tract in both normal subjects and a group of patients with spasmodic dysphonia. Measurements of laryngeal height and pharyngeal constriction were obtained in both groups during simple phonatory tasks. MRI is developing rapidly and promises to provide a valuable means of studying transient movements of the vocal mechanism.

Such developments represent the achievement of a third level of physiological investigation which will provide important benefits for the patient as well as underpinning much needed research. Baken (1987) describes the full scale of the currently available armamentarium of the voice therapist. He emphasizes, however, that none of the procedures individually or in combination can achieve a diagnosis 'that can be arrived at only on the basis of all the evidence – biological, physical, psychological and social – as interpreted by a professional who is well versed in theory and has wide ranging knowledge of how speech is produced'.

Damste (1983), having made considerable contributions to our knowledge of the physiological processes in phonation and pseudophonation, reminds his colleagues:

> In physiology we rarely discuss feelings; it is a hazardous subject we like to avoid because emotions cannot be quantified. However, since the voice is a very direct interpreter of feelings and a show window of emotional states, in any complete discussion of voice it is necessary to spend some time analysing the relation between feelings and voice.

When we understand more about the interrelationship between the physiological processes underlying learning and behaviour and the complex role of the emotions, we will begin to have greater insight into the process of phonation and the ways in which it can deteriorate in the dysphonic patient. More and more studies of vocal pathology are appearing which include a significant element of physiological evidence in the assessment of phonatory dysfunction and examination of the effects of intervention.

CHAPTER 2

Voice development and change throughout the life span

MARGARET FREEMAN

Introduction

The birth cry announces a child's arrival to the world. We can view this event from several different perspectives. Biologically, the birth cry is an audible indicator that the neonate's lungs and larynx are working, but like most of the neonate's early cries, it is an involuntary, whole body reaction. Acoustically, this a short, shrill utterance of around 500 Hz (Sataloff, 1991). From the perspective of communication, even though the new-born infant is not intentionally transmitting vocal messages, the listener's response and interpretation helps to set up a sequence of events which will eventually lead to spoken language (Locke, 1995). This is accomplished with little conscious awareness that we are developing a complex skill. Rather, the way we sound as adults

> is largely the result of speaking the same way, day after day, over a period of years. If you were lucky enough to develop a good-sounding voice, the luck was related to your having normal vocal equipment – lungs, vocal cords, throat, tongue, jaw, teeth, sinuses – plus being able to use this equipment in an easy, natural way (Boone, 1991, p. 2).

Biolinguists would argue that our vocal development is not just a question of luck. Our habitual vocal pattern is shaped by our social and cultural interactions and communication needs and uses, as well as by our individual anatomical and physiological characteristics. As we have learned more about the early stages of language development, it has become apparent that much of the motor control for speech, language and voice is at least primed, if not established, during the first two years of life (Studdert-Kennedy, 1991; Pinker, 1994; Locke, 1995). Morrison and Rammage (1994) also consider that control of voice is a skilled motor activity, but point out that it is highly probable that there are individual variations in the degree of mastery of this skill. A relatively small number of people make up the 'vocal elite', who seem to have naturally excellent vocal technique and may pursue 'vocally athletic careers without being trained or coached'. At the other end of the spectrum are the 'vocal yokels', that is, people whose 'vocal techniques are marginally adequate to get through the day' (Morrison and Rammage, 1994, p.113).

Most of the chapters in this book focus on people who are not quite so skilled with their use of voice, or for some reason the voice has caused them enough concern that they have sought help from doctors and voice therapists. Our clients often tell us that their vocal limitations have had quite a major impact on their day-to-day lives (Andrews, 1995; Smith et al., 1996). Before the voice changed, it had been taken for granted and was simply part of themselves; as a result of the voice problem, they may not be recognized by their vocal characteristics. People close to them cannot be so certain about the inferences we usually make about moods, emotions and physical health from the 'sound of the voice' (Scherer, 1995). Andrews (1995) reminds us that almost 40% of any verbal message comes from the vocal features. We all tend to make judgements about others, from our peers to politicians and people in the media, as a result of our social knowledge of vocal styles and stereotypes (Linville, 1996). This emphasizes the dual role of phonation. On the one hand, vocal features are part of the complex matrix of social behaviours which facilitate verbal and non-verbal communication; on the other, they are a product of biological function and, as such, will develop and change throughout our lives (Colton and Casper, 1996).

This chapter explores how vocal skills develop and change in relation to physical development and maturation, and in the more general context of social communication. For simplicity, the information is presented as a series of stages, but in reality, most people's voices follow the same gradual transition through each phase of lives, with moment-by-moment changes as well as those which are longer term (Colton and Casper, 1996). The aim of the chapter is to provide background information on normal development, which is an essential baseline for our understanding of voice disorder.

The neonate

A newborn human infant's vocal tract is initially quite different from that of its parents; in fact, there is more similarity between human neonates and adult primates than with adult humans (Lieberman, 1984). The neonate's tongue, for example, is positioned fully in the mouth; the larynx is high under the chin, almost underneath the back of the tongue (Sataloff, 1991). As the neonate swallows, the larynx can move vertically in the neck and during swallowing, it is tucked close to the back of the tongue, so that the airway is protected from liquids. Human infants, like primates, can breathe and swallow simultaneously (Laitman et al., 1977). In the early months of life, the infant's capacity for sound variations is limited by this anatomical 'safety device', but within three months the proportions will change as the baby grows. The larynx separates from the hyoid bone and begins a gradual descent from its original position, where it was parallel with the third and fourth cervical vertebrae. At five years, the vocal folds are typically parallel with the fifth cervical vertebra, and by age 20, they are closer to C7. As the dimensions of the vocal tract change, the potential for sound variation increases.

Despite the limited anatomical potential for sound variations in the first few weeks of life, newborn infants are active communicators. Although the birth cry is usually the first example of 'audible output' from a new baby, there are some reports of infants being heard to cry while 'still encapsulated' (Locke, 1995) in the birth canal. Locke (1995) suggests that these relatively rare examples of *vagitis uterinus* (Blair, 1965; Thiery et al., 1973) probably occur as a result of unusual conditions, but he cites them 'to reinforce the point that vocal experience may begin somewhat before "common sense" would have us believe' (Locke, 1995, p.133).

The evidence from child language research suggests that the foetus can hear parental voice *in utero*, so that a newborn infant is already tuned into voice and spoken language (DeCasper and Spence, 1986; Moon and Fifer, 1990). This may be the reason why newborn infants seem to respond more readily to the voices of their mothers and fathers within two days of birth (Fifer and Moon, 1989; Moon and Fifer, 1990) and show preferences for speech, rather than non-speech sounds (Eimas et al., 1971). Whatever the reasons, there is ample evidence that newborns tend to seek out and respond actively to voices and faces (Locke, 1995). Studies of carer–infant interaction have demonstrated that the infant's vocalizations are encouraged by faces that are smiling and by eyes that are looking into the baby's face. This led Sherrod (1981) to suggest that parents are not only caregivers and attachment figures, but are also part of the physical stimulus for communication development. As Locke (1995) points out, we can view the neonate's vocalizations as a means of setting up the stimulation they need for their vocal and linguistic development as well as a means of communication and bonding with his or her parents.

From vocalizations to spoken language

Young infants produce an extensive range of sounds. Although early sounds such as vegetative noises and crying may be involuntary, the sound inventory tends to move rapidly to include comfort and discomfort sounds and other vocalic utterances. Locke (1995) cites work that suggests that even within the first days of life, babies respond differently to replays of their own vocalizations, in comparison with sounds played from other newborns, and to other forms of feedback (Martin and Clark, 1982). This and other work (Eimas et al., 1971) indicate that infants have not only a capacity for discrimination of vocal sounds, but also some capacity for self-monitoring. In the early stages, the quality and quantity of vocalization tends to increase when their mother is nearby, even when compared to the presence of other adults (Tulkin, 1973; Delack, 1976). Between six and eight weeks, babies begin to produce quieter, lower pitched and more musical sounds, often in response to parental smiles and speech (Crystal, 1987).

By four to five months, infants can produce speech-like vocalizations similar to those of adults talking to them face-to-face (Kuhl and Meltzoff, 1988; Legerstee, 1990), which suggests that visible articulation and audible structure are beginning to be linked in the brain (Locke, 1995). Crying tends to decrease and the frequency of vocalizations increase (Lewis, 1969). Strings of sounds can be produced, although they are not produced rhythmically and lack intonation contours. Babies also begin to chuckle and laugh around this stage. Lip and tongue movements appear, in co-ordination with vocal fold activity. This seems to reflect both increased motor skill (Boliek et al., 1996) and self-monitoring. By nine months of age, most infants have some fairly clearly differentiated types of vocalizations, some of which seem to have deliberate communicative intent. D'Odorico (1984), for example, identified different patterns of 'call signs' associated with different contexts, which evoked different responses from the mother. As well as signalling intention, infants in the latter part of their first year begin to engage in active vocal play, with repetitions of consonant and vowel-like sequences, often starting at a high pitch and gliding down to lower pitches. Reduplicated babbling is followed by varie-gated babbling, with a movement towards the sound of the family's language. By the end of the first year, melody, rhythm and tone of voice are beginning to emerge. Parents can recognize the utterance patterns associated with questioning, wanting and greeting; the vocal games and rituals developed between parents and child show distinctive melodies (Crystal, 1987).

Locke (1995, p. 208) suggests that babbling is a 'working vocal guidance system...in which the ear monitors vocal tract activity and informs speech–motor control systems about targets and adjustments needed for mimicry of ambient speech'. This enables the child to develop mastery of the breath control, laryngeal activity and strings of articulatory movements which they will need to produce speech and speech-like utterances. By the end of the first year of life, the infant's vocal features, including fundamental frequency range, begin to gravitate towards the main language spoken around him/her (Boysson-Bardies et al., 1989; 1992).

Overall, the evidence from studies of early child language development suggests that babbling is a multi-function activity. For many parents, babbling is a form of speech (Locke, 1995), because at least some of it can communicate information about the child's focus of attention, mood and emotion. But most children also babble when they are alone, which tends to suggest that the activity is pleasurable *per se*. Locke (1995), like many others (Lewis, 1936; Crystal, 1981), points out that although infants may simply babble because they enjoy it, the vocal play itself helps to establish the neural integration of motor activity with auditory, tactile and kinaesthetic sensory feedback loops. The infant develops sound control and motor activity gradually, but not completely, during the first three years (Kent, 1976; Netsell, 1981; Boliek et al., 1996,1997).

Many different elements play their part in vocal learning. Some of this can be described as *vocal accommodation* (Locke, 1995, p.149), which comes from the interactions between the child and his/her caregivers; this includes vocal turn-taking and imitation by both partners. When the child begins to use words, it is clear that imitation plays a major role in the mastery of phonology, but Pawlby (1977), for example, showed that a large proportion of phonetic imitation between mother and child comes from the parent! By the time a child has an overt vocabulary of twenty words, he or she is also producing disyllabic stress patterns and is beginning to produce syllables that have the acoustic characteristics of adult-like speech, showing that they have at least primitive control over the vocal tract articulators (Boysson-Bardies et al., 1989; 1992). Locke (1995) suggests that this is *topographical learning* (p. 168), that is, being able to perceive differences between the sounds the child hears and can produce and moving to develop the articulatory control required to achieve more adult-like patterns. Although few parents give 'voice lessons', children gain some knowledge of the 'rules' of voicing through deduction and some through feedback from themselves and others as they try out their speech and language production. Although it has often been said that voice is an innate human characteristic, it is clear that a lot of learning goes into the mastery of the skills of vocal use – and some indication that the foundations of this skill development are built through active learning during our preverbal years.

Early school years to prepuberty

By the age of five years, most children seem to show mastery of vocal control through their use of voicing for phonological contrasts and ability to produce and imitate complex intonation patterns (Ingrisano et al., 1980; Ferrand and Bloom, 1996). Because their vocal anatomy is almost the same until the onset of puberty, boys and girls can produce the same vocal frequency range, which is around 200 Hz. (The vocal frequency range is the difference between the highest and lowest sounds that can be produced.) Ferrand and Bloom (1996) found, for example, that children between the ages of 3 and 10 years can generally produce their lowest sounds at a fundamental frequency (F_o) of around 150 Hz and a maximum Fo of around 350 Hz. Fortunately, few children (and even fewer adults) use this full range in conversational speech!

In fact, the 'choice' of pitch range used during conversational speech seems to be influenced by social factors from a fairly early age. Although their vocal anatomy is still very similar, measures of the range for conversational speech (or speaking fundamental frequency: SFF_o) shows us that boys and girls over the age of seven years begin to adopt different patterns of intonation and pitch use in connected speech. Ferrand and Bloom (1996), for example, found that boys tended towards the stereotypical male use of the lower end of SFF range (with a mean F_o range of 154.65 Hz), whereas girls followed a more typical female pattern, and had a mean Fo range of 194.58 Hz (Ferrand and Bloom, 1996). The boys also followed the adult male pattern of restricted intonation when compared with females, with proportionately fewer rise and fall intonation shifts.

It may be that children begin to show male–female differences in their uses of intonation patterns (Ferrand and Bloom, 1996) around the same time as they show understanding of the rules of prosody (Crystal, 1981), although Sederholm (1998) also found male–female differences in perceived voice quality in ten-year-olds. These changes seem to be more related to increased sociocultural awareness and, perhaps, gender identity than to physiological differences (Ferrand and Bloom, 1996). It seems significant from the voice therapy perspective, however, that Sederholm (1995) identified eight cases of chronic hoarseness out of a group of 33 ten-year-old boys, but no hoarseness among 22 girls of the same age.

Puberty

The major changes in voice occur during puberty, when both sexes show an increase in overall body height and weight, as the body moves towards full growth and sexual maturity (Spiegel et al., 1997). The timing of the onset of puberty varies, but the sequence of events tends to be similar (Andrews, 1995). Girls tend to begin the process earlier. Speigel et al. (1997) suggest that pubertal changes can begin between the ages of 8 and 15 in American females and between the ages of 9.5 and 14 years in American males. Aronson (1990) observes, however, that the onset of puberty tends to be related to climate; young people living nearer to the equator tend to begin puberty earlier than those living nearer the poles. The physical changes tend to occur quite rapidly; Aronson (1990) suggests that they may be completed within six months, although Spiegel et al. (1997) report that mutational voice changes may last longer and in some cases may take up to three years (Hagg and Tarranger, 1980).

The changes to the vocal tract are more dramatic in boys than in girls, although both sexes tend to show an increase in the dimensions of the vocal tract and changes in the relative size and shape of the vocal tract structures. In both males and females, the vocal tract begins to increase in length and circumference, and will continue to develop into adulthood; full growth is usually completed by 21 years (Spiegel et al., 1997). The epiglottis flattens, increases in size and is elevated. The tonsils and adenoids begin to atrophy, so that oropharyngeal and nasopharyngeal resonance may be altered. The connective tissues of the vocal folds will have been developing throughout childhood, but the superficial and intermediate layers of the vocal folds complete their development by age 16. The vocal folds increase in length. In males, the increase may be as much as 60%, or between 4 mm and 11 mm, to reach a final length of 17–23 mm. In females, the increase is nearer 34%, so that the adult length will be between 12 and 15 mm. During puberty, the female voice tends to drop about 2.5 semitones, so that average fundamental frequency is 220–225 Hz when the changes are complete (Spiegel et al., 1997). Typically, male voices drop by one octave, so by age 18, the average fundamental frequency is 130 Hz (Sataloff, 1991).

All the vocal tract changes are more apparent in males. Perhaps the most visible difference is the development of the 'Adam's apple', which becomes more pronounced when the angle of the male thyroid prominence has decreased to an angle of nearer 90 degrees. In comparison, the female thyroid cartilage remains at an angle of approximately 120 degrees. The growth spurt in puberty includes changes to both bones and muscles; again, males tend to have the greater increase in the length of their bones and in muscle size and strength (Andrews and Summers, 1991). Growth of the facial structures, including the sinuses, and completion of dental development add to the overall increase in size and shape of the vocal tract and increase the capacity for loudness and resonance. The chest wall enlarges and the muscles of the thorax and abdomen strengthen. When combined with an increase in lung size and volume in males this results in greater respiratory capacity and, potentially, respiratory control (Aronson, 1990; Andrews, 1995; Spiegel et al., 1997).

Spiegel et al. (1997) also point out that menstruation begins during puberty. Vocal changes can occur during the menstrual cycle, particularly around the 21st day when oestrogen levels drop and may cause laryngeal water retention, oedema, increased vocal fold mass and venous dilation (Abitbol et al., 1989). Singers in particular can find that this pre-menstrual phase may cause temporary loss of high notes, vocal instability, uncertain pitch and reduced vocal efficiency, huskiness and reduced vocal power and flexibility (Brodnitz, 1971; Spiegel et al., 1997). Andrews and Summers (1991) also observe that menstrual pain and stomach cramps can be a problem for some young women – as can the whole issue of adjusting to bodily changes while maintaining an active teenage lifestyle.

Andrews and Summers (1991) suggest that the sequence of physiological changes, which starts with genital development and continues through height spurt, growth of pubic and axillary (underarm) and finally facial hair in males, is a useful reference point for the speech-language pathologist when considering 'voice breaks'. A high-pitched voice is readily explained if a boy of 13 has not yet started a growth spurt, whereas a low-pitched voice in a ten-year-old with no signs of pubertal change may be more probably associated with vocal abuse or misuse. Andrews (1982) suggested that height may be a more useful index of vocal maturity than chronological age.

In some young people, the period of voice mutation may be relatively uneventful (Andrews and Summers, 1991). Often, the changes in girls' voices are not noticed, although some may be aware of changes in singing (as above). Boys may also make the transition to deeper voice with comparatively little concern (Andrews and Summers, 1991). Beery (1991, p. 163) suggests that the erratic pitch breaks and 'unusual vocal behaviours' can lead to teasing by peers or family members, causing some teenagers 'internal personal embarrassment or unexpressed anger, or both'. The voice changes are, however, part of a much bigger picture of individual physiological and psychosocial change. Beery (1991) also cites Erikson's (1963) view that, from the psychodynamic perspective, adolescence is one of the major stages of developmental crisis in the lifespan. In western society, it is recognized as a time when the young person will seek independence, challenge, question and test boundaries. Young people and their families react to this stage in varying ways, with many variations in their responses and coping strategies. Some of these variations are considered in considerable detail by Andrews and Summers (1991) and Beery (1991).

Adulthood: normal voice and its variations

After the many changes which occur during adolescence, the anatomy of the vocal tract tends to remain relatively stable for the next few decades. Voice use is, however, also influenced by many other factors, such as our cultural, linguistic, social and personal histories, as well as our current requirements. The aim of this section is to review some of the known factors which are part of 'normal voice'.

Male–female differences in voice and speech

It is generally accepted that the mean speaking fundamental frequency (SFF) for men is around 120 Hz at age 20; this gradually drops until the fifth decade, when it begins to rise again (Hollien and Shipp, 1972; Sataloff et al., 1997b). Similar measures for women indicate that mean SFF tends to be around 200 Hz, although the results of different studies tend to be rather more variable (Pemberton et al., 1998). As Ferrand and Bloom (1996) have observed, the variations in SFF for women may be influenced by the fact that women tend to use a greater variability of intonation patterns. In general, women tend to use more rising tones than men, who typically prefer falling tones.

In fact, although we may intuitively think that we can differentiate men's voices from women's voices on the basis of pitch, there is increasing evidence that it is the intonation patterns, rather than the basic SFF, which help us to make judgements about gender (Oates and Dacakis, 1983; Wolfe et al., 1990; Andrews and Schmidt, 1997). When we consider the *range* of the SFF, for example, we can see that men in their 20s have a range from 60 Hz to 260 Hz, whereas for women in the same age group, the lower end of the range is around 130 Hz and the upper end is over 500 Hz. The ranges for males and females therefore overlap considerably (Oates and Dacakis, 1983).

Voice quality seems to be another key influence in our portrayal and perception of male–female differences (Coleman, 1983; Klatt and Klatt, 1990). It is not yet clear whether this is due to sociolinguistic influences or physiological factors. Morrison and Rammage (1994) note, for example, that the voices of North American women are often described as 'breathy', but it also seems to be a widespread characteristic related to postural and vibratory characteristics in the larynx. Many younger women have a tendency to phonate with a posterior glottal gap (Sodersten and Lindestadt, 1987; Morrison and Rammage (1994).

Interestingly, there are some indications that the mean SFF of women's voices has changed over the past few decades. Pemberton et al. (1998) suggest that successive reports have shown a gradual decline in female mean SFF (Murray and Tiffin, 1934; Fitch and Holbrook, 1970; de Pinto and Hollien, 1982; Gilmore et al., 1992. These results may have been influenced by research design and methodology, but when Pemberton and her colleagues (Russell et al., 1993; Pemberton et al., 1998) compared data from young women in 1993 with similar data from an equivalent group, recorded in 1945, analysis showed that mean SFF was lower by 23 Hz. It has been suggested that this change is the result of psychosocial changes (Linke, 1973). There are a number of references in the literature to increased use of lower pitch among women who wish to portray a more serious or mature image (Cooper, 1984; Boone, 1991; Pemberton et al., 1998). It is of note, however, that some voice specialists have also suggested that this downward pitch shift may eventually link to dysphonia (Koufman and Blalock, 1988).

The effects of female hormones

As noted above, there are some indications that the hormonal changes associated with the menstrual cycle can have some effect on voice, either directly through changes around the pre-menstrual phase of the cycle or indirectly, as a result of menstrual pain (Sataloff et al., 1997a; Andrews and Summers, 1991). In general, the changes in voice are more noticed by singers. As Sataloff et al. (1997a) have observed, some professional women singers may have 'grace days' in their contracts, so that they avoid professional engagements at times when they can predict that hormonal changes may limit vocal control and loss of clarity on high notes. Monitoring singers and non-singers throughout two complete menstrual cycles, Chernobelksy (1998) found that there was a significant decrease in intrinsic laryngeal muscle tension in both groups. Interestingly, however, only three out of the 20 non-singers reported voice changes pre-menstrually and during menstruation, which was associated with hyperaemia and mild oedema of the vocal folds. By contrast, only four of the singers were asymptomatic during the two month period; in the rest of the group, hypotension occurred in 45% during premenstruation and menstruation, whereas similar changes were found in the remaining 35%, in whom hypotension was present outside the time of menstruation. This study seems to indicate that there are noticeable individual differences in physiological response, but, as Chernobelsky (1998) has observed, we need more information about the way that vocal effort interacts with the hormone-related changes.

It is also recognized that the physical changes during pregnancy may have a temporary effect on voice. Sataloff et al. (1997) report that occasionally marked increases in the oestrogen and progesterone levels during pregnancy can cause oedema to the superficial lamina propria of the vocal folds, which may be permanent (Flach et al., 1968; Deuster, 1977). There have also been some reports of vocal change as a result of oral contraception, particularly those which contain androgens; these are not available in the United States and are now rarely prescribed in Europe and the UK, however (Sataloff et al., 1997b).

Most women undergo the menopause some time after their late 40s. Essentially, the production of the female reproductive hormones, oestradiol and progesterone, gradually reduces to almost undetectable levels as ovarian activity ceases (Prevelic, 1996). Prevelic observes that the post-menopausal ovary then secretes the male hormone, androgen. This, combined with other androgens from the adrenal glands, leads to an excess of male hormones in the blood stream. The changes tend to be gradual, often starting with changes to the regularity of the menstrual cycle and vague feelings of increased irritability. As the process continues, however, the oestrogen deficiency causes other physiological changes such as hot flushes, unattributed feelings of anxiety and increased tendency to headache, insomnia, tiredness and decreased concentration. Despite the increase in general information about the menopause, many women find that the gradual onset means that they take time to recognize the symptom picture; this is often followed by the inevitable feeling that old age is creeping nearer. The psychosocial impact of this realization, especially when combined with the other physiological changes, can be quite devastating (Mathieson, 1997).

The loss of female hormones, combined with other age-related factors can have a direct effect on the larynx. These include atrophy of the laryngeal muscle, stiffening of the laryngeal cartilages, vocal fold thickening and loss of elastic and collagen fibres, as well as some potential virilization of the voice, due to the increase in androgenic hormones. A decrease in lung power as a result of inelasticity of the lungs can also occur (Prevelic, 1996; Sataloff at al., 1997a).

Changes in voice in later life

Sataloff et al. (1997a) have observed that: 'Like death and taxes, most people have considered ageing changes in the voice inevitable' (p. 263). As more research has been carried out, however, it has become more and more apparent that the ageing process is not a straightforward process of inevitable decline, but 'a complex conglomeration of biological events that change the structure and function of various parts of the body' (Sataloff et al., 1997a, p.157). We know that advancing age can eventually produce physiological changes that can alter the voice (Aronson, 1990; Sataloff et al., 1997). However, the clear message from professional voice user clinics and from other research into ageing is that physiological fitness and well-being – or 'biological age' (Sataloff et al., 1997b, p.157) – is a far more influential factor in the ageing process than actual chronological age (Ramig and Ringel, 1983; Ramig, 1986; Woo et al., 1992; Sataloff et al., 1997b).

As people live longer and maintain a healthier and more active lifestyle during their retirement, the cut-off point between being a 'mature adult' and an 'elderly person' is gradually being pushed back, which may mean that the data on fundamental frequency, some of which were collected over two decades ago (McGlone and Hollien, 1963; Hollien and Shipp, 1972), should now be reviewed. At present, however, it is generally reported that the mean SFF of men's voices gradually drops from around 120 Hz in their third decade to around 112 Hz by their early 60s, but begins to rise again gradually in subsequent years, to around 140 Hz in the 80–90 age group (Hollien and Shipp, 1972). The SFF of women's voice tends to drop after the menopause and to continue a slow decline in pitch, thereafter, to around 195 Hz in the 80–90 year age group (McGlone and Hollien, 1963).

The physical processes of ageing are the result of gradual slowing down of the endocrine, muscular, neural, skeletal and vascular systems (Boone, 1997). There is great variability among individuals in these processes, as well as in more specific laryngeal changes such as completion of the progressive calcification of the laryngeal cartilages, muscle fibre reduction and decrease in muscle tone (Kahane, 1987; Biever and Bless, 1989). Several voice experts have pointed out that singers, actors and others who have a long past history of voice training can maintain competent vocal function for a considerable time, and also that fit and active older people tend to maintain better vocal health and control (Boone, 1997; Sataloff et al., 1997b). Conversely, several clinicians have observed that some older people who notice reduced vocal function such as weaker voice tend to have become less active (Woo et al., 1992). Some of these people have gained considerable vocal and general physical benefit from enrolling in a 'wellness programme' (Woo et al., 1992, p. 143; Sataloff, 1997b).

There are, however, some aspects of ageing which can make a substantial difference to voice and speech changes. The first of these is the gradual decline in hearing, initially in the higher frequencies (Boone, 1997) which will influence self-monitoring in the individual and may influence vocal use if their partners and/or others demand amplification of the message; speaking over loud ambient noise may be another at-risk factor. Greene and Mathieson (1989) also point out that vision can be a major factor in controlling vocal volume, because of the individual's ability to judge speaker–listener distances. Other potential influences for older people include ill-fitting dentures which may affect articulation and thus reduce intelligibility and perhaps even compound other feeding or swallowing difficulties. Boone (1997) also observes that there is a greater prevalence of reflux oesophagitis-pharyngitis in older, rather than younger people; interdisciplinary liaison to ensure that swallowing is assessed and advice on diet or prescription of medication may alleviate some vocal symptoms.

Typically, there is some decrease in respiratory volume with increasing age. When combined with a general reduction of muscle strength and thoracic elasticity, this can alter respiratory control for voice. A history of smoking and/or increase in the incidence of respiratory problems with age may also impinge on breath control, and thus vocal control. Typical laryngeal changes such as atrophy of the laryngeal muscles, reduced elasticity of the ligaments and flaccidity of the vocal folds have been described in the literature (Aronson, 1990). These factors have been suggested as the explanation for increased breathiness, vocal fatigue, increase in tremor in the voice and variability of pitch control (Greene and Mathieson, 1989; Aronson, 1990).

The term *presbylaryngis* has often been used to describe some changes in the voices of elderly people. Typically, it has been assumed that bowing or weak adduction of the vocal folds was simply a result of reduced laryngeal muscle tone. In their review of 151 outpatients over the age of 60 years, however, Woo et al. (1992) reported that in otherwise healthy people there was 'a very low incidence of 'typical' age-related laryngeal findings. The finding of vocal fold bowing during sustained phonation is uncommon' (p.142). More usually, people with breathy weak voices had other physical problems which explained the changes in voice. These included vocal fold paralysis, weight loss, poor breath support and generalized weakness, often associated with other disease processes or dysfunctions. Although Woo et al. (1992) warn that their study was of a specific population, they noted that there was a higher incidence of multiple aetiologies as well as neurologic disorders and inflammatory conditions of the larynx among this patient group, when compared with younger populations. They also report that factors such as smoking, medication side effects and poor hydration were among the underlying causes of some inflammatory conditions such as non-specific laryngitis. Some of these problems can be alleviated by reviews of the medication, increased hydration and related vocal hygiene measures.

Overall, there is general agreement in the literature that healthy and active older people tend to maintain competent vocal function for longer, whereas people who have a more sedentary or less active lifestyle may be more prone to muscle weakness and reduced respiratory control and thus are more likely to develop vocal signs of ageing. Although other health problems are more likely to be present among the elderly population, many people may be able to maintain competent voice during their 70s and perhaps later. Perhaps the most important message, however, is that the individual person's own perceptions of functional deficit are important. As Woo et al. (1992) have observed, some older people can gain substantial benefit from specific goal-oriented approaches aimed at improving function, such as review of medication, ensuring that dentures, vision and hearing are optimized and, if appropriate, short-term voice therapy or other therapeutic activity.

Conclusion

Our understanding of the processes of vocal function has increased considerably during the past couple of decades, but it is clear from the literature that there is still more work to be done. There is a wealth of information on vocalizations in the infant language development, for example, but relatively little about normal voice development and vocal use in school-aged children, especially in comparison with our understanding of language and speech development. There is also a need for more information about a number of aspects of everyday voice use, such as the incidence of day-to-day voice change among adults who do not seek medical help for voice disorders (Enderby and Emerson, 1995). The results of recently published surveys, for example, suggest that many people may tolerate vocal symptoms which we, as voice therapists, may consider warning signals of vocal attrition (Sapir et al., 1990, 1993; Miller and Verdolini, 1995) or may live with chronic voice problems for some considerable time without referral to voice therapy (Smith et al., 1996).

It seems that much of the recent research has been driven by specific clinical need, in order to answer questions raised directly by our work with clients. There is a need to widen the scope of enquiry, however. Verdolini et al. (1998) have observed that there is a conspicuous absence of multicultural studies in voice therapy. Equally, there is a general lack of normative or comparative data on the phonatory function of speakers of different languages, or indeed of racial groups other than White speakers (Sapienza, 1997). Our understanding of normal and disordered vocal function should be based on the broadest possible studies of social, cultural and racial groups, so that we can gain a comprehensive understanding of human voice production in its many different modes.

CHAPTER 3

Surgical management of laryngeal disorders

ANDREW JOHNS

Introduction

The management of any medical condition involves the initial assessment by history taking, examination and investigations, which leads to a diagnosis, following which appropriate treatment can be given.

For those patients presenting with a change in voice quality, referral by their general practitioner is made to an Ear, Nose and Throat (ENT) surgeon. Because of the possibility that the voice change is caused by cancer of the larynx, this referral is, of necessity, urgent. It is a maxim that a patient with a hoarse voice that persists for three weeks should have the larynx inspected. Most ENT departments have flexible fibreoptic laryngoscopes available to supplement indirect laryngoscopy with mirrors, such that inspection of the larynx is possible in the majority of patients in the clinic setting. This examination, together with the history, allows a management plan for diagnosis and treatment to be established. Many ENT units now also run joint voice clinics with laryngologist and voice therapist working together. These clinics have often been regarded as tertiary referral repositories for difficult cases but more and more they receive direct referrals for initial diagnosis. In addition to this clinical role, voice clinics are an important forum for teaching trainee ENT Surgeons and Speech and Language Therapists.

The differential diagnosis of laryngeal disorders will include conditions primarily of organic aetiology. In these a pathological process such as inflammation, trauma or neoplasia produces an abnormal appearance in the larynx which is usually visible on simple examination in the clinic. Further investigation will then differentiate between the various pathological conditions. At the other end of the spectrum are the functional/psychogenic disorders of voice, and in these there is often no discernible change in the laryngeal appearances as seen with mirror or fibreoptic laryngoscopy. In the middle of this aetiological spectrum are those conditions primarily related to the misuse or abuse of the voice, which can result in organic pathology such as vocal fold nodules and chronic laryngitis.

The surgical management of laryngeal disease consists of procedures for diagnosis, procedures to establish and maintain an adequate airway, operations for the treatment of the disease process and finally, surgery primarily for the voice (or phonosurgery: see Chapter 17). Surgical treatment is often combined with other forms of treatment such as antibiotic therapy, chemotherapy, radiotherapy, voice therapy and counselling. In many instances, one of these modalities is all that is required and surgery plays no part in the management.

This chapter will concentrate on the conditions of primary and secondary organic pathology and the surgical aspects of their treatment. The assessment of the dysphonic patient is given a full account in Chapter 5 and the non-surgical aspects of management are left to other contributors who are experts in these fields.

Primary non-organic or functional disorders

In this group, the appearance of the larynx is normal to inspection with mirror or endoscope. The vocal folds are mobile during the phases of respiration and can be shown to adduct fully on coughing. However, adduction may not occur completely, or be maintained for phonation, and this is best demonstrated with stroboscopic illumination. Also shown well by the stroboscopic examination is overuse of supraglottic structures in voice production. Essentially, in these conditions the larynx is capable of normal function. An important result of the finding of normal appearances in the larynx is the reassurance that can be given to the patient that there is no serious pathology. A fear of cancer may add to the patient's anxieties and thus exacerbate the tension associated with this group of voice disorders.

These patients are managed by the voice therapist, first to identify areas of habitual misuse and abuse of the voice and/or stress and secondly, to help the patient overcome them. Very rarely, a deep-seated psychiatric disturbance will require referral to a psychiatrist or clinical psychologist. The patients will usually be reviewed in the voice clinic, and this is particularly important in cases where there is poor improvement, or at worst deterioration in the voice, to ensure that pathology has not been overlooked or arisen secondarily.

If a diagnosis of Spasmodic Dysphonia is made, the patient should be referred for a neurological opinion as the condition may be part of a generalized dystonia (see Whurr, Chapter 11). The surgical treatment of this condition is referred to in the second half of this chapter.

Failure of the normal transition to an adult male voice in adolescence is usually a functional condition. It is rarely due to hypogonadism and the majority of such cases will already have been diagnosed by a paediatric endocrinologist. This topic is fully described in Chapter 13.

Pathology secondary to functional disorder

In some conditions, in which the primary pathology may be said to be psychogenic, organic changes are produced in the laryngeal tissues. Examples of this are vocal fold nodules, vocal fold oedema and chronic laryngitis.

Vocal fold nodules

Vocal abuse is a major causative factor in the formation of nodules, which are therefore also known as singer's nodes in adults and screamer's nodes in children. Typically, they are found symmetrically on each vocal fold, at the midpoint of the free edge of the vocal fold between the anterior commissure and the vocal process of the arytenoid cartilage. (This is equivalent to a position in the glottic opening one third distant from the anterior commissure.) The rest of the larynx usually appears healthy. In the early stage of nodule formation, they consist of localized tissue fluid, but persistence leads to organization with fibrous tissue. The softer the nodule, the more easily reversible it is by a programme of voice therapy. Surgical removal of the nodules is not often required and will not offer lasting voice improvement if the patterns of voice abuse and misuse have not been corrected. This is much harder to achieve in children.

Vocal fold oedema

The accumulation of tissue fluid in the subepithelial space (of Reinke) of the vocal fold produces a very soft, floppy edge to the fold. Where this is diffuse, affecting the whole length of each vocal fold, it is also known as Reinke's oedema. Most often this condition arises in post-menopausal women, indicating an hormonal basis for the oedema, but there is often also a history of smoking and vocal misuse. Localized areas of oedema lead to the formation of simple benign polyps. These conditions are treated surgically, in conjunction with measures to remove the underlying causes. Early stages of oedema formation are best observed by stroboscopic examination and these will often be reversible without surgical incision of the fold and aspiration of the fluid.

Chronic laryngitis

Many factors are potential irritants to the larynx and include smoking, alcohol, vocal abuse, acid reflux, dusty, cold and dry atmospheres, poor dental hygiene, mouth breathing and chronic sinusitis. Following an acute laryngitis, usually viral, the presence of one or more of these irritants allows the persistence of inflammation, producing the clinical picture of chronic laryngitis. The changes in the laryngeal epithelium may be generalized and are seen as swollen, thickened, reddened mucous membrane coated with sticky secretions.

Attention must be paid to any irregular, white areas as these are indistinguishable to the naked eye from early cancers. Biopsy will demonstrate hyperplasia of the epithelium, with excess of keratin production. This process is called hyperkeratosis, and where it is found in regions of the larynx not normally lined with squamous epithelium, the change in cell type is termed metaplasia. The significance of these cellular changes is that they may represent steps in the development of a cancer, and hence these cases require careful follow-up examinations. Treatment aims at eliminating the causative factors and the role of surgery is generally only to provide tissue for histological examination.

Pathology of primary organic origin

Diseases may be the result of genetic abnormalities or the body's response to environmental influences. In any individual, the particular manifestation of disease is the result of the combination of the inherited genetic constitution and the external environment. When these factors operate before birth, a congenital abnormality is produced. Congenital abnormalities are often multiple, so a baby born with a laryngeal disorder may have abnormalities in other systems.

Congenital laryngeal disorders

In its early development, the entrance to the larynx ends blindly. Failure of canalization produces atresia of the larynx, which is incompatible with life. If the development is incomplete, the larynx may have a narrowed segment, usually the subglottis or a laryngeal web. The narrowed airway in subglottic stenosis will produce noisy breathing called stridor and this is heard in both inspiratory and expiratory phases of respiration. The embarrassment to respiration is often severe enough to require tracheotomy. Subglottic stenosis in neonates may also be an acquired condition, from endotracheal intubation used for ventilation of premature babies, or can result from the presence of a haemangioma in the subglottis, suspected when there is a cutaneous haemangioma. The further management of this condition is described below.

Laryngeal webs, if large enough, will cause airway obstruction, in which case surgical removal is carried out relatively early. This will enable removal of the tracheotomy tube. For those webs not severe enough to require an artificial airway, the main presenting symptom will be a harsh quality to the voice. Surgical removal of the web will still be needed, but can be left to a later, pre-school age.

The most noticeable difference in appearance of the infant larynx from the adult, apart from overall size, is the shape of the laryngeal inlet. The aryepiglottic folds are short and the epiglottis more curled. An exaggeration of this produces the commonest congenital laryngeal abnormality, that of laryngomalacia. The name suggests that the laryngeal cartilage is soft, providing inadequate support to maintain the airway. However, all infantile cartilage is very soft and the failure in development in laryngomalacia is the excessively short aryepiglottic folds. This creates an exaggerated omega shape to the epiglottis, and the arytenoid cartilages are tilted forward. On inspiration, the arytenoids prolapse further forward and the epiglottis flops backward producing airway obstruction, whereas on expiration the flow of air pushes the tissues apart. The noisy breathing (stridor) in this condition is therefore an inspiratory noise, musical in quality, while the expiratory phase is quiet. The obstruction would rarely be severe enough to require an artificial airway, but assistance is sometimes required to cover episodes of respiratory infection. The expectation is for the noisy breathing to decrease and stop over the first two years of life.

Congenital laryngeal disorders are often accompanied by feeding difficulties. The neonate receives an entirely liquid diet that the larynx must prevent from entering the trachea. Co-ordinated nerve and muscle function is needed to achieve this and immaturity of this function can lead to slow feeding and a tendency to cough and choke during feeds. This is a common feature of laryngomalacia and the difficulty can be eased by thickening the feeds which perhaps stimulates a more co-ordinated swallow reflex.

More serious incompetence of the larynx is found in posterior clefts of the larynx. The posterior wall of the larynx and trachea (which is also the anterior wall of the pharynx and oesophagus) may be congenitally deficient to a varying extent. This will leave the lower airways unprotected during swallowing and surgical repair of the posterior wall is required.

Malignant disease

The majority (95%) of malignancies arising in the larynx are squamous cell carcinomas (SCCs). Very few cancers therefore develop in the structural tissues such as cartilage. It is also evident that in sites of the larynx, which in the healthy state are lined by respiratory epithelium, the carcinoma that forms is of squamous cell type. The malignant cells spread locally superficially, but also invade the deeper tissues of the larynx including muscle and cartilage. Eventually, if untreated, the malignant cells gain access to the lymphatic channels and, less commonly for SCCs, blood vessels, allowing for distant spread of the disease. The first clinical sign of this will be the appearance of enlarged lymph nodes in the neck, which may be demonstrated by CT scan imaging before they are clinically palpable.

The only early symptom of carcinoma of the larynx is persistent and progressive hoarseness, which underlines the importance of urgent examination. The disease is commoner in males than females and there is a definite relationship to smoking. SCCs of the vocal fold will present in this way, whereas hoarseness may be later in the natural history of SCCs arising in other sites of the larynx. Late symptoms include pain often as referred otralgia, dysphagia, stridor, foetor and the development of a lump in the neck. Advanced disease is more common for those tumours arising in the supraglottis and subglottis, hence such cases have a worse prognosis compared to an early (T1) SCC of a vocal fold.

Diagnosis is made by biopsy of the suspicious lesion, the examination under anaesthetic allowing assessment of the extent of disease, together with information gained by CT imaging. The use of the stroboscope may demonstrate invasion by showing loss of fold vibration and may help in follow-up after radiotherapy, if a vocal fold does not regain vibration or subsequently loses it. This does not replace the need to biopsy any abnormal appearing epithelium.

Vocal fold paralysis

The clinical presentation of vocal fold paralysis depends largely on the position that the paralysed fold or folds adopt, and the accompanying loss of sensation. It remains a contentious issue as to the exact determinants which lead to a paralysed fold adopting a position near the mid-line (abductor paralysis) or a position away from the mid-line (adductor paralysis). Factors such as the unopposed action of the cricothyroid muscle (nerve supply external branch of superior laryngeal nerve), any remaining muscle tone and the actual mass of the vocal fold may be relevant in individual cases (see also Casper, Chapter 10).

The functions of the larynx, that is, phonation, part of the airway and airway protection in swallowing and coughing, are affected to varying degrees and can be considered under the four headings of unilateral abductor, unilateral adductor, bilateral abductor and bilateral adductor paralysis.

1 *Unilateral abductor paralysis:* Damage to one recurrent laryngeal nerve may result in the fold being near the midline. The non-paralysed fold will frequently compensate sufficiently to allow glottic closure in phonation producing a voice of acceptable quality. This compensation is aided by speech therapy and medialization of the paralysed fold may not be required. The other laryngeal functions are unaffected.

2 *Unilateral adductor paralysis:* A paralysed vocal fold lying in an abducted position will result from a vagus nerve injury, proximal to the level of the superior laryngeal branch, but is also seen in some apparently pure recurrent laryngeal nerve injuries, such as occur with carcinoma of the bronchus. The voice will be weak and breathy with air escape, the cough will also be reduced in power and there may be some tendency to inhalation during swallowing. There is no restriction to the airway. Improvement of the voice will require surgical medialization and this will also improve the cough reflex. It may be considered as an urgent procedure to improve the quality of the remaining life of a patient with terminal lung cancer.

3 *Bilateral abductor paralysis:* This is most likely to be the result of trauma, which is a risk of surgery to the thyroid gland. The main effect is on the airway, which may be severely compromised by the close approximation of both folds and their inability to abduct on inspiration. Tracheotomy relieves the obstructed airway; this can be an emergency requirement. Other cases are not so severely obstructed and can manage without tracheotomy, although the need for this can develop even years later, perhaps as a result of increased body weight and reduced fitness with age. The close relationship of the vocal folds allows for a good voice, in the case of a tracheotomized patient using a speaking valve fitted to the tracheotomy tube. Methods to relieve the airway obstruction in order to dispense with the tracheotomy are described below.

4 *Bilateral adductor paralysis:* This is a life-threatening condition, due to the incompetence of the larynx to prevent inhalation during swallowing, because of both the loss of sensation of the whole larynx and the inability to close the glottis. It is a rare situation and is often part of a severe neurological catastrophe affecting the brain stem, and thus the nuclei of both vagus nerves. The few patients who survive the neurological disaster require protection of the lower airway, initially by a tracheotomy tube with a cuff to make a seal with the tracheal wall. This can only be a temporary procedure and long-term protection may be by epiglottopexy, in which the epiglottis is sutured over the laryngeal inlet and could be reversed if there is neurological recovery. Total laryngectomy will also offer protection of the lungs and may be considered in these cases.

Pseudo bilateral adductor paralysis: dysphonia or aphonia of psychological aetiology is suspected if the folds do not adduct for phonation, but can be shown to have the neuromuscular ability to do so when the patient is asked to cough. The serious symptoms of laryngeal incompetence do not feature. Speech therapy combined with attention to underlying psychological problems may help, but some cases relapse. There is currently some debate about the nature of this condition, however (see Freeman, Chapter 8 and Oates, Chapter 7).

From the above descriptions it will be clear that the cause of the paralysis is obvious in some cases. Others need full investigation; this includes ENT, thoracic and neurological examination, together with examination of the aerodigestive tracts under anaesthetic and appropriate imaging of the thyroid gland and the whole region from base of skull to mid-thorax by CT scan or Magnetic Resonance. In about 15% of cases, no cause is found. Partial injuries to the recurrent laryngeal nerve may recover and therefore unless the nature of the injury is known to be complete, or division of the nerve or reliable electrical conduction studies indicate that recovery will not occur, surgical treatment for voice improvement should wait at least one year after the onset of the paralysis. This issue is also discussed by Casper (Chapter 10).

Superior laryngeal nerve injury: Isolated injury to this nerve, in particular the loss of supply to the cricothyroid muscle, may result in a change of voice noticed after thyroidectomy, where examination demonstrates that both folds do still abduct and adduct. In a unilateral injury, asymmetry of the glottis may be observed at stroboscopy. Compensation usually occurs with speech therapy.

Related conditions: Paralysis of the vocal fold may be mimicked by other conditions which affect the movement at the cricoarytenoid joint. The joint may be fixed as a result of inflammation perhaps secondary to endotracheal intubation or to primary joint disease such as rheumatoid arthritis. Muscle diseases, such as myasthenia gravis may also impair fold movement (see Ramig, Chapter 9).

Endocrine disorders

That the larynx is under the influence of the sex hormones is apparent from the changes that occur to the male voice at puberty. The mature larynx is – to a lesser extent – susceptible to changes in sex hormone status, but virilization of the female voice will occur with treatment for certain gynaecological conditions with androgenic hormones. Also, as mentioned above, is the development of Reinke's oedema in post-menopausal women. Hypofunction of the thyroid gland is characterized by thickening of the submucosal tissues leading to a husky voice together with the other features of myxoedema. Treatment is by oral administration of thyroxine.

Ageing

With advancing years, tissues lose their elasticity and muscles lose their bulk. It is by no means a universal feature of the elderly, but some do notice a change in pitch and power of the voice.

Inflammatory conditions

Apart from acute inflammatory conditions and non-specific chronic laryngitis, the larynx is vulnerable to certain specific infections and non-infective inflammatory disorders. Examples of the former are syphilis, which is now rare, and tuberculosis, which is on the increase. Sarcoidosis is a non-infective inflammation causing multisystem disease of which laryngitis may form one manifestation.

Other conditions

Disorders of the larynx which result from trauma and benign neoplasms are described under the relevant sections of surgical management below.

Surgery for diagnosis

Despite the availability of endoscopes in the out-patient setting, there remain a few patients where visualization of the larynx is not possible without a general anaesthetic. The procedure of direct laryngoscopy under general anaesthesia may be combined with use of the operating microscope for a magnified view of the interior of the larynx. This method has the disadvantage of not allowing observation of the movement of the vocal folds in phonation, but it may be possible to see gross abduction and adduction of the folds as the anaesthetic lightens. Where vocal fold movement is impaired, the mobility of the cricoarytenoid joint can be assessed by direct pressure.

The main diagnostic purpose of direct laryngoscopy is for the biopsy of lesions, for histological analysis. This is combined with an assessment of the extent of any disease process, with examination of related areas of the aerodigestive tract by oesophagoscopy and tracheobronchoscopy. These diagnostic procedures are completed with the accurate documentation of the findings.

Surgery for airway maintenance

Partial obstruction to the flow of air through the larynx will produce a noise termed stridor. In mild to moderate degrees of obstruction, this is an inspiratory noise, but more severe obstruction will produce the noise in both phases of respiration. Increased respiratory effort is used to overcome the increased resistance and, if the obstruction is not relieved, respiratory failure will follow.

Some obstructions will rapidly respond to medical treatment without recourse to an artificial airway. An example is the acute laryngeal oedema of an allergic reaction, which responds to high doses of steroids. Most instances where an artificial airway is required can be initially managed with endotracheal intubation, the tube splinting open the soft tissues of the larynx. If the underlying pathology is temporary, the tube can be removed following resolution of the obstruction. This would be the case in the acute obstruction, for example, in infants from supraglottitis caused by *Haemophilus influenzae*, a condition much rarer since the introduction of vaccination against this organism.

Tracheotomy

Long-term endotracheal intubation causes trauma to the laryngeal mucosa, with ulceration and a route for infection to damage the cartilage of the larynx. To prevent this – or in cases where intubation is not possible – a tracheotomy is performed. The track produced from the skin to the lumen of the trachea is maintained by a tracheotomy tube. Because all the expiratory air (as well as all the inspired air) now passes through the tracheotomy tube, the immediate effect of the procedure is to render the patient aphonic. Voice can be restored by the use of an expiratory valve fitted to the tracheotomy tube, which closes on expiration, thus directing air around the tube and up through the larynx. The valve opens on inspiration, allowing air to enter the lungs. The quality of the voice produced depends on the nature of the underlying laryngeal pathology and its effect on vocal fold function. In the case of bilateral vocal fold palsy with the folds in a static adducted position, a tracheotomy with speaking valve will allow an adequate airway on inspiration, and also a good voice.

Arytenoidectomy and cordectomy

An alternative approach to the management of bilateral abductor paralysis is to widen the glottic opening. There is an inevitable trade-off between the quality of the voice and the size of the glottic opening. In order to obviate the need for the tracheotomy, the patient will have to accept an inferior voice, while keeping the tracheotomy will maintain the good voice

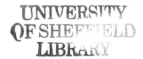

but with it the disadvantages of the tracheotomy. The choice rests with the patient after informed discussion.

The various techniques of widening the glottis involve removal of one arytenoid cartilage and lateralization of the vocal fold, or the removal of one vocal fold (cordectomy), or a combination of both arytenoidectomy and cordectomy. These procedures can be carried out endoscopically, using the carbon dioxide (CO_2) laser. By performing this in stages the optimum point of adequate airway with least detriment to the voice can be reached.

Airway maintenance in children

Tracheotomy is required in children for such conditions as congenital bilateral vocal fold palsy, severe laryngeal webs, subglottic haemangioma and stenosis. The tracheotomy will have been established in the neonatal period and therefore, before speech and language acquisition. Vocalization will occur if air is able to escape around the tube through the larynx on expiration. Children learn the trick of occluding the opening of the tube on expiration with their chin or finger, increasing the flow of air through the larynx. Alternatively, a valved tube can be used. Provided the other parameters (such as normal hearing) are intact, language and speech will be acquired. Although tracheotomy has a morbidity and a mortality, the necessary nursing skills can be taught to parents so that these children can live at home and attend normal school.

Methods are available to enlarge a narrowed sub-glottis, if examination under anaesthetic at three-monthly intervals has shown that insufficient growth is occurring naturally. Surgery is usually timed at 12–18 months of age. The larynx is exposed through the neck anteriorly and the thyroid cartilage split in the mid-line. The narrowed segment of the sub-glottis is identified and may be widened by a vertical split through the anterior wall of the stenotic area, usually the cricoid cartilage, and holding the two edges apart with a cartilage graft taken from a rib. Alternatively, a stepped incision is made through the cricoid cartilage and the upper tracheal rings, placing sutures to hold the edges apart (laryngotracheoplasty). A supporting stent is placed in the lumen of the larynx and upper trachea, above the level of the tracheotomy, and removed endoscopically about six weeks later when healing has occurred. By these means, earlier decannulation of the tracheotomy is possible.

Surgery for the disease process

In some conditions, most notably malignant laryngeal disease, surgery plays an important role in the cure or control of the disease. This is in contrast to surgical measures employed primarily for the improvement of voice, described below in the section headed 'Phonosurgery'. Surgery also plays a part in the management of some benign lesions and also in the management of laryngeal trauma.

Laryngeal cancer

Patients with laryngeal cancer require sensitive, lengthy and repeated counselling. There will be many fears that need to be allayed, in particular the commonly held belief that cancer has an inevitably fatal outcome. Explanations of the effects of radiotherapy and surgery are not readily taken in, especially at the time when a patient is confronted with the diagnosis of cancer, and therefore need reinforcing by doctor, nurse and speech therapist.

Radiotherapy and surgery both offer opportunity for cure of laryngeal cancer. The majority of patients in the UK are treated initially with radiotherapy, which for small glottic tumours has a cure rate of about 95%. An alternative approach for the treatment of T1 glottic tumours is surgical excision by CO_2 Laser. Very careful review is required during and after radiotherapy, to identify residual and recurrent disease which may then be treated surgically, usually by total laryngectomy. Laryngectomy may also be considered as primary treatment for advanced tumours in combination with radiotherapy.

Total laryngectomy: The operation of total laryngectomy aims to excise a sufficiently wide margin of healthy tissue around the tumour to ensure complete removal and yet restore the vital functions of respiration and swallowing. The former is achieved by the creation of a permanent tracheostomy and the latter by reconstruction of the pharynx. Vocal rehabilitation follows after healing has taken place, usually by ten days post-surgery, and may be by the acquisition of pseudo-voice, or by one of various techniques for surgical voice restoration.

Conservation (of the voice) surgery of the larynx, such as the partial laryngectomies, either supraglottic or vertical, has found limited application in the UK. These operations are rarely suitable for recurrent disease after radiotherapy and other cases are too advanced to make anything less than a total laryngectomy possible. Similarly, laryngectomy combined with construction of a neoglottis was never popular and has now been superseded by the much simpler tracheo-oesophageal puncture and valve procedures.

Benign swellings of the larynx

Many of the discrete lesions are easily recognized at indirect laryngoscopy. The majority require excision and this can be performed at microlaryngoscopy. The excised tissue is sent for histological examination.

In infants, a particularly challenging problem is that of juvenile papillomatosis. Papillomata have a propensity to seed throughout the respiratory tract. Judicious use of the laser offers the best local control, to maintain a patent airway with minimal scarring to the larynx. A tracheotomy may be necessary, but this increases the risk of seeding to the lower airways. There is a natural tendency for the papillomata to regress, suggesting the development of immunological defences. Many alternative treatments to surgery have been evaluated, including chemotherapeutic agents having antibacterial, antiviral or cytotoxic properties and the use of prepared vaccines. These have proved successful in individual cases but none offer a universal solution.

Laryngeal trauma

Blunt and sharp trauma to the neck may involve the larynx and its nerve supply. Disruption of the cartilaginous framework requires early repair with stenting and preservation of as much mucosa as possible. The airway is maintained via a tracheotomy. It may be possible to approximate the ends of a severed recurrent laryngeal nerve. The management of an established stenosis after trauma is very difficult and some patients will remain with a tracheotomy and speaking valve.

Phonosurgery

Surgery that has its aim in the deliberate alteration of voice is termed phonosurgery. This involves microlaryngoscopy, injection techniques and laryngeal framework surgery (see also Chapter 17). Also considered in this section is surgical voice rehabilitation after laryngectomy.

Microlaryngoscopy

The advent of the CO_2 laser, deliverable via the operating microscope, proved to be a false dawn in laryngeal microsurgery. It was used indiscriminately to treat vocal fold lesions previously excised with micro instruments. As more patients were assessed with stroboscopy, the scarring from laser surgery which inhibits the mucosal wave was recognized. In addition, lesions were more readily recognized as being submucosal, such as mucous and epithelial cysts, and therefore better excised via a cordotomy incision, which preserves the epithelial edge of the fold. Similarly, with vocal fold oedema, the practice of stripping the edge of the vocal fold should now be outlawed and be replaced by cordotomy and suction of the oedematous fluid, so preserving the vocal fold epithelium and promoting restoration of the mucosal wave.

Vocal fold medialization

In cases of unilateral adductor fold palsy, improvement in the quality of the voice may require positioning of the edge of the paralysed fold to the mid-line, in order to achieve glottic closure. This effect can be obtained by the injection of material to increase the bulk of the vocal fold. The substance that has been most associated with this procedure is a suspension of Teflon. It is injected deep into the muscle in the paraglottic space under general or local anaesthesia. It is essential to wait at least a year to allow for recovery of the paralysis before undertaking this procedure, unless there is certain knowledge of complete severance of the nerve by trauma or shown by EMG studies or where improvement in quality of life is sought in patients with terminal malignancy. Although uncommon, the risk of migration of the Teflon has led to the application of other materials. Collagen injection, apart from being very expensive, is not permanent and is a possible transmitter of disease. Autologous fat harvested from the patient does not suffer the latter risk but again is relatively temporary in its duration. A further development is the use of gelfoam (see Casper, Chapter 10; Bouchayer and Cornut, Chapter 17).

An alternative approach to the injection techniques is to push the vocal fold towards the midline, by cutting a window in the lamina of the thyroid cartilage at the level of the vocal fold and keeping it medialized by a plastic stent. This procedure is one of the types of thyroplasty.

Pitch alteration

Other types of thyroplasty have been devised, which aim to lengthen or shorten the vocal folds and thereby change the pitch of the voice. It is doubtful whether these procedures have any advantage over speech therapy.

Laryngeal reinnervation techniques

Attempts at re-establishing a nerve supply have met with limited success. The usual donor nerve is a branch of the ansa hypoglossi, which is anastomosed to the recurrent laryngeal nerve. Any return of innervation introduces tone to the paralysed muscle, but does return the power of abduction and adduction.

Surgery for spasmodic dysphonia

Injection of botulinum toxin into the vocalis muscle has improved the outlook for these unfortunate patients. Previously, surgical treatment had been by section of one recurrent laryngeal nerve. The transcutaneous injection is monitored by EMG and laryngoscopic visualization. The benefit of the injection lasts between three and six months after which time it can be repeated (see Whurr, Chapter 11 for more details).

Surgical voice rehabilitation after laryngectomy

The methods which offer the best voice restoration with the least disadvantage involve the formation of a tracheo-oesophageal fistula maintained by a valve. The valve (e.g. Blom-Singer) acts to direct air from the lungs into the oesophagus, while preventing flow of saliva and ingested food and drink in the reverse direction into the trachea. To direct the air through the valve, the stoma is occluded temporarily by finger closure or by an outer casing valve assembly covering the stoma and which opens on inspiration and closes on expiration. The air vibrates the P-E segment in the same way as in acquired oesophageal speech, but has the advantage of greater volumes of air to increase loudness of phonation and length of continuous phonation.

The fistula can be established as a primary procedure at laryngectomy. The feeding tube is passed through the fistula, to maintain it, and replaced by the valve when oral feeding is established. Secondary puncture can be undertaken in previously performed laryngectomies. This may need to be combined with cricopharyngeal myotomy if hypertonicity is demonstrated at videofluoroscopy.

The future

As a footnote to this chapter it is now possible to say that the future has arrived, with the first laryngeal transplant successfully performed in the United States of America. We watch this exciting development with interest.

CHAPTER 4

The causes and classification of voice disorders

MARGARET FAWCUS

Introduction

The wealth of words that can be used to describe voice is indicative of the important part it plays in our lives. A voice can be harsh, hoarse, strident, loud, soft, resonant, mellifluous, authoritative, reedy, weak ... the list is almost endless. Some of these adjectives are applied in a positive way, to suggest a voice which is pleasant to hear, and others are essentially negative. When it comes to an abnormal voice, however, the distinctions may be less clear. Ramig and Verdolini (1998) have defined a voice disorder as generally characterized by an abnormal pitch, loudness and/or quality resulting from disordered laryngeal, respiratory or vocal tract functioning. However, subjective opinions may differ on what is considered abnormal. Much will depend on who is listening, and the perceptions of a laryngologist, voice therapist or singing teacher may be very different from a 'non-professional' listener. In the final analysis, as Verdolini (1994) states, it is the patient's perspective that is the key to whether or not there is a voice disorder.

The chapter titles of this book indicate the wide range of possible causes of voice disorder. Basically, there are three conditions in which phonation can be affected:

1. The vocal folds may show structural abnormalities.
2. The folds may appear normal at rest but may demonstrate a disturbance of movement patterns.
3. There may be no apparent organic impairment in terms of either structure or function.

Causes of voice disorders

These three conditions will now be considered in more detail.

1. The larynx is vulnerable to physical stress which can result in the build-up of tissue reactions (vocal nodules, contact ulcers, or non-specific laryngitis). Physical vulnerability, upper respiratory tract infection and personality factors, as well as the demands of the situation, may all combine to produce a voice disorder. Where the vocal folds fail to present smooth vibrating edges, capable of full adduction along their total length, we may expect a voice characterized by air waste and a quality which may variously be described as 'rough', 'hoarse' or 'husky'.

   As indicated, such changes in the smooth appearance of the vocal folds may be a direct result of inappropriate voice use. In other cases there may be changes caused by physical trauma such as road traffic accidents or intratracheal intubation during general anaesthesia, causing haematoma or granuloma. Infection, benign or malignant new growths can also affect the structure of the vocal folds. In addition excessive alcohol consumption, smoking, chemical irritants, certain drugs, or hormone imbalance may also lead to tissue changes in the larynx. In many cases these factors occur in combination to have an adverse effect on voice quality.

2. The appearance of the vocal folds may be normal but the movement of the cords may be affected. Disturbed vocal function may be part of the dysarthrophonic syndrome (Peacher, 1949), where there is a disease process of the central nervous system, affecting both articulation and phonation. The dysarthrias associated with cerebellar, extrapyramidal, lower motor neuron and bilateral cortical lesions have associated voice problems involving all aspects of voice production (see Ramig, Chapter 9). At a peripheral level there may be interference with the nerve supply to one or both vocal folds. The most common of these is a unilateral recurrent laryngeal nerve lesion (see Casper, Chapter 10).

3. Voice disorders can exist in the apparent absence of any physical cause, although this may reflect the present state of investigation procedures rather than the true state of affairs. In some of these cases, more refined techniques such as laryngeal microscopy may reveal previously unidentified physical signs. This shift of emphasis from a psychogenic to a physical cause is demonstrated very clearly in the case of spasmodic dysphonia (see Whurr, Chapter 11). Generally speaking, however, wherever there are no apparent signs, the dysphonia is labelled as 'functional', 'psychogenic' or even 'hysterical'. Freeman (Chapter 8)

and Oates (Chapter 7) have indicated the complexities of the situation and the need for a careful evaluation of the variables involved.

There are two other areas where the client has a normal voice mechanism but the voice is perceived as abnormal: in cases of significant hearing loss and in transsexualism. Increasing interest has developed in recent years in the indirect but often very marked effects of profound hearing loss for the frequencies of voice production (see Wirz, Chapter 12). The speaker has a potential for normal voice production which is never realized due to his severely impaired auditory feedback mechanism and, in the case of acquired profound hearing loss, the continuous auditory monitoring that enables us to maintain consistent and appropriate intensity, pitch and intonation patterns.

In the case of the transsexual individual (see Chaloner, Chapter 14), we may indeed challenge the concept of a voice disorder, since vocal pitch (the only aspect of voice with which the transsexual person is normally concerned) may be entirely in keeping with the physical constraints of the laryngeal structure. There is, however, a mismatch between the modal range and the desired gender which he or she wishes to convey.

We must now consider what we mean by a voice disorder in more detail, and examine the ways in which interested voice therapists, laryngologists, and phoniatrists have attempted to classify the aphonias and dysphonias.

> A voice disorder exists [says Aronson (1980)] when quality, pitch, loudness or
> flexibility differs from the voice of others of similar age, sex, and cultural group.

It is on variants of these four perceived parameters of voice production that the listener judges the normality or otherwise of the voice he or she hears. Aronson considers that these judgements are made in relation to the listener's expectations regarding sex and age within a given cultural group. We must also consider the listener's individual preferences and biases, and his level of awareness of how voices sound and the differences between them. There is a continuum extending from the voice that is clear and audible to one which is unmistakably dysphonic.

Different listeners, asked to make a judgement about a speaker's voice, will not always place that voice at the same point on the continuum. For one listener, a voice may be acceptably 'normal', while for another judge the same voice may be noted as frankly abnormal. Wynter (1974) has emphasized the subjectivity of listeners' judgements, which has given rise to a confusing variety of terms to describe voice quality. 'Typically they are based on subjective auditory judgements rather than on objective observations of vocal function' (Reed, 1980).

Prevalence of voice disorders

Rather little is known about the prevalence of voice disorder, and any figures available must be regarded with some caution: not all speakers with a hoarse voice would regard it as pathological, and would therefore not seek medical advice. Dysphonia may be regarded as a problem only if it causes discomfort or interferes in some way with their life style. We do, however, know rather more about the relative prevalence of the different causes of voice disorder.

Herrington-Hall et al. (1988) carried out a retrospective study of 1262 patients seen by eight otolaryngologists over a two-year period. The total population was approximately 2.3 million. The purpose of the investigation was to look at the occurrence of laryngeal pathologies across three variables: sex, age and occupation. They also looked at the residential environment of the patient population (rural or city). Herrington-Hall et al. identified 22 laryngeal pathologies (Table 4.1). Of these the most common was vocal nodules (21.6%) followed by oedema (14.1%), polyps (11.4%), carcinoma (9.7%), vocal fold paralysis (8.1%), and dysphonia with no apparent pathology (7.9%).

In taking the variable of age into account, it is clear that laryngeal pathologies occur most frequently in the older age group (carcinoma and vocal-fold paralysis being the most commonly found causes of vocal dysfunction in the elderly). Females presented with laryngeal pathologies at a slightly younger age. In the total population, nodules and oedema were more common in early adulthood (25–44 years), with polyps and dysphonia with a normal larynx occurring in middle age (45–64 years) (Table 4.2) .

It is interesting, but not altogether surprising, that nodules occur most frequently in males under the age of 14 years when we might well expect abusive vocal behaviour (ratio of males to females was 2.7:1). In contrast, nodules and oedema are found most commonly in females between the ages of 25 and 44 years. This is a period when many women are raising young children, and may also be facing the additional demands of being a working mother. Psychogenic voice disorders, perhaps for some of the same reasons, also showed an increased incidence in early adulthood.

When Herrington-Hall et al. looked at the influence of occupation, they found that the presence of laryngeal pathologies tended to reflect both the amount of voice use and the conditions under which voice was used (including noise and stress). Of the 73 occupations identified in the study,

Table 4.1 The prevalence of laryngeal pathologies and their percentage of occurrence

Total number (1262)	n	%	Cincinnati (580)	n	%	Dayton (578)	n	%	Small town/ rural (104)	n	%
Nodules	272	21.6	Nodules	110	19.0	Nodules	147	25.4	Normal on exam	41	39.4
Oedema	179	14.1	Oedema	97	16.7	Cancer	90	15.6	Nodules	15	14.4
Polyps	144	11.4	Vocal-fold paralysis	59	10.2	Polyps	86	14.9	Oedema	10	9.6
Cancer	122	9.7	Polyps	53	9.1	Oedema	72	12.4	Leukoplakia	8	7.7
Vocal-fold paralysis	102	8.1	Laryngitis	40	6.9	Vocal-fold paralysis	41	7.0	Polyps	5	4.8
Normal on exam	100	7.9	Leukoplakia	37	6.4	Normal on exam	28	4.8	Functional	4	3.8
Laryngitis	53	4.2	Normal on exam	31	5.3	Functional	16	2.7	Papilloma	4	3.8
Leukoplakia	52	4.1	Cancer	29	5.0	Vocal-fold paresis	11	1.9	Granuloma	3	2.9
Psychogenic	34	2.6	Psychogenic	22	3.8	Bowed vocal fold	11	1.9	Cancer	3	2.9
Functional	31	2.4	Bowed vocal folds	19	3.3	Hyperkeratosis	11	1.9	Laryngitis	3	2.9
Bowed vocal folds	30	2.4	Neurogenic	11	1.9	Laryngitis	10	1.7	Vocal-fold paralysis	2	1.9
Neurogenic	18	1.4	Functional	11	1.9	Psychogenic	10	1.7	Cyst	2	1.9
Hyperkeratosis	16	1.2	Laryngeal trauma	11	1.9	Leukoplakia	7	1.3	Psychogenic	2	1.9
Papilloma	15	1.2	Ventricular phonation	9	1.5	Neurogenic	7	1.3	Vocal-fold paresis	1	0.9
Ventricular phonation	15	1.2	Contact ulcer	9	1.5	Stenosis	6	1.0	Contact ulcer	1	0.9
Contact ulcer	14	1.1	Cyst	7	1.2	Papilloma	6	1.0			
Vocal-fold paresis	12	1.0	Granuloma	5	1.0	Ventricular phonation	6	1.0			
Granuloma	12	1.0	Papilloma	5	1.0	Granuloma	4	0.7			
Cyst	12	1.0	Hyperkeratosis	5	1.0	Contact ulcer	4	0.7			
Laryngeal trauma	11	0.9	Spastic dysphonia	5	0.9	Cyst	3	0.5			
Spastic dysphonia	7	0.5	Cricoarytenoid arthritis	4	0.5	Spastic dysphonia	2	0.3			
Stenosis	6	0.5	Hormonal	1	0.07						
Cricoarytenoid arthritis	4	0.3									
Hormonal	1	0.07									

Table 4.2 Distribution of laryngeal pathologies across age groups for the total sample and for males and females separately

	0–14 years			15–24 years			25–44 years			45–64 years			Over 64 years		
	Total	Male	Female	Total	Male	Female	Total	Male	Female	Total	Male	Female	Total	Male	Female
Nodules	74	54	20	35	2	33	103	26	77	51	12	39	9	2	7
Oedema	5	3	2	17	8	9	67	29	38	57	21	36	33	15	18
Polyps	3	2	1	8	5	3	46	16	30	61	24	37	26	6	20
Cancer							2		2	60	46	14	60	46	14
Vocal-fold paralysis	2	1	1	3	2	1	13	7	6	39	15	24	44	22	22
Normal on exam	4	2	2	7	4	3	27	11	16	42	11	31	20	7	13
Laryngitis	1	1		4	1	3	21	7	14	17	7	10	10	4	6
Leukoplakia				2	2		14	7	7	29	22	7	7	6	1
Functional	2	1	1	2	2		9	2	7	11	3	8	7	3	4
Psychogenic				3	2	1	18	2	16	9		9	4	1	3
Bowed vocal folds				1		1	2		2	7	3	4	20	15	5
Neurogenic							1		1	4	3	1	13	5	8
Hyperkeratosis							3	3		7	6	1	6	5	1
Papilloma				2	2		6	6		7	3	4			
Ventricular phonation	1	1		2		2	2		2	7	2	5	3		3
Contact ulcer							7	4	3	4	2	2	3		3
Vocal-fold paresis				1		1	2		2	2		2	7	4	3
Granuloma				2		2	3	1	2	5	3	2	3		3
Cyst				2		2	2	1	1	5	3	2	5	3	2
Laryngeal trauma				4	4		4	4		2	1	1	1		1

Table 4.2 (contd)

	0–14 years			15–24 years			25–44 years			45–64 years			Over 64 years		
	Total	Male	Female	Total	Male	Female	Total	Male	Female	Total	Male	Female	Total	Male	Female
Spastic dysphonia							4	2	2	3	1	2			
Stenosis	1	1								4	1	3	1	1	1
Cricoarytenoid arthritis										2	1	1	3	2	1
Hormonal													1		1
Total	93	66	27	93	32	61	356	128	228	435	190	245	285	146	139

the most frequent were retired persons, homemakers, executives/ managers, teachers, students, secretaries, singers and nurses. Since we generally regard professional voice users as at risk of voice disorders, some of these occupations may seem surprising. The retired group are normally the elderly group, and we have already seen that laryngeal problems are more common in the ageing population, although the rarity of vocal nodules suggests that vocal abuse is seldom a cause of voice disorder in the elderly.

'Homemakers' may be coping with a number of sources of anxiety and stress and, as Herrington-Hall et al. have pointed out, many more women are now working and therefore face additional pressures and responsibilities. We may therefore assume a complex of factors in any client described as a 'homemaker'. Eighty-five per cent of voice disorders described as 'psychogenic' occurred in women. Herrington-Hall et al., in surveying a number of previous studies, noted a marked increase in the number of women presenting with voice disorders. Whilst this may be related to changes in life style and the increased number of women now working, Herrington-Hall et al. mention studies showing that women are now more aware than men of the need for health care and may therefore be referring themselves for a medical opinion on their voice problems.

More recently, research has focused on the prevalence of voice disorders amongst professional voice users. Smith et al. (1997) compared a group of teachers with a control group of individuals employed in other occupations. They found that teachers were more likely to have a voice problem than subjects in the control group. Furthermore, 20% of the teachers had missed days from work because of their voice problem, whereas none of the control group had done so. They came to the conclusion that teaching was a high-risk occupation for voice disorders, with the possibility of significant work-related consequences. In a study of 125 teachers of singing (Miller and Verdolini, 1995) 21% reported on current and 64% on past voice problems. Harvey (1997) has commented that 'the young adult and middlescent professional voice user is often over-worked, over-tired and over-extended'.

Sapir et al. (1993) have used the term vocal attrition, which they define as wear and tear of the vocal mechanism, with overall reduction in vocal abilities. They consider that teachers as a group are at risk of vocal attrition, not only because of the excessive demands on their voices, but also because of the unfavourable acoustic environment in which they work. This opinion was confirmed by the results of a questionnaire survey of 237 female teachers. Over half of these reported multiple symptoms of vocal attrition. Of this group, one-third found that their ability to teach effectively was impaired, and nearly one-third had to miss work because of voice problems. Moreover, nearly one-fifth of the teachers studied had found their voice a source of chronic stress and frustration.

Classification of voice disorders

It is inevitable that problems occur in devising a satisfactory classification of voice disorders, because they often represent the culmination of a number of predisposing, precipitating and maintaining factors. Perkins (1971) has commented that we are 'mired in a terminological swamp, with terms whose lineage is physiological, anatomical, acoustical and psychological'. While most writers are agreed that there is a need to strive for a greater objectivity, we must remember that descriptive labels may be important and meaningful to the voice user himself. As Thurman (1977) observes, the client's own terms may be inaccurate and difficult to define, but they may have more relationship to what he is doing vocally than the usual professional terms: 'The clinician should pick up the terms the client uses and attempt to identify the problem as the client sees it and to relate it to normal voice production.'

Dysphonia, Aronson (1980) reminds us, is a disorder of communication and has 'personal, social and economic significance'. In judging the normality of voice he poses the following questions:

1. Is the voice adequate to carry language intelligibly to the listener?
2. Are its acoustic properties aesthetically acceptable?
3. Does it satisfy its owner's occupational and social requirements?

The answers to these questions provide an effective way of judging, in the first place, whether the patient actually has a voice problem. Secondly, the answers may help us to evaluate the efficacy of our remedial procedures.

There is, however, one further dimension of voice disorders that has received scant attention in the literature: how does the voice feel to the patient? The degree of discomfort experienced is a vital and sensitive barometer of the condition of the larynx and the state of voice use. However normal the voice may sound to the therapist, or to anyone else for that matter, if it does not feel comfortable to the patient then we have failed in our task of vocal remediation. Absence of physical awareness of the voice is the target to be achieved.

Verdolini (1994) has suggested that the degree of effort subjectively involved in speaking and singing is another important aspect of the severity of the voice problem. Again, such a 'scaling of phonatory effort' would be useful as a pre- and post-treatment measure.

Before considering some of the ways in which voice has been classified, we must remember that labels may be applied at a number of different levels. Brackett (1971) has discussed this problem in a very comprehensive contribution on the parameters of voice quality. Much will depend on who is applying the label: the patient describing his problem, the laryngologist reporting on the appearance or movement of the vocal folds, the therapist noting the perceived symptoms, or the physicist measuring certain acoustic phenomena of voice production. In other words, are we making some sort of classification on the acoustic, anatomical, physiological, or psychological correlates of voice disorder? As Brackett says, 'the nature of the disorder remains the same, although different labels may have been used in its descriptions'.

Classification based on acoustic phenomena

Wilson (1979) has observed that voice problems are 'traditionally' classified under the aspect of voice affected (quality, loudness and pitch problems). While this is a useful and apparently simple form of classification, we are immediately faced with the fact that in the majority of dysphonic patients all aspects of voice production are affected.

As Van Riper and Irwin (1958) observe, 'seldom does the abnormal variation exist along one dimension of voice alone'. Classically, the dysphonic voice is weak in intensity, restricted in pitch and 'hoarse' or 'husky' in quality. While we may encounter conditions where a single feature of voice is affected, such as the level of intensity in the early stages of Parkinson's disease, these cases are relatively uncommon. Furthermore, such a classification does not tell us all we need to know about the causes underlying the disturbed acoustic features. There are, of course, exceptions: the overloud voice in an elderly person may suggest a fairly marked degree of presbycusis, and persistent monotony may be associated with depression. Such exceptions are scarcely sufficient to justify the use of a classification system which is more appropriate as an assessment tool.

The majority of voice cases present as 'weak', 'hoarse', or 'husky' (or whatever words we may choose to apply in place of these terms) and demonstrate a disorder along all parameters. It is also important to consider those cases referred with a voice that appears essentially normal, but where the problem may be one of vocal fatigue and discomfort, with as yet little effect on the way the voice sounds.

When we examine the many terms used to describe voice quality there are three that occur most frequently: harsh, hoarse and breathy. While they represent an essentially subjective judgement of voice, there does appear to be surprising agreement in their use.

The term 'breathy' implies that there is a degree of air waste during phonation. Moore (1971) described the breathy voice as a combination of vocal fold sound and whisper noise produced by turbulent air. 'The quality of the breathy voice', he says, 'varies over a wide range that is determined by the ratio of breath noise to phonatory sound.' Air waste occurs when there is incomplete adduction of the vocal folds, which may have an organic cause (bowing of the cords or vocal nodules), or may be a habitual pattern of voice in the absence of organic changes.

The harsh voice, by contrast, implies that the vocal folds are adducting normally, but that the speaker is employing excessive tension. A synonym for harsh is strident, again a term that occurs frequently in the literature. Van Riper and Irwin (1958) state categorically that the essential feature of the harsh voice is tension. Brackett (1971) describes a study in which inflammation of the vocal folds was achieved experimentally by the deliberate use of harsh voice. They state that the intensity of the harsh voice appears louder than normal, but consider that this may result from the effect on resonance of tension in the oral and pharyngeal cavities. It is commonly characterized by a hard glottal attack.

Brackett (1971) has described this as hypervalvular phonation – 'the vocal folds strike each other vigorously at the beginning of the closed phase and separate violently when the opening phase is initiated'. In addition, 'the vocal folds offer increased resistance to air flow with subsequent increase in subglottal air pressure'.

The harsh voice has been described as generally lower in pitch than normal. Bowler's (1964) study found a mean fundamental frequency of 94 Hz for harsh voices compared to 127 Hz for normal adult male voices. Depending on the physical vulnerability of the vocal folds, such habitual vocal misuse may eventually lead to tissue changes of chronic laryngitis, vocal nodules or contact ulcers. The voice therapist, hearing a harsh, strident quality, is alert to the risk of vocal abuse, particularly if the patient complains of local discomfort after voice use, or periods of vocal weakness and pitch breaks.

The majority of dysphonic voices, however, present as 'hoarse' and this is the label most often encountered. Wilson (1979) states that 'hoarseness in its simplest definition is a combination of harshness and breathiness, with the harsh element predominating in some hoarse voices and the breathy element in others.' In addition to the turbulence created by air waste, there is also an aperiodicity of fundamental frequency. Van Riper and Irwin (1958) describe an experiment in which a husky (breathy) voice and a harsh voice were blended in simultaneous recording of the same sentence. Eight of the ten judges listening to the resultant recording described the voice as hoarse. The tension present in hoarse phonation may represent the patient's physical effort to compensate for a weak, breathy voice. In some cases this tension may represent a long-term pattern of vocal behaviour (hyperfunction) which resulted in a weak (hypofunctional) voice (Brodnitz, 1959). On the other hand, tension may have been of more recent origin – for example, occurring after an attack of acute laryngitis, where the patient was trying to make himself heard. Boone (1977) wrote of these 'temporary laryngeal changes which cause compensatory vocal behaviours that persist and become the individual's particular set for subsequent vocal behaviour'. As we have already said, one important constraint of a classification based on perceptual factors is the limited information it offers about the condition of the larynx in terms of muscle movement and tissue change, and the causes of the voice disorder. Clearly we have to look elsewhere for a more satisfactory classification, leaving the areas of pitch, intensity, intonation and quality to be the focus of careful assessment and evaluation.

The functional versus organic dichotomy

The traditional approach to classification is the broad one of a functional versus organic dichotomy, but as Van Riper and Irwin (1958) comment, 'both organic and functional factors are often present and it is difficult or impossible to weigh their influence properly'. Aronson (1980), who gives a comprehensive survey of organic voice disorders, describes the cause as organic 'if it is caused by structural (anatomic) or physiologic disease, either a disease in the larynx itself or remote systemic illnesses which impair laryngeal structure or function'.

Brackett (1971), in discussing some of the theoretical difficulties involved in using such a classification, makes three important points: in the first place, a speech structure may be used in a variety of ways and therefore we may use the normal voice mechanism to produce a number of different acoustic effects; secondly, the way in which a structure is used may have an effect on that structure (It is well documented that hyperfunctional voice use leads to vocal nodules, inflammation and oedema); thirdly, certain structural anomalies, such as laryngeal web, will place constraints on voice use. 'Present understanding', says Brackett, 'does not permit a clear differentiation between the two terms functional and organic since both the condition and the use of the structure are determinants in the assessment of the disorder.'

The condition of vocal nodules is a very clear example of the oversimplification which the organic/functional dichotomy represents. The essential element in the development of nodules is the manner in which the patient is using his voice. Van Riper and Irwin (1958) provide a graphic picture of the 'repeated impact of highly tensed vocal cords hitting each other under conditions of excessive strain' which eventually leads to a tissue reaction in the epithelium of the larynx. It is these organic changes, in the form of small, bilateral, localized fibrous growths, that prevent full adduction of the free edges of the vocal folds. This results in a voice characterized by air waste, and, in most cases, by the hoarse quality that indicates the excessive effort the patient is making to overcome the vocal weakness. The organic problem is indeed having its effect on the voice, but initially it was the way in which the vocal mechanism was used which created the tissue changes.

This same patient may experience considerable anxiety about his dysphonic voice and its effect on his career or social activities. This can lead to still further localized or generalized tension. He may try to compensate for his weak voice by making greater vocal efforts, which inevitably lead to a worsening of the organic condition. This illustrates the complex interaction between functional and organic factors, and under-lines the essential limitations involved in using this form of classification. As Wilson (1979) says, 'the continuum (between organic and functional) is a two-way path because a pathology can result in a poorly functioning mechanism, or a poorly functioning mechanism can result in organic changes or an organic condition'.

This brings us to a more careful consideration of the term 'functional'. Brackett (1971) says that functional applies to the physiology or use of the structures in attaining particular objectives. Aronson (1980) takes a very different view in claiming that functional is a synonym for psychogenic, and that psychogenic voice disorders are caused by psychoneuroses, personality disorders, and faulty habits of voice use. The voice is abnormal 'despite normal anatomy and physiology'. Wilson (1979) uses 'functional' as an umbrella term to include both vocal misuse and emotional disturbances.

In using the word 'functional' in clinical practice, it is clearly important that we define our meaning. For many speech pathologists, the term implies a psychogenic voice disorder, in the apparent absence of vocal misuse. However, the concept of 'vocal misuse and abuse' (Van Thal, 1961) may also be properly regarded as a functional problem. It is obviously essential, in the management of voice disorders, to be clear what we mean by the term. To complicate the issue still further, functional is frequently used synonymously with hysterical, but as Van Thal observed, 'strictly speaking, hysterical aphonia is one form of functional voice disorder, and not all functional disorders are hysterical'.

The fact that the term 'hysterical' is mentioned rather rarely in current literature on dysphonia, reflects a considerable shift in the appraisal of functional voice disorders and the changing attitudes on the subject of hysteria. Luchsinger and Arnold (1965) suggest that it is better to avoid the term hysterical 'because of its derogatory characterological and sociolog-ical connotations'. It is all too easy to label a condition as 'neurotic' or 'hysterical' when it fails to respond to traditional treatment methods.

We have seen that the terms 'functional', 'psychogenic' and 'hysterical' have been used synonymously, and have been applied to those patients who exhibit a voice problem in the absence of any apparent organic symptoms on indirect or direct laryngoscopy. The use of the word 'apparent' is important: as Freeman (Chapter 8) has stressed, increased knowledge of laryngeal function and the physical effects of stress have made us aware of the need to investigate for hitherto unexpected causes of laryngeal dysfunction.

We know, for example, that dysphonia (manifest by a lowering of pitch and a roughness of quality) is an early symptom of hypothyroidism, which may be overlooked on laryngeal examination. Damste (1967) has warned that the administration of androgens and anabolic steroids can result in vocal symptoms, such as 'unsteadiness of timbre', before changes are revealed by laryngoscopy or even stroboscopic examination. In a four-year period (1962–66) 10% of women referred to the ENT clinic at the University of Utrecht had disturbances of vocal function due to virilizing agents. The therapist must be aware of possible discrete physical changes which are not visible on what may have been a superficial examination (for example, indirect laryngoscopy of a patient whose larynx has been difficult to view).

In summary, functional is an umbrella term which can be used to describe a number of vocal behaviours:

1. It can refer to those cases where abuse and misuse of the vocal mechanism is clearly indicated.
2. We may propose that it is used for all 'learned' patterns of maladaptive vocal behaviour (for example, a compensatory mode of voice production which develops during a period of acute infective laryngitis).
3. The umbrella must be large enough to cover an apparently psychogenic cause where there is a cumulative history of emotional stress and tension, but the patient does not present with a recent history of vocal-fold pathology or evidence of misuse. Sudden onset can be associated with emotionally traumatic events.

We might further divide such apparently psychogenic cases into two groups:

1. patients who present with a (sometimes long) history of psychosomatic conditions and a positive psychiatric history, who seem to be particularly vulnerable to physical and emotional stress;
2. patients who appear to have a stable personality, and an absence of psychiatric history, but where the voice problem is a reaction to prolonged and increasing stress and tension in their domestic or work environment.

It is not within the scope of this chapter to discuss the possible mechanism of sudden or even more gradual voice loss in psychogenic voice disorder, or to consider the personality and physical variables involved in response to stress. It is obvious, however, that we need to be very clear in our own mind what we mean when we describe a voice case as functional, since this will inevitably have considerable implications for treatment.

It has been demonstrated that the functional/organic dichotomy is not an entirely satisfactory form of classification. As Murphy (1964) said, they represent 'an untenable dichotomy'. He went on to say, however, that it is a convenient classification despite the imprecision of the terms, since most therapists recognize that in many functional cases subtle organic factors exist, and that in most, if not all, organic cases functional factors can be found.

Greene and Mathieson (1989) have proposed an interesting and useful alternative to the organic/functional dichotomy by classifying voice disorders under the headings behavioural and organic. Changes in the laryngeal mucosa resulting from hyperfunctional voice use (e.g. vocal nodules and contact ulcers) are grouped within the behavioural category. Organic conditions are grouped under the four headings of structural abnormalities, neurological conditions, endocrine disorders, and laryngeal disease (Table 4.3). Greene and Mathieson stress, however, that while the classification is conveniently tidy, the clinical reality is likely to be more complex. Nonetheless, their classification is appealingly simple for the voice clinician.

Hyperfunctional and hypofunctional voice use

Some attempts have been made to classify voice on a continuum of overadduction or underadduction. Greene (1980) prefers the term 'hyperkinetic' which she equates with vocal strain. Brackett (1971) introduces the concept of hypovalvular and hypervalvular phonation, which can clearly be used synonymously with hyperfunctional and hypofunctional and hyperkinetic and hypokinetic. He describes optimal laryngeal valving as a degree of valving which 'offers sufficient resistance to air flow to accomplish unhampered vibrations of the vocal folds at the desired intensity for speech'.

Luchsinger and Arnold (1965) used the term 'hypokinetic' to describe inefficient laryngeal movements, 'reflecting the passive breakdown of laryngeal function'. Hyperkinetic refers to excessive laryngeal movements, which 'express the subconscious, aggressive protest of the patient against the difficulties encountered in his life'. They viewed both these problems as dysphonia of psychogenic origin.

Table 4.3 Classification of voice disorder

Behavioural	Organic
1. *Excessive muscular tension* No changes in laryngeal mucosa	1. *Structural abnormalities* Laryngeal web Cleft palate Nasal obstruction Trauma
2. *Excessive muscular tension* *– changes in laryngeal mucosa* Vocal nodules Chronic laryngitis Oedema Polyps Contact ulcers	2. *Neurological conditions* Recurrent laryngeal nerve paralysis Pseudobulbar palsy Bulbar palsy Cerebellar ataxia Tremor Parkinsonism Chorea Athetosis Apraxia Multiple lesions, e.g. motor neuron disease, multiple scerosis
3. *Psychogenic* Anxiety state Neurosis Conversion symptoms Delayed pubertal voice change (puberphonia) Transsexual conflict	
	3. *Endocrinological disorders* Thyrotoxicosis Myxoedema Male sexual mutational retardation Female virilization due to adverse hormone therapy Adverse drug therapy
	4. *Laryngeal disease* Tumour – benign/malignant Hyperkeratosis Papillomatosis Cyst Laryngitis – acute/chronic Cricoarytenoid arthritis Granuloma Fungal infection

Aronson (1980) uses the term 'kinesiologic' for this form of classification and comments that although this idea is not without merit, if used exclusively it 'oversimplifies the complexities of the laryngeal pathologies, placing excess emphasis on the degree of approximation of the vocal edges rather than on the multiple causes of such approximation defects'.

The aetiological classification of voice disorders

A classification that looks at the causes of voice disorder 'encourages the deepest understanding of dysphonia or aphonia' (Aronson, 1980). Such a form of classification, based on the physical condition of the larynx, tends to have been developed by laryngologists. It implies the need for a careful investigation of the physical factors that may be involved, embodying such diverse disciplines as otolaryngology, neurology and endocrinology. Indeed, while referrals normally come via the ENT department, both surgeons and voice therapists need to be alert to the possibility of both endocrine and neurological pathology as causative factors. Oates (Chapter 7) and Freeman (Chapter 8) in this volume have emphasized that apparent absence of observable signs cannot always be assumed to indicate a psychogenic voice disorder.

Simpson's (1971) classification of voice disorders provides a systematic and comprehensive framework for the study of voice disorders and has clearly facilitated co-operation between laryngologists and speech therapists. Simpson wrote that 'dysphonia in the absence of gross laryngeal pathology has in the past received scant attention from the orthodox laryngologist, whose very training has concentrated his interest on gross pathology and life-threatening disease'. Such a statement has been less true in other parts of Europe, with emergence of the specialist area of medicine known as phoniatrics. Most, but not all, phoniatrists were originally otolaryngologists with a special interest in voice.

Luchsinger and Arnold (1965) gave the following system of classification:

1. dysplastic dysphonia: voice disorders of constitutional origin;
2. vocal nodules and polyps: primary dysphonia and secondary laryngitis;
3. endocrine dysphonia: vocal disorders of endocrine origin;
4. paralytic dysphonia: vocal disorders from laryngeal paralysis;
5. dysarthric dysphonia: vocal disorders of central origin;
6. myopathic dysphonia: vocal disorders of myopathic origin;
7. the influence of the neurovegetative system on the voice (in which they included vasomotor monochorditis and contact ulcers);
8. traumatic dysphonia: vocal disorders following laryngeal injury;
9. alaryngeal dysphonia: voice without a larynx;
10. habitual dysphonia: vocal disorder of habitual origin;
11. psychogenic dysphonia: vocal disorders of emotional origin.

Aronson's (1980) aetiology of voice disorders is broken down under three main headings: organic, psychogenic, and those of indeterminate aetiology (under which he wisely places spastic dysphonia!). Under the organic heading he lists the following causes:

* congenital disorders
* inflammation
* tumours
* endocrine disorders trauma
* neurological disease.

The psychogenic voice disorders are listed as follows:

* emotional stress – musculoskeletal tension;
* voice disorders without the secondary laryngeal pathology;
* voice disorders with secondary laryngeal pathology (vocal nodules and contact ulcer);
* psychoneurosis; conversion reaction – mutism, aphonia, and dysphonia;
* psychosocial conflict – mutational falsetto (puberphonia), dysphonias associated with conflict of sex identification;
* iatrogenic.

His classification of psychogenic voice disorders tends to assume causes which may not be demonstrated so easily – puberphonia may have a number of causes, and psychosocial conflict is not necessarily one of them! Not everyone would accept that hyperfunctional voice use should be classified as psychogenic. Aronson's classification remains, however, a useful and simple way of classifying voice disorders, devised by an experienced speech pathologist.

The aetiological classification attempts to locate the precise area of breakdown in the vocal mechanism and the cause of that breakdown. It is the most essential aspect of assessment of vocal dysfunction, since we may find that there is a condition which requires medical and surgical treatment. Management of the voice disorder may therefore be irrelevant in some cases, or follows only after appropriate treatment from a laryngologist or endocrinologist.

Attempts to classify voice continue, and one of the more recent has been suggested by Verdolini (1994). She has grouped voice disorders into the following four categories: discrete mass lesions, distributed tissue changes; organic movement disorders and non-organic disorders (see Table 4.4). This provides a useful framework for the clinician and also overcomes some of the pitfalls encountered in other classification systems.

Table 4.4 Classification, after Verdolini (1994)

Category	Description	Presumed primary cause and possible contributors	Primary effect on voice
Discrete Mass Lesions			
Membranous Folds			
Nodules	Protrusions at midpoint of membranous folds; edematous and/or collagenous	High vocal fold impact force High vocal fold tissue viscosity	Hoarseness
Polyps	Protrusions at midpoint of membranous folds; edematous, possibly vascularized	High vocal fold impact force. High vocal fold tissue viscosity	Hoarseness
Cysts	Protrusions along membranous folds, often at midpoint, fluid-filled sacs of epithelium	Glandular blockage	Hoarseness
Papilloma	Laryngeal warts	Virus (presence of vaginal warts in mother, and vaginal delivery)	Hoarseness
Keratosis leukoplakia	White plaque-like lesions	Irritants (smoke)	Hoarseness
Cancer	White grainy lesions	Smoke and alcohol	Hoarseness
Posterior glottis Contact ulcers	Protrusions on medial surface of arytenoids, possibly with contralateral concavity	Gastric reflux; 'pressed' phonation Low pitch	Phonatory effort
Distributed Tissue Changes			
Reinke's edema	Distributed edema along membranous folds	Irritants (smoke)	Low pitch in speech
Laryngitis	Distributed inflammation	Bacteria, virus Chronic heavy voice use	Hoarseness Weak voice
Bowing	Persistent bowing of folds (muscular deformation?)	Elderly age	Weak voice
Sulcus vocalis	Groove parallel to vocal fold margin	Congenital, development Heavy voice use	Weak voice
Trauma	(Appearance depends on type of trauma)	Mechanical, thermal or chemical trauma	Variable

(contd)

Table 4.4 (contd)

Category	Description	Presumed primary cause and possible contributors	Primary effect on voice
Organic Movement Disorders			
Peripheral paralyses	Limited (medial) movement of affected fold	Local trauma (including surgery) Virus Heart Disease	Weak voice
Central paralyses	Resistance to movement	Cerebral cortex lesions (Stroke)	Tight voice
Extrapyramidal disease (e.g. Parkinson's Disease)	Small range of motion	Dopamine deficiency	Monotone voice in speech Weak voice
Nerve-muscle junction dysfunctions (myasthenia gravis)	Rapid fatigue in function	Rapid depletion of chemicals sustaining vocal fold contaction	Rapid voice fatigue
Spasmodic dysphonia	Abrupt adductions during speech (adductory) Abrupt abductions during speech (abductory)	Undetermined	Spasmodic voice
Non-Organic Disorders			
Mutational falsetto	Persistent high pitch in postpubertal male, with normal-appearing larynx	Psychological conflict Learned behaviour	High pitch (falsetto)
Ventricular phonation	False (ventricular) vocal folds vibrate and produce sound	Sometimes compensation for poorly functioning true vocal folds	Gravelly voice
Conversion aphonia/dysphonia	Lack of voice (aphonia) or hoarse voice (dysphonia), with normal-appearing larynx	Psychological	No voice or hoarse voice
Muscular tension dysphonia	Persistent posterior glottal gap during phonation, and complaints of voice problems	Simultaneous contraction of laryngeal adductors and abductors	Breathy voice Phonatory effort

A developmental perspective

The incidence of voice disorder and the prevalence of different types of voice problem might be expected to vary with different age groups. As research into voice disorders gains momentum, we are beginning to learn more about voice problems in children, adolescents, adults and the ageing population. To take the developmental perspective even further, Sataloff (1995) has suggested that we should be looking at the genetics of voice and the relationship between the structure of the vocal tract and its function, and the transmission of both normal and abnormal voice characteristics.

In looking at the incidence of childhood dysphonia, Silverman and Zimmer (1975) studied a group of 162 school children. Chronic hoarseness was found in 20% of the group and over half of these presented with vocal nodules. With the onset of puberty, females may experience vocal changes in the premenstrual phase. Oedema of interstitial tissues and increased vocal fold mass may lead to a more restricted pitch range, particularly for high notes and huskiness (Spiegel et al., 1997). These symptoms can, of course, persist until the menopause, but may be a problem only for the serious or professional singer.

Spiegel et al. (1997) have suggested that upper respiratory tract infections (which will include laryngitis) are common in younger age groups because of 'multiple and frequent personal contacts'. Allergies are also reported to be more common and 'multiple allergic manifestations can affect voice'. Allergic laryngitis, usually associated with allergic rhinitis or asthma, will obviously affect voice quality. Spiegel et al. also list the potential effects of gastro-esophageal reflux and bulimia on the vocal folds.

In Harvey's (1997) experience, most of the voice disorders encountered in young adults and the 'middlescent' are hyperfunctional (musculoskeletal tension dysphonias). She goes on to observe that 'many patients have a concomitant disorder that may significantly complicate treatment and recovery'. She lists such conditions as endocrine dysfunction, asthma and multiple chemical sensitivity, as well as HIV and AIDS.

A study by Boltezar et al. (1997) of 51 adolescents (age range from 10 to 17 years) found that the main characteristics of the adolescent voice were instability of amplitude and more specifically the instability of pitch.

Gastro-oesophageal reflux can continue to be a problem in adult life (Verdolini, 1994), as can a susceptibility to allergies and upper respiratory tract infections, all of which can lead to the onset or maintenance of a voice problem.

Sataloff et al. (1997b) have listed the effects of ageing on the larynx, which may lead to a loss of vocal efficiency, with breathiness and loss of volume being characteristic of the ageing voice. These physical changes include atrophy of ligaments, muscle and neural tissue, so that the vocal folds thin and lose their elasticity. We may also find arthritic changes in the larynx.

A chart review of 151 dysphonic patients over the age of 60 (Woo et al., 1992) came to the conclusion, however, that ageing-related voice disorders were more likely to be due to disease processes associated with ageing rather than with the ageing process alone. These included central neurological disorders affecting laryngeal function, such as cerebral vascular lesions and Parkinson's disease; benign vocal fold lesions; inflammatory disorders, including the effect of medication; laryngeal neoplasia and laryngeal paralysis. They found what they called 'typical laryngeal findings of presbylaryngis' (indicated by bowing of the vocal folds and breathiness) in only six patients.

Conclusions

Perhaps we have worried too much about getting the words right. Ultimately it is the patient, and those who have to listen to him or her, who will judge whether the voice is normal or not, whatever the 'experts' may say about the matter. The experts, however, continue to discuss the problem of describing voices, and continue to search for a more satisfactory way of doing so. We have seen that it is possible to look at voice disorders in a number of different ways: happily these are not mutually exclusive and each one may yield not only different information about the voice disorder but also a different way of looking at it. Perceptually we may describe the acoustic features of voice production in terms of pitch, intonation, intensity and quality; we recognize the variables involved in the development of voice disorders by attempting to describe the cause as functional or organic; the concept of underadduction or overadduction indicates the degree of tension involved, which has important implications for treatment procedures; and finally, it is the laryngologist and other medical specialists who give us a precise account of what is wrong (if anything) with the condition of the larynx and provide an essential opportunity to assess the efficacy of our treatment.

A developmental approach to voice disorders is becoming increasingly relevant as our understanding of the physiological changes in the larynx becomes more sophisticated.

CHAPTER 5

The speech and language therapist's assessment of the dysphonic patient

PAUL CARDING

Introduction

Comprehensive assessment of the dysphonic patient is important for a number of reasons. First, it enables the clinician to determine the nature of the dysphonia, to understand the cause and to consider all the relevant 'precipitating, predisposing and perpetuating factors' (Morrison and Rammage, 1994. p.50). Secondly, it allows for an evaluation of the degree and severity of the presenting dysphonia, from the perspective of both the clinician and the patient. Thirdly, full assessment helps the voice therapist to decide what type of therapy to embark upon, where to start and what aspects to cover. Fourthly, the assessments can be used to establish a baseline against which voice change can be measured (Carding and Horsley, 1992). For these reasons, comprehensive voice assessment is probably the most important aspect of the speech and language therapist's management of any patient with a voice problem.

Voice is a multi-dimensional phenomenon and therefore requires a multi-dimensional approach to assessment. No individual assessment can provide anything other than a part of a complex whole. The perceptual, anatomical, physiological, psychological and acoustic aspects should complement each other in providing a full understanding of how and why a particular voice sounds the way that it does.

For convenience, the assessments discussed below are divided into three broad categories: the case history interview, perceptual judgements and instrumental measurements. Together, this battery of assessments can provide a full picture of the voice problem: how the voice sounds, what the larynx looks like, how the laryngeal structures move, what characterizes the vocal output signals and how the dysphonia has affected the individual. Each of these three categories is discussed in detail below.

69

Wherever possible, the reader is referred to source texts, since each aspect of voice assessment is a large topic within itself and it is not possible to do justice to all of the techniques in one chapter.

The case history

Taking a good case history is a skilled and practised art form. There are as many ways of doing it as there are successful voice therapists. Experienced clinicians often prefer their interview to be led by the patient's responses, to let the discussion flow, so that the information is gathered in an informal and relaxed manner. Less experienced therapists prefer to follow an established format to be sure that all the relevant areas are covered. There are some good examples of a standard case history format in the literature (Stemple, 1984; Greene and Mathieson, 1989; Colton and Casper, 1996; Harris, 1998). Some clinicians may prefer to ask the patient to fill in a questionnaire (Martin, 1986) and then use this as a basis for the interview and discussion. Morrison and Rammage (1994) identify the importance of open-ended questions and non-judgemental questions (i.e. 'Tell me about your voice problem' is probably better than 'How long has your voice been this bad?'). They suggest that the response to an open-ended question may be more genuine, and hence more revealing. In general, it is better to go from the general question ('How's your voice been?') to the specific question ('What exactly has changed since the last time?'). By using an increasingly specific series of questions, the clinician is helping the patient to focus on the main issues of the problem. Questions should avoid professional jargon and should use the patient's terminology wherever possible (as long as it is mutually understood).

There are some main areas that need to be covered in the dysphonia case history and these are addressed below.

History of the voice problem √

It is important to establish the chronological progression of the disorder (i.e. from the onset to the time of presentation). The patient should be asked to consider all aspects which may have contributed to the onset of the voice problem. It is likely that there will be a number of factors that have combined to make the dysphonia occur (Morrison and Rammage, 1994; Colton and Casper, 1996; Harris, 1998). Sudden onset of voice problems for no organic reason has traditionally been considered an indicator of psychogenic aetiology (but see Freeman, Chapter 8 of this volume). The voice loss may be severe (including total aphonia) and has been seen as an unconscious reaction to high levels of stress or a dramatic life event (Aronson, 1985b). Gradual onset is generally considered a symptom of prolonged habitual misuse or abuse of the voice. Gradual increase in severity is usually an indicator of mechanical or hyperfunctional dysphonia (this is discussed in more detail by Oates, in Chapter 7).

The patient should also be encouraged to explore all the possible factors which might have contributed to the maintenance of the problem. The maintenance factors may not be the same as the causative ones; for example, a period of acute dysphonia following an upper respiratory tract infection may result in dysphonic symptoms. However, excessive voice use at that time may lead to the patient trying to compensate for poor voice quality. This may result in maladaptive vocal behaviours, which then develop into a habitual mechanical or hyperfunctional dysphonia.

Intermittent dysphonias are difficult to assess. The patient describes symptoms that can be very variable. It is important to establish how severe the patient's vocal symptoms are at the time of consultation, in comparison with their extremes of variability. Very variable voice problems are often seen as a reaction to external influences – for example levels of stress or as a reaction to specific voice abuse. However, it has been suggested that some cases may be early presentations of vocal abuse or misuse (Kotby, 1995). Intermittent dysphonias are often best assessed over a period of time and often involve the patient keeping a vocal diary (Boone and McFarlane, 1988; Freeman, Chapter 8, this volume) and tape-recording his or her voice at home at different levels of severity.

Medical history

Relevant medical problems can be important in establishing the cause or maintenance of a voice problem. Medical conditions that coincide with the onset of the dysphonia should obviously be investigated thoroughly. Upper respiratory tract infections are the most common medical condition to cause a voice problem. Although these infections can be self-limiting, many dysphonias begin with an acute episode and then develop into a chronic problem of vocal mismanagement, voice abuse or misuse. However, voice problems can also be caused by a huge variety of medical conditions including diseases of the head and neck; diseases and disorders of the nervous system; endocrine disorders; hormonal imbalance; arthritis; allergy; asthma; gastro-oesophageal reflux and acquired immune deficiency syndrome. The effects on voice disorders produced by most of these conditions are briefly described by Johns (Chapter 3) and Oates (Chapter 7). More detailed descriptions can be found in chapters of the excellent book edited by Sataloff (1997).

Because numerous medical conditions may lead to dysphonic symptoms, it is important to ensure that a 'voice clinic team approach' is used in the diagnosis and management of voice disorder (Morrison and Rammage, 1994). Pharmacological treatment of the underlying medical condition may result in an alleviation of the dysphonic symptoms. More commonly, however, pharmacological treatment is required in conjunction with voice therapy, which is aimed at optimizing vocal function.

Psychological and personality factors

Understanding the influence of a patient's individual personality and psychological state on his or her voice problem is crucial to the management of it. Particular psychological states such as anxiety, stress, depression, or personality traits (including the patient who is over-assertive or extremely nervous) may help explain the cause or maintenance of a voice problem (Aronson, 1990). In a small number of cases, severe psychological problems may be the cause of the voice disorder (Baker, 1997), while in others psychological difficulties may be a significant contributing factor (Butcher et al., 1993). In almost all cases, a voice disorder can have psychosocial consequences (Andrews, 1995; Butcher, 1995). The clinical skill is trying to determine what is cause and what is effect (see Freeman, Chapter 8, for further discussion).

There is also some evidence to suggest that personality factors may have a bearing on the effects of voice therapy. Patients who are able to introspect and analyse the influences on their own voice problem of life style, stress factors and other personal responses have a better prognosis than those who cannot (Carding and Horsley, 1992; Ritchie, 1996). Clinicians vary in the way they assess these factors. The Voice Handicap Index (Jacobsen et al., 1997) can help to gain insights into the patient's current view of the problem; the General Health Questionnaire GHQ-60 (Goldberg and Williams, 1988) is also used in some voice clinics (White et al., 1997; Butcher and Cavalli, 1998).

Occupation and social life

Finally it is important to understand the patient's vocal use and environment. It is very relevant to discover the levels of background noise, the air quality (i.e. dusty, smoky, dry) and acoustic environment of the patient's workplace. Similarly, it is important to determine the amount and nature of vocal demands such as telephone talking, giving presentations or shouting. The clinician should also ask similar questions about the patient's social life and hobbies. This information not only enhances the understanding of the vocal demands on the patient and identifies areas of potential misuse and abuse but also helps the clinician to understand the likely consequences for the patient of being dysphonic in terms of disability/activity and handicap/participation (see Oates, Chapter 7 and Freeman, Chapter 8, for further discussion).

A set of questions that may form the basis of the case history is in Appendix 5.1. All of these areas may require further investigation depending on the particular needs and problems of the individual patient.

Perceptual judgements

This section describes three subjective assessment techniques: (a) auditory perceptual judgement of voice quality, (b) visual perceptual judgement during laryngoscopic examination and (c) the patients' judgement of their own voice problems. Auditory judgement and laryngoscopic examination are still the most commonly used voice assessment procedures by which most dysphonic patients are diagnosed and monitored (Hirano, 1989). This is despite criticisms that these techniques are too subjective and open to individualistic interpretation (Bless, 1991; Gould and Korovin, 1994).

(a) Auditory voice quality ratings

Auditory voice quality evaluation requires a listener to judge a voice sample, usually consisting of sustained vowels and/or connected speech, on various parameters such as overall severity, roughness, breathiness. The listener usually rates these voice parameters using one of a number of rating scales (Darley et al., 1969b; Hirano, 1981; Laver et al., 1981; Bassich and Ludlow, 1986; Hammarberg et al., 1986; Wilson, 1987; Eskenazi et al., 1990; Kreiman et al., 1993). Each of these rating scales has been devised in order to overcome a perceived deficiency in the others. It is important for any practising clinician to choose a rating scale which he or she fully understands and feels comfortable with, because this tends to improve reliability.

Gerratt et al. (1993) have observed that patients and clinicians use their judgements of how the voice sounds to decide the nature and severity of the problem and to evaluate whether treatment has been successful. Despite this, there are known problems with perceptual measures of voice quality, because:

1. there are potential problems with intra- and inter-judge reliability (Ludlow, 1981);
2. they do not provide objective measures (Liss and Weismer, 1992);
3. there is no commonly accepted set of perceptual scales (Yumoto et al., 1982).

There is a wealth of literature on the problems of judging perceptual voice quality, a lot of which is contradictory and confusing. Kreiman et al. (1993) provide an excellent review of the major issues pertaining to this complex topic, which include the following.

1. The voice quality parameters of 'breathiness', 'strain' and 'vocal stability' are most commonly used and are the most reliably judged (Hammarberg et al., 1986; Kreiman et al., 1993).
2. Ratings of overall dysphonic severity, that is judgements of how 'normal' or 'abnormal' the voice and voice quality sounds, are relatively consistent (Hammarberg et al., 1986; Dejonckere et al., 1993; Kreiman et al., 1993). Overall severity may be seen as a generic term, which relates to the general impression created by a voice quality.
3. A rating scale with a visual analogue is probably the most familiar and simplest design to use (Eskenazi et al., 1990; Kreiman et al., 1993).

It is possible to review some of the existing rating scales with these considerations in mind. According to Greene and Mathieson (1989), the three most commonly used voice rating scales are the Buffalo III Voice Profile (Wilson, 1987), the GRBAS Scale (Hirano, 1981) and the Vocal Profile Analysis (Laver et al., 1981). The Buffalo III Voice Profile requires the listener to rate 12 aspects of the voice, on a five-point scale (1 = normal; 5 = very severe). The scale includes common aspects of voice quality such as resonance and pitch, although other aspects are included under one general heading of 'laryngeal tone'. The Buffalo III Voice Profile also includes items that are not strictly related to how the voice sounds, such as ratings of 'speech anxiety' and 'amount and degree of voice abuse'.

The Committee of Phonatory Function of the Japan Society of Logopedics and Phoniatrics proposed the GRBAS scale for the perceptual analysis of dysphonia (Hirano, 1981). Voice quality parameters of 'roughness', 'breathiness', 'aesthenia' (or weakness) and 'strain', together with an overall severity grade are rated on a five-point scale. This committee acknowledged that the GRBAS scale is not comprehensive because, for example, the scale does not include any parameters for vocal pitch. However, it represents a realistic approach to voice quality judgement and recognizes that there must be a compromise between comprehensiveness and reliability; the GRBAS scale is therefore still used by some clinicians.

The Vocal Profile Analysis (Laver et al., 1981) is a comprehensive schema which enables the listener to rate each aspect of the vocal apparatus as it contributes to a speaker's characteristic voice quality. It includes a number of supralaryngeal features as well as aspects from the laryngeal level. There are a large number of parameters to judge 9 voice quality features, 3 prosodic features and 5 general features, with a series of sub-categories for each parameter. Use of the Vocal Profile Analysis is demonstrated by Wirz, in Chapter 12, this volume.

(b) Visual laryngoscopic judgements

Visual examination of the larynx may be performed in a variety of different ways. Indirect laryngoscopy involves the examination of the larynx via a mirror placed in the nasopharynx. Light is reflected off the mirror, enabling the examiner to view the larynx (Hirano, 1981). Rigid endoscopy involves the use of a powerful light source, which is built into the endoscope, to provide an illuminated view of the larynx. Traditionally, these techniques have been performed by laryngologists; very few speech and language therapists have acquired the skills to do these procedures. Because instruments are placed into the mouth during indirect laryngoscopy and rigid endoscopy the patient's tongue and jaw movements are restricted, which means that movements of the larynx can be observed only during sustained phonation.

In recent years, flexible fibreoptic nasendoscopy has proved a very useful technique for examination of the larynx during phonation (this procedure is sometimes also called 'flexible fibreoptic laryngoscopy'; see Johns, Chapter 3). A growing number of speech and language therapists are being trained to perform this technique for use in therapy. The flexible fibreoptic scope is passed transnasally, to sit just above the larynx; because it does not restrict tongue movements, it allows examination of voice production during connected speech. The speech and language therapist can therefore observe the laryngeal and supralaryngeal structures in action, to determine how they contribute to the abnormal vocal sound, and is therefore in a better position to devise a treatment programme to develop a more appropriate manner of phonation.

Endoscopic procedures may also be used with a stroboscopic light source, which flashes pulses of light in relation to the vibratory speed of the vocal folds during phonation (Bless et al., 1987; Bless, 1991). If these light flashes are slightly asynchronous with the vibratory pattern, the movement of the vocal folds is perceived in 'slow motion'. The advantage of this technique is that it allows careful examination of the laryngeal mucosal waveform during phonation.

In the normal vocal fold, waves travelling on the mucosa from the inferior to its superior surface are observed during vocal fold vibrations. This wave is called the 'mucosal wave' or 'travelling wave' on the mucosa. Existence of a soft pliant superficial layer of vocal fold tissue is considered to be essential for the occurrence of the mucosal wave (Hirano and Bless, 1993). Stroboscopic examination of the mucosal wave may have significant value for the early diagnosis of organic laryngeal pathology (Hirano, 1981, Hirano and Bless, 1993; Harris et al. in Chapter 18 of this volume). Experienced voice clinicians can use the information from stroboscopy to describe the closure and configuration of the vocal folds, vibratory behaviour and other features of laryngeal activity. As Colton and Casper (1996) have observed, however, judgements of the stroboscopic images are mainly based on the skills of the clinicians and therefore there are still a number of unresolved issues with respect to this process.

If neither indirect laryngoscopy, rigid endoscopy nor fibreoptic endoscopy is possible, then laryngeal examination under a general anaesthetic may be performed by the laryngologist. Direct laryngoscopy is unable to provide any information with regard to laryngeal movement and co-ordination during phonation. It is not therefore the examination method of choice in order to characterize features of dysphonia.

(c) The patient's opinion

Formalizing the patients' opinion of their voice problems (as opposed to interpreting their comments at interview) can be very valuable in determining how the problems have affected their communication in everyday life (Carding and Horsley, 1992). There are no standardized questionnaires for patients' descriptions of their voice problems. Jacobson et al. (1997) have recently published the Voice Handicap Index, which provides a general overview of the impact of the voice disorder. Carding and Horsley (1992) devised a Patient Questionnaire of Vocal Performance which enables patients to consider aspects of their own voice and rate the severity of each aspect with regard to their normal voice usage. The questionnaire uses a continuous judgement format which involves the ranking of items in a hierarchy of best to worst, or most to least. The patient therefore responds to a particular question with a qualitative judgement, marking the item which most agrees with their own opinion. The use of graded answers (such as levels of severity) means that the patients' opinion of their own voice performance can be quantified. The Patient Questionnaire of Vocal performance is in Appendix 5.2.

(d) Posture and alignment

Posture and body alignment should be observed throughout the case history interview. Poor posture can result in a restriction in the function of (1) the breathing mechanism, (2) the laryngeal structures and (3) the vocal tract resonators. A common body misalignment involves adduction of the scapulae so that the shoulders are positioned in an unnatural posterior position. Another common pattern is retraction of the head onto the neck so that the jaw protrudes upwards and forwards (Morrison and Rammage, 1994). The first misalignment would produce considerable restriction in airflow for phonation as well as the development of neck and laryngeal hyperfunction. The second misalignment would also result in laryngeal hyperfunction, but would in addition impair natural resonance in the supralaryngeal, pharyngeal and oral spaces (see also Oates, Chapter 7).

It is important to enquire about injuries or illnesses that may have contributed to postural problems and may be ongoing, especially osteo-arthritis and whiplash injuries. It is also important to discuss with the patients their habitual postures at work, such as: at their desk, on the telephone, while singing or during verbal presentations. Obviously, not all postural problems are exhibited during a one-to-one interview, which is often conducted in comfortable chairs.

(e) Performance measures

A number of measures have been proposed which aim to provide indications of laryngeal and respiratory function. Measures such as Maximum Phonation Time (MPT: Hirano et al., 1968); the s/z ratio (Eckel and Boone, 1981; Colton and Casper, 1996) and high-quiet singing (Bastian et al., 1990; Verdolini, 1994, p. 304) have been suggested as indicators of the degree of closure of the vocal folds. It has also been suggested that laryngeal diadochokinetic rates, in which the patient is asked to produce rapid, repeated glottal plosives, can help the clinician to make inferences about the efficiency and neural control of the larynx (Verdolini, 1994, pp. 279 and 305). Performance on this test is based on (1) the rate of production (the number of glottal plosives per second); (2) the strength of the plosives and (3) consistency or steadiness of the productions across time.

There is a considerable amount of literature relating to MPT and the s/z ratio in particular. It has been recognized that performances on these measures can vary for a number of different reasons (Stone, 1983; Kent et al., 1987; Verdolini, 1994). Factors such as rehearsal effects, fatigue, motivation, the number of trials and the role of demonstration have all been identified as potential influences. Despite these potential hazards, experienced clinicians can find some or all of these measures useful indicators in assessment of phonatory activity (Verdolini, 1994; Andrews, 1995; Colton and Casper, 1996).

I did not use these.

Instrumental voice measurements

There has been a long-standing desire in the field of voice disorder to develop measures that would be less subjective and provide more reliable assessment than the perceptual judgements described above (Hillman et al., 1989, 1990). The term 'instrumental' is often used synonymously with 'objective' with respect to voice measurement techniques. However, 'objective' measures of voice still require interpretation and in some cases, correlation to other measures, in order to be of value. Hirano (1989) conducted a world survey and identified over fifty instrumental techniques that were used in measuring different aspects of voice quality and vocal function. There is a vast amount of literature in this area; this chapter is confined to only the most commonly used instrumental techniques.

Laryngographic measurement of vocal function

Laryngography (also called Electroglottography and Electrolaryngography) is a technique which is used to measure aspects of vocal fold contact during voiced phonation (Fabre, 1957; Fourcin, 1974; Abberton et al., 1989). The Laryngograph operates by sensing the electrical conductance between two electrodes which are placed on the skin, one on either side of the speaker's thyroid prominence. The Laryngograph (Fourcin, 1974) or Electroglottograph (Colton and Casper, 1996) monitors the varying electrical conductance between the two electrodes during the vibratory cycle of the vocal folds. Current flow will be at a maximum when the vocal folds are in contact, and at a minimum when the folds are apart. The output waveform (Lx) can be viewed on an oscilloscope, but it is more commonly used as part of a computer interface system; such as PCLX (Laryngograph Ltd.) and interfaces for the Computer Speech Lab (Kay Elemetrics) voice analysis systems.

There is some controversy about the way that the Lx waveform can best be used as a measure of voice. Abberton et al. (1989) suggested that the Lx waveform may be of value in the examination of aspects of abnormal vocal function. They described a number of Lx trace patterns in relation to auditory perceptual qualities and laryngeal examination findings. Furthermore, they suggested that the opening phase and closing phase measurements, in particular, may be of value in detecting and quantifying aspects of abnormal laryngeal movement. In contrast, however, Baken (1987) stated that 'quantification of phases of the Lx cycle is of questionable validity' (p. 224) because of the very limited information about the open phase of the vocal fold vibratory cycle. Baken (1987) suggested that it may be best to interpret Lx traces qualitatively, with our current level of knowledge.

Several other authors provide examples where the Lx traces have been 'read' to provide an estimate of normality. Titze (1990) and Motta et al. (1990) have concentrated on interpreting the Lx waveform in relation to expected norms. Titze (1990) described an 'ideal Lx image' of glottal configuration and then illustrated a number of Lx traces which correspond to various theoretical movements of the vocal folds as they make contact during phonation. Fourcin (1981) and MacCurtain and Fourcin (1982) have made the following observations about the 'normal', idealized Lx waveform (see Figure 5.1):

1   There is a regular pattern to the Lx waveform over time; each complete cycle's shape is uniform with each corresponding vibration.
2. There is an identifiable point of maximum closure for each Lx cycle (that is, a peak to each cycle).
3. There is a steep rising edge which corresponds to the closing phase of the vibratory cycle. The closing phase begins abruptly and has a very short rising time; a rapid and sharply defined closing phase correlates with good vocal tract acoustic excitation and efficient vocal production.
4. The closing phase takes less time than the opening phase.
5. The falling edge of the trace (the opening phase) is smooth and longer in duration than the closing phase.
6. There is usually a trough in the trace which is essentially constant with the time when there is no contact of the vocal folds, along their whole length.

Lx traces can show signs of dysphonia by the absence of normal features. For example, the absence of an identifiable point of maximum closure may indicate poor glottic closure and may illustrate the vocal fold vibratory pattern of a particularly breathy voice quality. This may or may not constitute pathological voice. Carlson (1993) provides a useful case study which includes clinical interpretations of laryngograph signals.

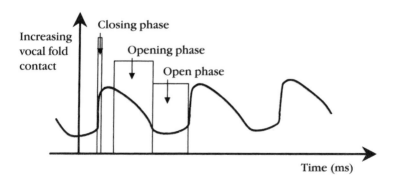

Figure 5.1 Laryngograph waveform (Lx).

Mean speaking fundamental frequency

Abnormal vocal pitch is considered by many authors to be an important aspect of dysphonic voice (Stone and Sharf, 1973; Prater and Swift, 1984; Gordon, 1986). However, listeners' perceptions of vocal pitch may be unreliable (Montague et al., 1978) and some form of instrumental measurement of speaking fundamental frequency is therefore preferable (Baken, 1987). There is some debate in the literature about whether the mean or the modal speaking fundamental frequency should be used (Baken, 1987). Similarly, some authors have highlighted the difference between 'reading speaking fundamental frequency' and 'conversational speaking fundamental frequency' (Hollien and Jackson, 1973; Ramig and Ringel, 1983). These issues have not yet been fully resolved.

Despite the known limitations, using a standard reading passage ensures that fundamental frequency measures from a sample of connected speech can be directly compared with published data and that baseline voice samples can be compared with post-therapy results. Most of the published normative data for mean speaking fundamental frequency (SFF_o) has been based on 'reading speaking', often using a standard passage. There is a considerable amount of normative data for age and sex matched normal values for mean speaking fundamental frequency of normal adults, based on American Caucasian speakers reading 'The Rainbow Passage' (Fairbanks, 1960).

These studies are described in detail by Baken (1987); there is also a brief discussion of some of the issues related to frequency measures in Freeman (Chapter 2). A summary of the findings of those studies is presented in Table 5.1.

Table 5.1 Summary of findings of mean fundamental frequencies for adult males and females

	Mean	Range of means	References
Males	112Hz	84–151 Hz	Mysack, 1959
			Michel, 1968
			Horii, 1975
Females	192 hz	168–221 Hz	Saxman and Burk, 1967
			Hollien and Paul, 1969

Aerodynamic measurements

Measurements of air pressure and air flow that result from speech activity may permit the clinician to infer a great deal about the nature and degree of vocal disability. Clinically based aerodynamic assessment of vocal function primarily involves measuring average glottal airflow rates (litres per second) and average subglottal air pressures (cm H_2O). The reader is referred to Baken's excellent book *Clinical Measurement of Speech and Voice* (1987) for a more complete review of this subject. Both airflow rates and subglottal pressures are obtained via a face mask during well-controlled utterances. Mean phonatory flow rates are usually measured in steady-state vowel utterances to provide estimates of glottic impedance since resistance of the oral cavity is minimal. Because of the complex relationship between phonatory flow rates and vocal intensity and fundamental frequency, these measures should be made under a variety of intensity and frequency conditions (Morrison and Rammage, 1994). Low mean flow rates may be indicative of breath holding during attempts to phonate (as in some psychogenic aphonia patients) or underlying respiratory disease. Estimates of subglottal air pressure is calculated from the utterance of strings of (bi-labial + vowel) syllables. Excessive subglottal air pressure during phonation means an excessive subglottal driving pressure which may have a physiological (spasmodic dysphonia) or functional (i.e. vocal hyperfunction) basis.

The Phonetogram

A Phonetogram is a graph on which is plotted the sound pressure level versus fundamental frequency of voice (Gramming, 1988). To plot the graph, the patient is presented with stimulus tones at graded frequencies and is required to sustain a vowel at a matching vocal pitch. Minimal sustainable intensity is elicited by instructing the patient to say the vowel as softly as possible without whispering; maximal intensity is generated by having the patient shout it as loudly as possible without screaming. Several trials of each minimum and maximum are done. A microphone placed at a fixed distance from the lips is connected to an intensity measurement system. The extreme values for each condition are the data and determine the vocal 'space'' for the patient. This graph or space can be a useful visual tool in explaining the vocal limitations of a speaker. Phonetogram measurements have been used to infer laryngeal physiology in several papers (Gramming, 1988; Gramming and Akerlund, 1988; Gramming et al., 1988; Akerlund et al., 1992). However, these inferences have not been substantiated. There is, as yet, no convincing evidence to correlate phonetogram findings with particular types of laryngeal function (or dysfunction). However, clinicians report that it can be a useful way of comparing pre- and post-therapy vocal range.

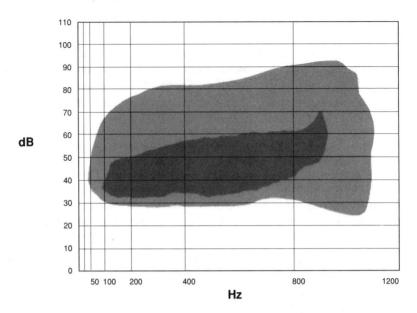

Figure 5.2 An example of the phonetogram's value in illustrating the difference between the pre- and post-therapy voice capabilities of a patient with hyperfunctional dysphonia.

Acoustic analysis of the speech waveform

Acoustic analysis of the waveform is based on the fact that laryngeal pathology alters the normal vibratory pattern of the vocal folds; there is a relationship between the vibratory patterns at the glottal source and certain parameters of the acoustic waveform generated by this vibration.

The use of acoustic techniques to analyse dysphonic voice has been the subject of considerable attention from researchers. Most techniques concentrate on measuring either aperiodic noise in the signal (i.e. noise as seen in the spectrogram) or cycle-to-cycle variability in the waveform (perturbation: i.e. 'jitter' and 'shimmer'). These techniques fall into two main categories: those that analyse sustained vowel samples and those that analyse continuous speech (Laver et al., 1992). The analysis of isolated vowels is simpler to process than connected speech, because it does not have to take into account intonational changes, phonetic irregularities, and voiceless and speech pause segments. The analysis of connected speech has to be able to recognize and process these segments appropriately. For this reason, the analysis of connected speech is more likely to produce results with artefactual distortion (Laver et al., 1992). Therefore, most of the published techniques appear to favour the analysis of single vowel utterances. There are many different ways of calculating the acoustic parameters within a speech waveform. The most common forms are described below.

Calculating 'Noise' in the speech signal

The identification of noise in the speech signal is seen by many authors as central to the acoustic measurement of dysphonic voice (including Kim et al., 1982; Yumoto et al., 1984; Baken, 1987). The larger the noise component, the more this reflects diminished regularity of phonatory vibration (Sorenson et al., 1980). Comparisons of pathological and non-pathological voices (as diagnosed by laryngeal examination) have demonstrated greater amounts of noise in the pathological group (Hartman and von Cramon, 1984; Zyski et al., 1984).

There are many different techniques that have been devised to measure the noise in the speech signal. These include measurement of the intensity of harmonic peaks (Hiraoko et al., 1984), various measures based on a long-time-averaged spectral representation (Hammarberg et al., 1986), comparison of the original spectrum with a reconstructed harmonic spectrum (Klingholz, 1987), quantification of the relationship betwwen the harmonic structure and the inter-harmonic noise (Yumoto et al., 1982; Hiraoko et al., 1984). Despite the different calculation methods, all of these authors recognize the value of expressing noise levels in relation to periodic structure and all have found it a valuable index of the level of dysphonia.

Frequency perturbation

Frequency perturbation (commonly called 'jitter') is defined as the degree of cycle-to-cycle variability of the fundamental frequency. In steady vowel phonation (i.e. with constant pitch and volume) the degree of jitter may also provide an index of the stability of the phonatory mechanism. Jitter is usually concerned only with short term variation – how much one period differs from the period that immediately follows it. It would appear that jitter is a measurement of some aspects of dysphonic voice. However it is only one component of the complex acoustic characteristics of a dysphonic waveform (Hammarberg et al., 1986; Bielamowicz et al., 1996; Colton and Casper, 1996).

There are many different ways of defining and calculating frequency perturbation (Laver et al., 1992). Liberman (1961) established the fundamental principle of calculating the variability (in his case – the distribution of the magnitude of the differences) between adjacent periods of the waveform. Since then several variations of perturbation calculation have been proposed including directional perturbation factor (Hecker and Kreul,

1971), relative average perturbation (Koike 1973), jitter factor (Hollien et al., 1973), frequency perturbation quotient (Takahashi and Koike 1975), period variability index (Deal and Emanuel, 1978) and jitter ratio (Horii, 1979). Most fundamental frequency perturbation measures appear to be sensitive to phonatory pathologies, although comparison across studies that have used different jitter calculation techniques can be problematic.

Amplitude perturbation

Measurements of amplitude perturbation ('shimmer'), like frequency perturbation, are also indications of short-term variability in the vocal signal. However, amplitude perturbation is a measurement of the amount of peak amplitude variability from one cycle to the next cycle (Wendahl, 1963; Takahashi and Koike, 1975; Horii, 1980). Again, in a phonatory task where voice amplitude is intended to be constant, cycle-to-cycle variation may well be indicative of a disordered or inadequate phonatory mechanism. Similar to jitter measurements, there are a number of different calculation methods for shimmer. These include directional perturbation (amplitude) factor (Hecker and Kreul, 1971), amplitude perturbation quotient (Takahashi and Koike, 1975) and amplitude variability index (Deal and Emanuel, 1978).

Conclusions

A comprehensive assessment of the dysphonic patient involves a combination of case history factors, visual and perceptual judgements and instrumental measurements. This information should combine to produce a composite picture to explain how and why a voice sounds like it does. As other chapters in this book demonstrate, the information obtained from clinical assessments using various methods of description, objective measurement and instrumentation has been used to explore vocal impairments and increasingly as a way of evaluating the outcomes of therapy (Carding and Horsley, 1992; Ramig and Verdolini, 1998).

Equally, if the evidence from the different assessments do not complement each other, then the experienced clinician will see this as good reason to recommend further, more detailed evaluation. However, in a large majority of cases the combination of information will mean that the speech and language therapist is in an excellent position to understand the presenting condition, to explain it to the patient, to establish a number of baseline measures against which voice change can be compared, and to design a voice therapy programme which is tailored to the specific needs of the patient, in order to remediate the problem.

Talk about evidence based practice

Appendix 5.1 Basic case history questions

History of the voice problem

What is the problem? What has changed in the voice? When and why did it happen? Is the problem acute, chronic, constant, intermittent? Is this the first episode? If not, how frequently have previous episodes occurred? If there are variations in the voice, what might explain them? Is the problem getting worse, better or remaining the same? What has made the patient do something about it? Is there a discrepancy between the patient's and the clinician's view of the voice problem?

Medical factors

Are there any medical factors which coincide with the onset of the voice problem? Any related surgery? What medications is the patient on and what side-effects do they complain of? Is there any evidence of mental illness (including depression)? Ask particularly about asthma, oesophageal reflux, osteoarthritis, allergies and hormonal changes.

Social and occupational factors

Ask about tobacco, alcohol and recreational drug consumption. Ask about dietary habits, caffeine intake and exercise levels. What are the vocal demands at home and at work? What are the personal, social and economic consequences of being dysphonic? How does the patient relax? What other pressures (i.e. family) is the patient facing?

Psychological considerations

Is there a history of mental health problems? Is the patient's reaction to their dysphonia proportionate to the disability and handicap? Are there any recent life events that may have contributed to the voice problem? Have recent problems or circumstances elevated stress levels? Is there a family history of throat cancer or other health concerns?

Appendix 5.2 A patient questionnaire of vocal performance

Paul Carding
Department of Speech
University of Newcastle upon Tyne

Name   Date

1. How do you think your voice sounds now (compared to before your voice problems started)?

    (a)   No different from usual voice
    (b)   Only slightly different from usual voice
    (c)   Quite different from usual voice
    (d)   Very different from usual voice
    (e)   Totally different from usual voice

2. Does your voice give you any physical discomfort when you talk?

    (a)   No discomfort
    (b)   Slight discomfort
    (c)   Moderate discomfort
    (d)   A lot of discomfort
    (e)   Severe discomfort

3. Does your voice get worse as you talk?

    (a)   Not at all – it stays the same
    (b)   Occasionally when I talk
    (c)   Often gets worse when I talk
    (d)   Often gets a lot worse when I talk
    (e)   Always gets a lot worse when I talk

4. Do you find it an effort to talk?

    (a)   No effort at all
    (b)   Slight effort sometimes (e.g. at the end of the day)
    (c)   Quite an effort sometimes
    (d)   An effort most of the time
    (e)   A constant effort to talk

5. How much are you using your voice at present?

    (a)   As much as I usually would
    (b)   A little less than I usually would
    (c)   Somewhat less than usual
    (d)   A lot less than usual
    (e)   Hardly at all

6. Does your voice problem stop you doing what you would otherwise normally do?

    (a)   Doesn't stop me doing anything that involves me using my voice
    (b)   Stops me doing a few things that involve using my voice
    (c)   Stops me doing a lot of things that involve using my voice
    (d)   Stops me doing most things that involve using my voice
    (c)   I can hardly do anything that involves me using my voice

7. In your opinion do you think that your voice is ever difficult to hear or understand?

    (a)   Not at all
    (b)   A little difficult
    (c)   Quite difficult
    (d)   Very difficult
    (e)   Extremely difficult

8. Do OTHER people (e.g. close family) ever comment that your voice is difficult to hear or understand?

    (a)   No comments
    (b)   Occasional comments
    (c)   Quite often there are comments
    (d)   Frequent comments
    (e)   Very frequent comments

9. Since your voice problem started has your voice...

    (a)   Improved a lot?
    (b)   Improved a little?
    (c)   Not improved at all?
    (d)   Deteriorated a little?
    (e)   Deteriorated a lot?

10. Since your voice problem started have OTHER people (e.g. close family) commented that your voice has improved?

   (a) Other people say that my voice has improved a lot
   (b) Other people say that my voice has improved a little
   (c) Other people say that my voice has not improved at all
   (d) Other people say that my voice has got a little worse
   (e) Other people say that my voice has got a lot worse

11. Would you say that the sound of your voice was ...

   (a) Normal?
   (b) Not quite normal?
   (c) Mildly abnormal?
   (d) Quite abnormal?
   (e) Very abnormal?

12. How much do you worry about your voice problem now?

   (a) Not at all
   (b) Hardly at all
   (c) Quite a lot
   (d) A good deal
   (e) Almost all of the time

By assigning a numerical value of 1 for every (a) answer, 2 for every (b) answer and so on, a total severity score can be calculated for each patient. The range of possible total scores is 12 (normal voice functioning as perceived by the patient) to 60 (severely limited voice functioning).

CHAPTER 6

Children with voice problems: a perspective on treatment

MOYA L. ANDREWS

Introduction

Voice problems negatively affect an individual's performance and comfort level in many areas of life. However, the effects of voice problems are often insidious and not always fully understood by the individual or by teachers and relatives. Yet, severe penalties for voice problems may be exacted even though lack of understanding or politeness results in no explanation being offered. For example, no one is going to tell a child, 'Your voice makes me feel irritated with you and therefore negatively affects our interactions.' Thus children and families may be totally unaware that voice handicaps, seemingly minor and subtle, nevertheless restrict options and limit achievement. Incidence studies in the United States (Wilson, 1979) indicate that 6–9% of young school children have voice disorders but that only about 1% receive treatment.

Clinical experience suggests that children seem to enjoy and benefit from voice therapy if it is tailored to fit their developmental stage, lifestyle, interests and needs. They enjoy experimenting with different ways of using their voices, inappropriate habits are not yet ingrained and unacceptable compensations have not been overlearned. Since young children are eager for genuine attention from adults and are anxious to please adults, it seems an optimal time for them to learn appropriate voice use. It seems sensible to teach them positive vocal behaviours that enable them to get and hold listeners' attention and that also protect them from the effects of negative physiological and interpersonal strategies.

While voice treatment for children poses some challenges it also, in my experience, brings many rewards. Some clinicians seem anxious about how to approach planning programmes for children with voice disorders. It is probably important for them to remember that clinical knowledge and experience in planning programmes for children with other types of disorders is applicable and relevant also to voice cases. Many of the same principles apply. However, there are some significant aspects of voice treatment with children that need to be kept in mind. Let us begin with an examination of these aspects and how they affect what clinicians plan and implement in voice programmes.

General principles

First of all we have to remember that children, unlike most adults, do not have much general knowledge or awareness about what voice is and how its use affects themselves and others. They also do not have much specific knowledge or awareness about their own voice habits. They often lack the basic concepts and linguistic terms necessary for successful comprehension of a need to change behaviour and the benefits of changing. They lack the perceptual skills needed to focus on and discriminate between specific vocal behaviours and their features. Thus, they usually have a lot to learn before we can expect them to make changes in their own voices. We must pay close attention to children's developmental stages and provide the prerequisite knowledge and skills they need to succeed. If we fail to plan this part of their programme carefully, they do not automatically know what it is we expect them to do. For example, we may ask a child to use a 'higher' voice when he does not know what 'high' means. Even if he does know 'high' in relation to spatial referents because of climbing in gym, he may not understand its application to auditory referents. Even if he is aware of 'high' in relation to auditory events, he may still have trouble with the comparative. 'Higher than what?' he may wonder (Andrews and Madiera, 1977). Thus, our first principle is always to provide the knowledge base necessary for success, before the production phase of the programme plan. This means we need general and specific awareness phases in the treatment plan. During these phases we put the cognitive and perceptual framework in place. A metaphor for this is the way a builder uses a scaffold. Our scaffold must be well designed and firm enough so that the child is not balancing precariously on abstractions when we proceed to the production phase of the programme.

Secondly, we must never forget the important link between voice and meaning and feeling. We must make that link explicit at all stages of our programming. This can start in the pre-school years whenever songs and stories are presented. For example, 'Mother duck felt so happy when she found her baby ducks. Let's make her quack with a happy voice. Put a smiley face beside mother duck.' Happy and sad facial expressions can be easily paired with happy and sad voices. Simple yet important vocal contrasts such as these, used in a general kindergarten classroom or with a language stimulation group are invaluable to focus children's attention on how feelings are conveyed through metalinguistic cues. Many developmentally delayed children, learning disabled children and others at risk in terms of pragmatic learning do not make this critical connection themselves. For children with diagnosed voice disorders, we especially need to teach awareness of a range of vocal options that differentiate meanings and feelings. This provides the basis for later teaching of the effects of vocal behaviour on interpersonal relationships. In voice therapy for adults, we frequently must engage in cognitive restructuring as part of our psychodynamic aspects of treatment. With children, we also have psychodynamic goals related to learning about how others react to our voice use and how others have different perceptions from ours. We know from the social psychology literature that perspective taking is an important part of social learning. Children with voice problems must learn about cause and effect in relation to voice use.

A third principle to bear in mind is the importance of the multidisciplinary and team approach to voice assessment and treatment. With children, the team often includes not only physicians and psychologists, but also school personnel who provide valuable insights and support. Family members and other significant adults are often also critical to the overall success of the intervention. It is important, however, that we do not ask these individuals to serve only as watchdogs who constantly remind children of poor voice use. Rather, we want these people to reinforce appropriate behaviours and to understand the dynamics inherent in the context in which the child operates. Parents often benefit from observing voice therapy and from the assignments sent home. Our models, counselling sessions and worksheets frequently enable them to learn important new concepts and help them make changes in their own behaviour. Positive reinforcement of parents and other team members is often equally important as reinforcement for the child. We must carefully analyse and use the key players in the child's environment in order to create a positive context in which the child can achieve success.

With the exception of mutational falsetto in adolescents, the types of voice disorders we see in children are no different from those seen in adults. It is our approaches, activities and materials that differ. Children need more concrete, developmentally matched activities. They need structured practice and tangible documentation of progress. In every phase of the programme they need more varied activities and structure. There needs to be more care taken to intersperse tasks requiring physical activity with tasks requiring quiet sitting. Children have shorter attention spans and we factor this in, when planning our sessions and our carry-over activities.

Additionally, children's motivation must be tied to the present gratifications rather than long-term effects of their vocal behaviours. There are certain themes that are useful in this regard. All children seem to be interested in vocal techniques that result in success interacting with parents teachers and siblings. They are interested in getting what they want, e.g. their fair share of the attention, toys and sweeties. They want to avoid being misunderstood, embarrassed or unfairly treated and punished. They don't want others messing with their stuff. Stories and activities that use these themes with respect to the costs/benefits of voice strategies seem to have motivational appeal (Andrews, 1994). Our fourth principle, therefore, is that the child's present lifestyle should provide the themes for the rationale that is inherent in the programme as it is implemented.

The majority of children we treat exhibit patterns of hyperfunctional behaviour. A smaller number may have hypofunctional patterns related to congenital or acquired laryngeal anomalies or impairment and neuromuscular constraints. Sometimes an overlay of hyperfunctional symptoms is seen together with hypofunctional behaviours (see Casper, Chapter 10). In the process of identifying hyperfunctional and hypofunctional patterns, we usually look at key behaviours subsumed under the four areas of respiration, phonation, resonance and pyschosocial behaviour. These areas are not discrete, of course, but merely categorized for convenience in assessment and programme planning. (It should be noted that in cases where the problem is primarily a resonance disorder we should refer to sources such as Kummer and Lee, 1996.) However when dealing with laryngeal disorders, we frequently find goals for behavioural modification drawn from all four areas noted above. Hypertonicity or hypotonicity frequently affect both respiratory and phonatory behaviours. In the case of excessive tension and effort, we will use reflexes and images and facilitating techniques that relax the muscles and create a more open respiratory tract. Conversely, when there is too little muscle tone and/or strength we will need to facilitate improved respiratory control and vocal fold adduction. This may involve reflexes that tighten and images of constriction. In both instances however, improved resonance (i.e. more facial buzz) may be employed to improve the quality and carrying power of the voice. In a hyperfunctional case the emphasis on the 'facial buzz' may serve as a distraction from the laryngeal effort. In a hypofunctional case, it may provide a much needed increase in audibility. Therefore, our fifth general principle is that a goal from the area of resonance may be appropriate, even for children who have no resonance problem and very different respiratory and laryngeal symptoms. Stated another way, improved resonance is often useful as a compensatory behaviour in the presence of atypical respiratory and phonatory behaviours.

Researching the aetiology of the voice disorder

A variety of developmental, medical, behavioural and psychosocial factors may have been or may be contributing to the problem with which a child presents. Some years ago, it was believed that most voice problems in children were due to vocal abuse. Now we know that it is not quite that simple. We do see many examples of abusive behaviours in children, but frequently those behaviours are responses or coping mechanisms adopted because of other underlying factors. The effortful vocal strategies of the child with chronically swollen vocal folds is an example of this. Until the reason for the swelling of the folds is found and treated the overlay of hyperfunctional behaviours is not easily addressed. We have to examine not only the laryngoscopy findings but also the medical history and interview data to discover information that will allow us to develop clinical hypotheses that can be tested during assessment. Let us take a hypothetical case.

> Billy, aged five years, is referred because of a severely hoarse voice and frequent periods of aphonia. The medical history reveals that Billy was a premature infant who spent time on a respirator in the intensive care unit following his delivery. He suffers from allergies and digestive problems. His mother also reports he has frequent upper respiratory infections. He is the youngest of six children and his father, a heavy smoker, is congenitally hearing impaired. Billy's teacher says that he is 'high strung and disruptive' at school. The otolaryngologist was not able to get a good look at the larynx as Billy was uncooperative.

Hypotheses concerning possible contributing factors would include:

Medical

- congenital laryngeal anomaly or damage acquired as a result of intubation;
- allergic oedema of the folds;
- gastro-oesophageal reflux;
- chronic infectious laryngitis;
- dehydration;
- hearing impairment;
- developmental delay;

Psychosocial

- noisy, competitive family environment;
- atypical or immature social skills;
- emotional neediness (e.g. excessive bids for attention related to father's problem);
- secondary gains from atypical voice use;

Obviously there are certain questions that will need to be asked to obtain information to support or refute these hypotheses. Patterns of behaviour will need to be identified. Generally, it is helpful to avoid yes/no questions and to use open-ended statements such as 'Tell me about Billy's allergies' and 'How does Billy interact with his father?'. It is important to find out if Billy's voice ever sounded clear. If so, the periods when the voice sounds best will help establish possible cause/effect relationships. If Billy has been consistently hoarse ever since infancy his problem may be iatrogenic, i.e. due to a previous medical procedure such as intubation. If his hoarseness is intermittent, we can establish if it is related to seasons of the year, time of day and so on. A child who sounds best first thing in the morning is probably not severely affected by gastro-oesophageal reflux (Pope, 1994) or dehydration of tissues as a result of nocturnal mouth breathing. Adequate hydration, however, is important for all children with voice disorders, especially those who take medication that may dry the mucosa, such as antihistamines and decongestants. So it is always sensible to ask questions such as 'Tell me about Billy's medications ...' and 'About how much water does Billy drink a day ...?'. While most voice symptoms seem to worsen in the course of the day because of the interaction between vocal fold swelling/irritation and amount/type of voice use, some systemic medical conditions result in increased swelling at night. These include hypothyroid problems (Isselbacher et al., 1994) and renal problems (Kereiakes, 1996). Any systemic condition requiring anaesthesia during treatment (Thomas, 1993) also carries with it the risk of intubation trauma.

Referrals may be necessary to obtain additional information to support or refute hypotheses. Depending on the results of the hearing screening, Billy may need a referral for audiologic evaluation. There may also need to be a referral to an allergist or a request for a report from an allergist or physician who has treated him previously. If the information from the interview warrants it, a referral to a psychologist or a report from a school psychologist may also be requested. It is often necessary to obtain additional laryngological examinations if there is any uncertainty about the current status of the larynx. Vocal fold paralysis, for example, is frequently not identified during a fleeting glimpse of the larynx and yet has been cited as one of the most common laryngeal anomalies in children (Harvey, 1996).

Assessing the child's vocal capabilities

We are interested not only in a child's expressive vocal behaviour, but also in what we might describe as his receptive abilities or vocal competence. Can he 'read' the voices of others appropriately? Is he aware of the effects his vocal behaviour has on others and if so, how does he adjust his own voice accordingly? Vocal decoding and encoding play a major role in overall pragmatic success. It is also essential that we find out whether the young child has the language concepts necessary to understand the instructions we might give him when we are presenting tasks to assess expressive voice use. One key concept is that of continuity. During tests involving prolongations of sounds (e.g. MPT and S/Z ratio) we use instructions such as 'Keep going as long as you can.' We need to make these tasks less abstract (Champley and Andrews, 1993) if we are to obtain accurate information. If a child does not demonstrate an awareness of key receptive concepts, this information allows us to teach them at the beginning of treatment (Flynn and Andrews, 1990).

During assessment we must also be concerned about stimulability. Under what conditions can we elicit changes in the voice? What models, auditory, visual and tactile cues appear to evoke improvements in the vocal pattern? During a task such as Maximum Phonation Time, for example, we are interested in a number of pieces of information. We provide a number of trials to time the length of a prolonged vowel. We learn whether successive trials result in increased length, what cues are needed and whether the vibratory pattern can be sustained more evenly at certain times or not at all. Are there episodes of diplophonia, aphonia and pitch breaks? Are these consistent or intermittent?

Voice quality on tasks such as high-quiet singing and vowel prolongation are usually compared with loud, mid-range singing and vowel prolongation. When the folds are swollen or if additive lesions such as nodules are present, the quality is poorest when the voice is soft and high, and best when it is loud, at mid range or lower and effortful. A more comprehensive account of voice stimulability techniques is found in Andrews (1991). It is important to obtain detailed information about stimulability, as this provides us with the information to design treatment goals effectively. The status of the child's awareness of key concepts and knowledge of relevant linguistic terms leads us to develop appropriate general and specific awareness goals. The child's responsiveness to voice stimulability tasks guides our formulation of the voice production goals for behavioural modification. (For a sample pre-test/post-test for children see Appendix 6.1.)

Let us look now at some of the behaviours a child like Billy may demonstrate.

Respiration

1. Quick shallow inhalation (shoulder movement)
2. Inefficient exhalation phase (3 secs duration)

3. Inappropriate use of replenishing breaths (taken at random when air is depleted)

Phonation
1. Hard glottal attacks (on vowel initial words)
2. Hoarse effortful quality (severe and constant)
3. Inability to prolong an even vibratory pattern (frequent aphonia)
4. Vocal variability limited to loudness increases (observable tension)

Psychosocial
1. Talks too much; does not take turns
2. Gets attention by loud talking
3. Does not adjust voice to situation or feedback

Making decisions about treatment

When designing the treatment programme, the clinician considers the child's current status and level of function and develops a rationale and a plan. Children, unlike most adults, will usually need to be taught some specific reasons why they need to work on their voices. In most cases this must be preceded by some general awareness training, so that they understand exactly what voice is. If we plunge directly into the production phase without first focusing attention, the child does not have a cognitive or perceptual framework that will support the new learning. A child like Billy, for example, does not automatically know that voice is the raw material from which words are fashioned. Nor could he understand that description. We would need to begin with some activities about the distinctive features of voices that allow us to identify the user. Birds chirp, dogs bark, cats meow (see Flynn and Andrews, 1990) and the sounds they make help us to identify them. Similarly, even when human speakers say the same words, we can tell who they are by the way they say those words. For instance, the baby brother and the grandfather may both be saying 'Bye bye' but if Billy is asked to point to the picture of the person talking he can demonstrate his awareness of voice differences between those two speakers. After learning that people have different voices, and that voices are unique, Billy can then be taught to attend to some specific characteristics of voice that are relevant to his own behaviour. This is the specific awareness phase of the treatment programme. It usually works well if a child learns the key concepts (e.g. tight/loose; easy/hard; rough/smooth; shoulders up/shoulders down) by focusing first on other people's behaviours. It seems effective to teach new information and to contrast appropriate versus inappropriate behaviours in a story format. See, for example, stories where one character, the hero, embodies a set of positive behaviours compared with an anti-hero who demonstrates the negative ones. The child learns to identify the differences specifically, as well as some of the reasons why appropriate behaviours are effective (Andrews, 1991, 1994).

Clinical experience suggests that stories need to be simple, with developmentally appropriate language concepts and themes. The rationale for changes in behaviour are illustrated through the effects of the positive behaviours on the characters themselves and on others. The hero should be a powerful figure who gets what he or she wants, who is listened to and liked, who feels and sounds good and so on. As a child absorbs the information in the stories and learns to describe why certain results occurred because of the behaviours used, the link between cause and effect is established. This is part of the scaffold that is then in place before the production phase of the programme plan is implemented.

Now let us see how we can translate this information into goals for Billy. We first must decide on an approach. Shall we work on each area separately or shall we try to teach Billy about the overall pattern of behaviours, combining information from all three areas? Since Billy is only five years old, a gestalt approach may work best, as we can integrate various manifestations of the effort he expends and relate it to behaviours subsumed under our three areas. We can use a story format to teach the information and help him to perceive the differences in effortful versus non-effortful behaviours. Shall we use the terms 'easy' and 'tight' for our basic contrast? We could apply those terms to the neck, shoulders, voice, breathing and so on. We could demonstrate the meaning of those words with reference to relaxed or tense arms, neck muscles, word onsets, etc. Also, the phonetic configuration allows for the words themselves to be produced smoothly ('easy') and jerkily ('tight'). Thus, these terms seem to be flexible enough and simple enough for us to use them to achieve what we need. Let us now formulate a general awareness goal. The general awareness phase of therapy is where we orient the child to the overall area we want to address. It also includes learning the language concepts to be used in the specific awareness and production phases of therapy. We will formulate only one illustrative example of a general awareness goal although, of course, more than one would be used in Billy's treatment programme.

General Awareness Phase

Goal: Billy will identify 'easy' versus 'tight' arm movements with 100% accuracy when the clinician demonstrates.

See Appendix 6.2 for pictures of arms.

Strategy: Today we are going to read a story about arms. Look at these pictures of children playing. Look at their arms. How many arms does each child have? How many arms do you have? Yes, you and I both have two arms and aren't we lucky we do? We use our arms a lot. One thing we do with our arms is to hug. I bet your mother hugs you a lot as you are a very huggable boy. Mums like to hug their children. Sometimes we get a tight hug and sometimes a kind of easy hug. Watch while I give myself a hug. This is a tight one, see my arm muscles are tight. Now I'll give myself an easy hug. Look at these pictures of lots of different people hugging. Notice that some are very tight hugs and some are loose, easy hugs. Different kinds of hugs make us <u>feel</u> different things.

See Appendix 6.3 for pictures of hugs.

Now let's look at some other ways we use our arms. Here is a woman waving. Who is she waving at I wonder? Is that the Queen? Some of these people are making big, easy waving movements. They seem very laid back and relaxed. But look here, this person is waving in a very tight sort of way. Watch me make a tight wave, I think I am trying to stop someone doing something I don't like. See the frown on my face? It makes my face look tight too. I have a tight arm and a tight face. I'll even make a tight mouth and jaw. Don't I look as if I'm in a bad mood!! Someone needs to tell me to 'take it easy'. Here is a picture of a soldier. Doesn't he have tight arms? Let's both stand up and make tight arms like the soldier.

See Appendix 6.4 for pictures of people waving.

Now I will play a guessing game with you. I will do things with my arms and fingers and you guess whether I *feel* 'easy' or 'tight'. I don't think I'll be able to trick you.

The preceding example of a general awareness goal and strategy shows how we begin to build the scaffold to support the learning we hope to produce when we begin specific awareness activities.

In the specific awareness phase we begin to focus the child's attention on behaviours relevant to his own voice pattern. At first we direct his attention to what others are doing. Note that, by design, they are demonstrating behaviours Billy himself exhibits. Although it seems obvious to us Billy will probably be totally unaware of this similarity.

Specific Awareness Phase

Goal: Billy will identify 'easy' and 'tight' breathing during inhalation, modelled by the clinician (100% accuracy).

See Appendix 6.5 for pictures of Hal and Ed.

Strategy: Here is a story about Hal and Ed. Look, here is a picture of Hal and here's one of Ed. Everyone likes Hal. He's friendly and easy-going and he has a very happy face, don't you think? He's a good runner and swimmer too. He says it's because he takes very big deep breaths so he always has plenty of air. When his friends ask 'How do you do it, Hal?' he just smiles his easy smile and says, 'I just take deep easy breaths like this. See my chest and tummy move easily in and out. The trick is not to move your shoulders. I never have tight shoulders.' The other boys were glad that Hal shared his secret about easy breathing with them. They tried it and it worked for them too. It even made them *feel* good too – easy and calm. The only boy who couldn't get it right was Ed. Poor Ed, he tried and tried, but his shoulders were so tight and he kept moving them higher and higher when he breathed in. What advice would you give to poor Ed?

Now I will do some breathing and you tell me if it is easy breathing like Hal, or tight breathing like Ed. Let's make it a guessing game.

After Billy has learned to discriminate between 'easy' and 'tight' breathing and can also describe the specific characteristics of each pattern, we can proceed to the production phase, i.e. asking Billy himself to produce the behaviours. Since we are using a gestalt approach we might tie some hard attacks into the next activity since we have chosen the names 'Hal' and 'Ed' to allow for this. Because 'Hal' begins with the high glottal air flow /h/ and 'Ed' begins with a vowel, it will be a maximal contrast.

Production Phase

Goal: Billy will imitate respiratory and phonatory patterns associated with the characters Hal and Ed. (Given instructions, model and cues and with 70% accuracy.)

Strategy: Let's play a game today where we act like Hal and Ed. Remember them? Hal is the great runner and swimmer who taught the other boys his easy breathing trick. He says the best thing is never to move the shoulders. 'Don't ever have tight shoulders,' Hal says. Ed couldn't do it, could he ? Do you remember all the trouble Ed had? I'll be Ed. Tell me again what I should do to breathe like Hal. Yes, that's right, easy deep breaths down low, not high tight shoulders. Oh, that feels better. I feel calm when I do Hal's sort of breathing. I'll say 'Hello Hal' as I breathe out. It feels tickly when I feel it on my hand. Can you do that? Of course you can. You breathe just like Hal. Even your voice sounds easy. Listen while I imitate Ed. When he breathes out he says *'Ed'* all tight and jerky. He sounds uptight too. Let's do it together Hal's way. It *feels* good when it's easy. Now we'll do 'Hello Hal' three times and see if we can do easy breathing each time. I'll go first and you catch me if I'm tight. Watch carefully and help me.

Substituting appropriate vocal options

In the preceding section there are examples of some goals and strategies for Billy to illustrate how we teach young children the background information they need to support successful modification of their own behaviour. The approach we adopt with children is different from that used with adults but the modification techniques are, of course, similar. Examples of stories that can be used with children are presented in Andrews (1994). In this section we will explore some of the appropriate vocal patterns that can be presented to Billy as alternatives to inappropriate behaviours.

Whenever there is a need to improve the carrying power of the voice, and as an alternative to increased laryngeal effort, it is wise to substitute improved resonance. This is why a child like Billy, with a laryngeal constraint, is taught the 'front of the mouth' voice. The 'facial buzz' is emphasized both as a distraction from effortful laryngeal behaviour and as a resonance booster.

Practice materials loaded with voiced continuants are used so that chanting and continuous smooth vibration throughout an entire utterance can be achieved. See Andrews and Summers (1991) and Andrews (1995).

It is also helpful to remember that depending on the child's symptoms we can use reflexive behaviours in order to facilitate vocal tract adjustments. Once the vibrating column of air leaves the larynx it is modified by the shape of the acoustic tube it passes through. Voice training depends to a large extent on how an individual can be taught to make positive adjustments to the vocal tract. Reflexive movements are used as triggers to create an awareness of these adjustments. Swallowing, for example, lowers and relaxes the larynx, lengthening the tract. Yawning relaxes and widens the pharynx and a yawn-sigh facilitates openness and relaxation. The size of the oral cavity, tongue position and velar movement are also critical to vocal tract configuration and ultimately the appropriate balance of vocal resonance. This is why mouth opening, jaw relaxation and specific phonetic combinations in practice materials are frequently employed in the production phase of therapy.

A child like Billy also needs to be taught to expand his vocal options with regard to vocal variety. Getting and holding attention are often limited to increasing effort and loudness by many hyperfunctional voice users. If we want him to avoid effortful loud voice use, we must give him more acceptable ways to be expressive. The clinician may expand his vocal repertoire by teaching him about 'voice pictures' (Andrews, 1991). The use of variation of rate, duration, pauses, pitch changes, facial expression and body language ensures he isn't limited to high risk methods of getting attention.

Additional production goals and practice materials for Billy

These may include:

Goal: Billy will focus his voice ('front of the mouth' voice) by humming and feeling the facial buzz when given a model and instructions (95% accuracy).

Goal: Billy will produce words loaded with voiced continuant consonants when presented with flash cards (85% accuracy on 10 word list) emphasizing frontal tone focus.

Goal: Billy will complete a sentence using the carrier phrase 'My mom mails me —' given picture stimuli (85% frontal tone focus on 15 words).

Warm-ups to practise (mouth gym)

Miami	Miami	Miami
millionaire	millionaire	millionaire
yummy	yummy	yummy
oh me	oh me	oh me
my mum	my mum	my mum
mellow yellow	mellow yellow	mellow yellow
jelly lolly	jelly lolly	jelly lolly

Phrases (link words to avoid hard onsets on vowel initial words)

My name is:	Alan	Oliver	Omar	Evil
	Ian	Ozzie	Izzie	Morrie
	John	Jim	Jonah	Liam
	Neville	Reggie	Neil	William

Word List (no devoicing of buzzy sounds)

melons	lemons	razors	rings	wellies
mail	jam	mirrors	leaves	jelly
maize	jewels	nails	lions	rain
raisins	roses	wings	money	meals

Carry Over Phase

Goal: Billy will use his frontal tone focus every time he answers the phone at home and says the word 'hello'.

Strategy: Family members will phone him and reinforce him.

Goal: Billy will identify words in his school reading book that are easy to say in his 'front of the mouth' voice. He will write them down and bring them to his therapy session.

Strategy: Teacher will ask Billy to say the words in class (after clinician has worked on them with him) and reinforce him appropriately.

Goal: Billy will practise a short joke in therapy (to share with family and friends) using his 'front of the mouth' voice.

| *Strategy:* | Question: | Why does a witch ride a broom? |
| | Answer: | A vacuum cleaner is too heavy (emphasize the vowels and voiced continuants). |

The brief illustrative example of Billy's goals and strategies shows how a child with either chronic or acute vocal fold changes could be helped to produce his voice using improved 'facial buzz' to supplement a less than optimal laryngeal buzz. This is the type of positive compensatory technique that is frequently effective with children with a variety of laryngeal and/or respiratory constraints. By substituting a positive compensatory technique the clinician is able to reduce the negative compensations of increased effort and tension in the laryngeal mechanism. Throughout the entire programme Billy would also work concurrently on respiratory and psychodynamic goals.

Conclusion

Therapy for children with laryngeal disorders, like all types of therapy for children, works best when it is tailored to fit the individual child's developmental level, needs and lifestyle. There are many approaches that work well and the most important aspect is to design each treatment programme so that it is relevant to each individual child and his or her own special world. In this chapter the example of Billy has been used to provide one perspective on the clinical problem-solving process we go through as we build an individualized voice treatment plan for a young child.

Appendix 6.1: Pre-Test/Post-Test Items

Respiration

Length of exhalation

Blows through a straw in water to make bubbles	_____ secs
Prolongs s	_____ secs

Inspiratory patterns   Yes   No

Observational tension   ☐   ☐
Lower chest expansion   ☐   ☐
Raises shoulders   ☐   ☐
Replenishing breaths
   appropriate frequency   ☐   ☐
   appropriate placement   ☐   ☐

Phonation

Prolongations

Prolongs voiced and unvoiced cognates s/z	_____ secs /s/
	_____ secs /z/
Prolongs vowel /a/	_____ secs

Quality during prolongation of /a/ (Circle items that apply.)

voice breaks	hoarse
pressed	clear
continuous	harsh
breathy	diplophonic

Loudness

Adjusts loudness levels   ☐ Yes   ☐ No (when cued)
                                             ☐ Yes   ☐ No (spontaneously)

Sustains soft phonation   ☐ Yes   ☐ No (prolonged sounds)
                                             ☐ Yes   ☐ No (phases)

Vocal abuse (Circle items that apply.)   ☐ Yes   ☐ No

      hard attacks   tension

      habituated loudness   other practices

Pitch

Adjusts pitch levels	☐ Yes	☐ No (when cued)
	☐ Yes	☐ No (spontaneously)
Uses pitch variability	☐ Yes	☐ No (contrastive words)
	☐ Yes	☐ No (reading)
	☐ Yes	☐ No (speaking)
Sings 'Happy Birthday'	☐ Yes	☐ No (melodic accuracy)
	☐ Yes	☐ No (monotone)
	☐ Yes	☐ No (some pitch variations)

Duration/Rate/Rhythm

Sings 'Happy Birthday'	☐ Yes	☐ No (correct timing and beat)
Phrases appropriately	☐ Yes	☐ No (spontaneous speech)
	☐ Yes	☐ No (reading)
Uses variation for meaning	☐ Yes	☐ No (spontaneously)
	☐ Yes	☐ No (when cued)

Number of syllables produced in one breath group _____ syllables
Rate during speech sample   _____ words per minut

Resonance

Adequacy of velopharyngeal mechanism   ☐ Yes   ☐ No
(note medical documentation)

Nasal emission on oral productions (Circle items that apply). ☐ Yes ☐ No

      plosives   fricatives   affricatives

      words   phrases   vowels

Nasal emission on nasal consonants   ☐ Yes   ☐ No

Resonance pattern during connected speech (Circle items that apply.)

        hypernasal   hyponasal

        appropriate balance   weak resonance

Maximizes resonance	☐ Yes	☐ No (vowels)
	☐ Yes	☐ No (voiced continuants)
	☐ Yes	☐ No (projected speech)
	☐ Yes	☐ No (conversational speech)
Assimilated nasality (regionalisms)	☐ Yes	☐ No

Psychodynamics

Adjusts vocal behaviour	☐ Yes	☐ No (effect on listeners)
	☐ Yes	☐ No (context)
	☐ Yes	☐ No (when cued)
Discusses vocal options	☐ Yes	☐ No
Lists rules for vocal hygiene	☐ Yes	☐ No
Balances talking/listening time	☐ Yes	☐ No
Demonstrates conversational skills	☐ Yes	☐ No (turn taking)
	☐ Yes	☐ No (question asking)
	☐ Yes	☐ No (topic maintenance)

Significant factors related to voice use (Circle items that apply.)

abusive habits	mouth opening	loudness level
role in family	amount of talking	posture
attitude	relationships	self-esteem
hydration	environment	pollutants

Comments

Lifestyle modifications

Behavioural modifications

Role of significant others

Appendix 6.2: Arms

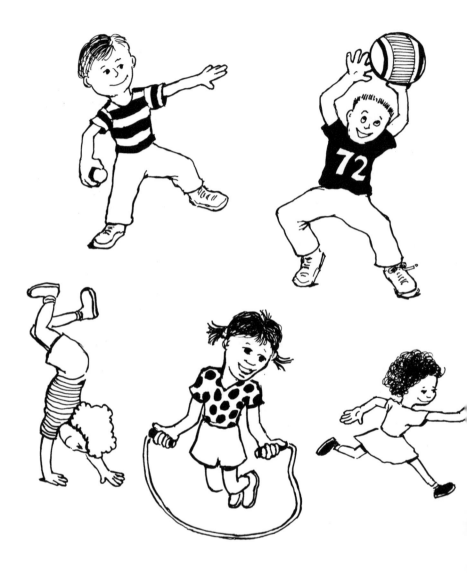

Appendix 6.3: Hugs

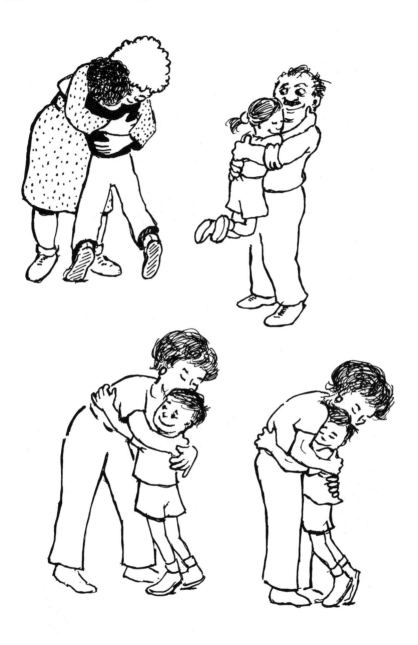

Appendix 6.4: People waving

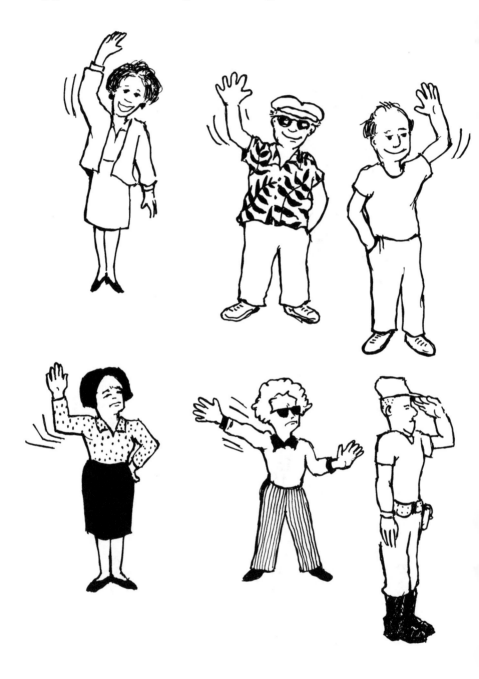

Appendix 6.5

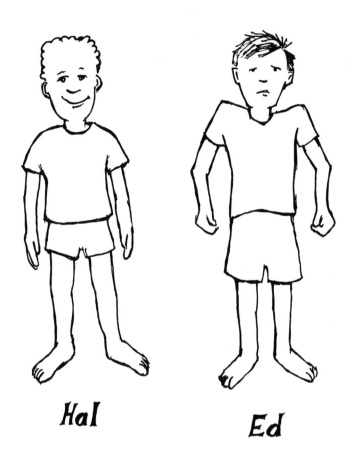

Hal   Ed

CHAPTER 7

Voice disorders associated with hyperfunction

JENNIFER OATES

Introduction

One of the most common themes in the literature on voice disorders is that hyperfunction of laryngeal musculature underlies the majority of vocal disorders (Boone and McFarlane, 1994; Morrison and Rammage, 1994; Stemple, Glaze and Gerdeman, 1995; Colton and Casper, 1996). Although vocal hyperfunction may take many forms (Hillman et al., 1989), this term generally refers to the use of levels of laryngeal muscle tension, force and constriction which are in excess of those required for efficient voicing. The many alternative terms used to refer to vocal hyperfunction in the literature include vocal misuse and abuse, phonotrauma, vocal trauma, mechanical stress, hyperkinetic phonation and musculoskeletal tension. Voice problems associated with vocal hyperfunction are similarly referred to as hyperfunctional voice disorders, muscular tension dysphonias, musculoskeletal tension disorders, or mechanical voice disorders (Hillman et al., 1989; Aronson, 1990; Boone and McFarlane, 1994; Morrison and Rammage, 1994). The signs of vocal disorder which are most commonly associated with hyperfunction include vocal fatigue, throat discomfort, impaired voice quality, and pathological changes such as vocal fold oedema, inflammation, nodules, polyps or haemorrhage.

Although there is little direct evidence that hyperfunction is behind most voice disorders, this contention has considerable face validity. Epidemiological studies of the prevalence of vocal disorders in the general population, as well as reviews of otolaryngology and speech pathology caseloads, indicate that the majority of voice problems do not originate from psychological conversion processes or from structural lesions of the larynx, primary laryngeal disease, neurological conditions or endocrine dysfunction (e.g. Cooper, 1973; Herrington-Hall et al., 1988; Yiu and Ho, 1991; Fritzell, 1996). In the absence of such conversion disorders or organic conditions, the most likely aetiological candidate is vocal hyperfunction. Further, the increased prevalence rates of vocal disorders among people who have vocally demanding occupations and lifestyles indicate that hyperfunction is likely to be a common denominator (e.g. Calas et al., 1989; Sapir et al., 1990; Fritzell, 1996). Indeed, in a comparison of the vocal intensities used by teachers and nurses, Masuda et al. (1993) demonstrated that teachers spent more of their phonation time using loud speech and screaming intensities, suggesting that this hyperfunctional vocal behaviour may underlie the higher prevalence rates of voice disorders among teachers than nurses. Similarly, the disproportionate number of higher pitched voices (i.e. young children and adult females) among those with voice disorders suggests that the frequency of collision between the vocal folds is instrumental in the development of voice problems (Titze, 1994).

The typical location of pathological changes assumed to arise from vocal hyperfunction provides further support for the role of excess muscle tension and force; the common pathologies of vocal fold nodules and polyps, for example, occur in the centre of the membranous part of the vocal folds where the mechanical impact of vocal fold vibration is greatest (Hirano et al., 1983). In addition, investigations of the structural alterations to the vocal fold cover which occur in these vocal pathologies, in concert with studies of the effects of mechanical trauma on canine vocal folds, demonstrate that vocal hyperfunction is likely to cause damage to the epithelium and lamina propria of the vocal folds (e.g. Gray and Titze, 1988; Gray, 1991; Dikkers et al., 1993; Gray et al., 1993). Such damage may include loss of surface microvilli, epithelial desquamation, rupture of subepithelial blood vessels, subepithelial oedema, disruption of the basement membrane zone, and increased collagen production.

Direct evidence for the negative effects of vocal hyperfunction in humans is scarce, but a small number of experimental studies have been conducted to examine the effects of hyperfunctional vocal behaviours such as loud talking, speaking at high pitch levels, and prolonged voice use at high intensity and/or high pitch (e.g. Stone and Sharf, 1973; Gelfer et al., 1991; Scherer et al., 1991; Stemple et al., 1995b). Although such investigations have not generally simulated the vocal hyperfunction which can occur in a naturalistic environment, and although the findings are inconsistent, there is certainly some evidence that such vocal behaviours can lead to vocal fatigue and throat discomfort, alterations in glottal configuration, and negative effects on various measures of vocal quality and pitch.

peaking of secondary

The susceptibility of the human larynx to vocal hyperfunction is not surprising. To fulfil its primary biological functions of protecting the lower airways from aspiration of food, liquid and foreign bodies and of facilitating defecation, childbirth, heavy lifting and coughing, the larynx must reflexively rise in the neck and close off the airway (Brodnitz, 1959; Aronson, 1990). This reflexive pattern of closing down, or constricting, takes precedence over the phylogenetically more recent role of the larynx in speaking and singing (Boone and McFarlane, 1994). With a predilection for constriction in the vocal tract, it is no wonder that vocal hyperfunction creeps into human speech patterns so readily.

Taken together, these considerations suggest that hyperfunction or mechanical stress on the vocal mechanism will be a primary focus in the evaluation and management of clients with voice disorders.

The nature of vocal hyperfunction

The description of vocal hyperfunction as the use of excessive levels of laryngeal muscle tension, force and constriction is useful as a broad definition, but is not sufficiently specific to guide clinicians in the evaluation and treatment of hyperfunctionally related voice disorders. Specification of the types of vocal behaviours that are hyperfunctional, classification systems for differentiating the various forms of hyperfunction, and approaches to the quantitative measurement of vocal hyperfunction are also required if clinicians are to provide effective management for clients with these voice disorders.

All of the major textbooks on voice disorders outline examples of vocal behaviours which are considered to be hyperfunctional (e.g. Wilson, 1987; Aronson, 1990; Boone and McFarlane, 1994; Morrison and Rammage, 1994; Andrews, 1995; Stemple at al., 1995a; Brown et al., 1996; Colton and Casper, 1996; Dworkin and Melecca, 1997). There is considerable consistency in the examples provided in these texts and controversy as to what constitutes hyperfunctional voicing is rare. The most commonly cited hyperfunctional behaviours include:

- speaking or singing with excessive loudness levels;
- speaking or singing with excessively high or low pitch levels;
- persistent use of glottal fry in speaking;
- speaking or singing with excessive intrinsic laryngeal muscle tension and constriction (e.g. hyperadduction of the vocal folds and/or ventricular folds);
- speaking or singing with excessive extrinsic laryngeal muscle tension (e.g. holding the larynx rigidly in a raised or lowered position);
- yelling and screaming;

- speaking with hard glottal attack;
- excessive coughing and throat clearing;
- crying, laughing and sneezing with excessive laryngeal muscle tension and constriction;
- phonation during effort closure of the glottis in non-speaking activities such as weightlifting.

Whether or not hyperfunctional vocal behaviours will lead to signs of vocal dysfunction such as vocal fatigue, throat discomfort, impaired voice quality, or pathological changes such as vocal fold oedema, inflammation, nodules, polyps or haemorrhage will depend on the frequency and extent or severity of the hyperfunction. Occasional throat clearing with low levels of laryngeal muscle tension and constriction, for example, is unlikely to lead to vocal impairment or vocal fold pathology. Similarly, it is likely that some of these behaviours can be used even for long periods, without resulting in voice disorders, if the individual uses a vocal technique which protects them from vocal damage. Although there is considerable controversy surrounding the use of belting in singing (see Van Lawrence, 1979; Miles and Hollien, 1990; Schutte and Miller, 1993, for example), it is clear that some singers can employ this type of high-intensity voicing with little or no ill effect (Estill, 1988). Ethel Merman, Barbra Streisand and Liza Minelli are prime examples of singers who have maintained effective voices despite the use of very loud singing.

In addition to the use of vocal techniques which are protective, it may be that certain individuals have laryngeal structures which are less susceptible than others to the negative effects of vocal hyperfunction (Child and Johnson, 1991). We are all aware of individuals who appear to be able to use potentially hyperfunctional voicing such as loud talking, yelling and screaming without developing any vocal pathology or vocal impairment. As long as three decades ago, Arnold (1962) proposed that genetically determined cellular composition of the laryngeal mucous membranes and overall configuration of the larynx may result in differing degrees of susceptibility to pathologies such as vocal nodules and polyps. More recently, Child and Johnson (1991) have suggested that genetic differences in vocal fold histology may predispose some individuals to hyperfunctionally related voice disorders. That certain people are predisposed to voice problems related to vocal hyperfunction has received some early empirical support from the landmark work of Stephen Gray and his colleagues at the University of Iowa. Gray's investigation of the detailed structure of the vocal folds has indicated that the make-up of the basement membrane zone between the outer epithelial layer and Reinke's space may determine susceptibility to pathologies such as vocal nodules (Gray, 1991; Gray et al., 1993).

Why does vocal hyperfunction occur?

Before treatment programmes can be designed to reduce or eliminate the negative effects of vocal hyperfunction, it will be important to try and elucidate the factors which underlie this vocal behaviour. A purely symptomatic approach to treatment, which does not address the underlying reasons for vocal hyperfunction, is unlikely to be maximally effective. Consider, for example, the person who persistently clears the throat because of chronic laryngopharyngeal reflux disease. A behavioural method for reducing throat clearing is likely to be inadequate in this case; medical treatment of the reflux disease will often be required before the hyperfunctional behaviour can be eliminated.

Posture and respiratory patterns

It is important to recognize first that, because of the interconnections between the muscles and cartilagenous framework of the larynx and other skeletal and muscle systems of the body, hyperfunctional vocal behaviours may arise from impaired function or posture of areas of the body, rather than the larynx. An individual may therefore display hyperfunctional voicing because of postural misalignments such as hyperextension or hyperflexion of the neck and mandible, slumping of the spine, raising of the shoulders, exaggerated positioning of the pelvis (e.g. tucked under or pushed forwards), uneven distribution of body weight and locking of the knees (Morrison and Rammage, 1994; Andrews, 1995). Similarly, restricted mobility of the temporomandibular joint, excessive muscle tension of the suprahyoid muscles, the pharyngeal constrictors and the tongue, and excessive tongue retraction may lead to excess tension and constriction within the larynx (Laver, 1980; Morrison and Rammage, 1994; Colton and Casper, 1996). Finally, inefficient respiratory patterns such as initiating speech at very low or excessively high lung volumes, speaking on reserve air, holding the breath before beginning to speak, speaking for too long on one breath group, and failing to support high subglottal pressures with sufficient inspiratory muscle engagement are likely to result in laryngeal hyperfunction (Morrison and Rammage, 1994; Sapienza and Stathopoulos, 1994; Colton and Casper, 1996;).

Situational and learning factors

The myriad of contributors to the development of vocal hyperfunction can be broadly categorized as situational, faulty learning, medical, laryngeal irritant, compensatory and psychogenic factors. The types of *situations* that are conducive to vocal hyperfunction are self-evident and include communicating over large distances without amplification or in environments with poor acoustics, speaking or singing over background noise, being required to sing pieces which are beyond a comfortable vocal range, speaking to people with poor attentional skills, participating in or observing at sporting events, performing vocally while dancing or adopting misaligned body postures, speaking to people with severe hearing impairments, performing with the use of character voices, playing while using the voice as a noise maker, using automatic speech recognition devices and singing over loud bands without fold-back speakers. *Learning factors* include imitating other people's faulty voice production in childhood, adopting suboptimal vocal features in order to create a particular personal image (e.g. use of a low pitch and glottal fry to convey authority), developing excess laryngeal muscle tension and constriction in order to increase pitch in male–to–female transsexuals, and learning of ineffective vocal techniques in singing, acting and public speaking. This category also covers the learning of hyperfunctional voice behaviours that may be associated with severe hearing impairment (Boone, 1966; Wirz et al., 1980; Wilson, 1987; Andrews, 1995).

Medical factors and laryngeal irritants

A number of *medical* conditions are associated with a propensity to vocal hyperfunction. Viral or bacterial infections and allergic reactions of the vocal tract, chronic sinusitis, laryngopharyngeal reflux and certain respiratory conditions may lead to vocal hyperfunction. In cases of infective laryngitis, for example, where the vocal folds are inflamed and oedematous, the sufferer is likely to increase vocal effort and clear the throat or cough in an attempt to reduce throat discomfort and to improve the effectiveness of the voice (Child and Johnson, 1991; Colton and Casper, 1996). The inflammation and oedema of the vocal folds associated with this condition is also likely to increase the vulnerability of the vocal folds to vocal hyperfunction (Child and Johnson, 1991; Colton and Casper, 1996). Chronic sinusitis with purulent discharge and laryngopharyngeal reflux may also irritate vocal fold mucosa and lead to excessive coughing and throat clearing (Stemple et al., 1995a; Colton and Casper, 1996; Koufman et al., 1996; Shaw et al., 1996), although there is not yet consensus about the role of reflux in dysphonia (e.g. Kjellèn and Brudin, 1994). In addition, respiratory conditions such as chronic obstructive airways disease, whooping cough, lung cancer and asthma can result in hyperfunctional behaviours, particularly coughing and throat clearing (Stemple et al., 1995a).

A propensity towards persisting vocal hyperfunction may develop even when medical conditions such as infective laryngitis, sinusitis and whooping cough have resolved. Although there is little direct evidence for such effects, it may be that the sufferer is left with an increased reactivity or hypersensitivity of the larynx (Stemple et al., 1995a). In this situation, vocal tract sensations that would normally go unnoticed (e.g. throat sensations produced by drainage from the nasopharynx or breathing in cold air), would stimulate the hyperfunctional response of coughing, throat clearing or laryngeal muscle constriction.

There are many *laryngeal irritants* which, in addition to their direct effects of vocal fold inflammation, oedema and mucosal drying, can induce hyperfunctional vocal behaviours such as throat clearing and laryngeal constriction. Common laryngeal irritants are tobacco and marijuana smoke, alcohol, caffeine, chemical fumes, dust and other air pollutants, excessively dry air, recreational drugs such as cocaine, and a long list of medications (Mueller and Wilcox, 1980; Van Lawrence, 1987; Child and Johnson, 1991; Stemple et al., 1995a; Colton and Casper, 1996). The types of medications which are known to irritate laryngeal tissues include inhaled corticosteroids, antihistamines, decongestants and cough suppressants, antipsychotic agents and antidepressants, antihypertensive drugs, large doses of vitamin C and anticholinergics prescribed for diarrhoea and motion sickness (Martin, 1988; Reed Thompson, 1995). Although the effects of these medications vary depending on individual responsiveness and dosage, the major mechanisms underlying negative vocal responses are increased viscosity of upper respiratory tract secretions (thickened and sticky secretions) and increased viscosity and drying of the vocal fold mucosa. The laryngeal irritation effects of these changes in fluid balance and viscosity may in turn lead to increased laryngeal tension and constriction, throat clearing and coughing. While the antihypertensive drugs do not have a direct effect on laryngeal mucosa, the associated release of prostaglandins causes bronchial hyperreactivity; chronic coughing is then a likely result. The influence of corticosteroids on vocal fold structure is as yet unknown, but coughing and throat clearing are common side effects of these asthma medications and it may also be that the voice quality deterioration sometimes associated with inhaled corticosteroids leads the asthma sufferer to adopt hyperfunctional behaviours in an effort to improve vocal effectiveness (Watkin and Ewanowski, 1985; Williamson et al., 1995).

Compensatory mechanisms

Vocal hyperfunction also frequently occurs as a *compensatory mechanism* in individuals with organic pathologies of the larynx and vocal tract (Aronson, 1990; Stemple et al., 1995a; Brown et al., 1996; Colton and Casper, 1996). In an attempt to improve vocal output and/or the symptoms of throat discomfort in the presence of an underlying organic pathology, many patients develop hyperfunctional behaviours which in turn may exacerbate the vocal problem. Such compensatory hyperfunction is commonly associated with pathologies such as vocal fold palsy, infective laryngitis, abductor spasmodic dysphonia, vocal fold scarring and velopharyngeal incompetence.

Psychogenic factors

The notion that *psychogenic factors* can contribute to the development of hyperfunctional voicing patterns is one of the most common themes in the major textbooks on voice disorders (e.g. Wilson, 1987; Aronson, 1990; Morrison and Rammage, 1994; Andrews, 1995; Stemple et al., 1995a; Colton and Casper, 1996). These authors contend that personality characteristics (e.g. aggressiveness, use of emotional coping strategies), emotional reactions to acute or chronic life stressors and dysfunctional interpersonal relationships (e.g. anger, hostility, resentment), and emotional disturbances (e.g. chronic anxiety and difficulty in expressing negative affect) result in increased levels of intrinsic and extrinsic laryngeal muscle tension and hyperadduction of the vocal folds and/or ventricular folds.

The evidence for the relationship between psychogenic factors and vocal hyperfunction comes from large numbers of clinical case studies (e.g. Morrison and Rammage, 1994), empirical investigations of the personality, coping styles, psychobehavioural characteristics and interpersonal relationships of people with hyperfunctionally related voice disorders (e.g. Green, 1989; Goldman et al., 1996; McHugh-Munier et al., 1997; Roy et al., 1997b) and studies which demonstrate that discrete emotions are associated with changes in pitch, loudness, voice quality and laryngeal constriction (see Aronson, 1990 for a review). Current understanding of the neurological control of the human voice has also provided some evidence for the likely role of emotion in vocal behaviour. The anterior cingulate gyrus, the subcortical limbic system and the periaqueductal gray are now thought to control emotional vocalization and this neural mechanism may explain why laryngeal constriction is a common response to emotional stress (Aronson, 1990; Larson, 1992). Although there is little disagreement that psychogenic factors can induce vocal hyperfunction, it is important to remember that direct research evidence is not always consistent with this contention and that the psychophysiological mechanisms which lead to hyperfunctionally related voice disorders have yet to be clearly identified (Rollin, 1987; Rosen and Sataloff, 1997a). A more complete discussion of psychogenic aspects of voice disorders is provided by Freeman, Chapter 8 of this volume.

Classification and measurement of vocal hyperfunction

The terms 'vocal misuse' and 'vocal abuse' appear frequently in discussions of voice disorders related to hyperfunction. For some authors and clinicians, these terms refer to two different categories of vocal hyperfunction (e.g. Brown et al., 1996; Colton and Casper, 1996). In this classification scheme, vocal abuse is defined as hyperfunctional behaviours which are extreme enough to lead to laryngeal tissue changes such as nodules, polyps, oedema, haemorrhage and non-specific laryngitis, or to changes in glottal configuration such as a persistent posterior glottal chink. Vocal misuse, on the other hand, is considered to constitute faulty vocal technique and less extreme forms of hyperfunction which are less likely to alter vocal fold structure or glottal configuration. In this categorization, vocally abusive behaviours would include screaming and excessive coughing whereas misuse would include persistent use of a high pitch and glottal fry. Discrepancies abound, however, with certain vocal behaviours such as loud talking categorized in some cases as misuse (e.g. Brown et al., 1996) and in others as abuse (e.g. Colton and Casper, 1996).

Other authors employ a variation on this categorization of abuse and misuse and consider misuse as an overarching term for both vocal abuse and what is referred to as 'inappropriate vocal components' (e.g. Stemple et al., 1995a). In this scheme, inappropriate vocal components are similar to the vocal misuse behaviours described by Colton and Casper (1996) and include the use of inappropriate pitch levels and glottal fry. Vocal abuse again refers to activities such as shouting and screaming.

In general, the distinction between abuse and misuse is not clear-cut and the definitions given in the literature are not sufficiently operational-ized to provide a useful classification system for the various forms of hyperfunction. As Colton and Casper (1996) suggest, abuse and misuse are probably best considered as existing on a continuum of hyperfunc-tional behaviour rather than as discrete categories. Very little is gained in the diagnosis and treatment of hyperfunctionally related voice disorders from making a distinction between abuse and misuse.

Morrison and Rammage (1994) have developed an alternative system for classifying vocal hyperfunction which does not require a distinction to be made between vocal abuse and misuse. These authors describe three main types of muscle tension dysphonias (MTD); laryngeal isometric pattern (MTD Type 1), lateral contraction (MTD Type 2), and anteroposterior supraglottic contraction (MTD Type 3). These types of muscular tension dysphonia may co-exist and are therefore not mutually exclusive categories. MTD Type 1 refers to the creation of a posterior glottal chink due to excess and sustained contraction of the posterior cricoarytenoid muscle and increased tension of the suprahyoid muscles. Morrison and Rammage state that this laryngeal isometric pattern is most common in professional voice users. Psychological factors such as anxiety are also said to be secondary contributing factors to this type of MTD. These authors also suggest that the laryngeal isometric pattern may be a precursor to vocal fold pathologies such as nodules, polyps and non-specific laryngitis. The mechanism proposed here is that the high degree of vocal hyperfunction required to overcome the posterior glottal chink results in excessive shearing stresses on the vocal fold cover.

MTD Type 2 denotes medial compression of the true vocal folds and/or ventricular folds (Morrison and Rammage, 1994). Again, Morrison and Rammage associate this pattern of muscular tension with poor vocal technique and psychogenic factors. A distinction is made between hyperadduction at the glottic and supraglottic levels, with the former being linked primarily to vocal misuse and the latter to 'unresolved psychological conflict'. Morrison and Rammage list normal appearing vocal folds, erythema or diffuse thickening of vocal fold mucosa, an increased closed phase of vocal fold vibration and reduced amplitude and mucosal wave as the possible signs of MTD Type 2 at the glottic level. The resulting voice features are said to include harshness, vocal fatigue and throat discomfort. MTD Type 2 at the supraglottic level is described as involving compression of the ventricular folds over either tightly adducted true vocal folds or over incompletely adducted true vocal folds where there would be a gap between the membranous and cartilagenous glottis. The former pattern is said to result in a 'high-pitched squeaky voice' whereas the latter is associated with a breathy voice or a 'tense whisper'.

MTD Type 3 with anteroposterior supraglottic contraction refers to the use of a laryngeal posture where the distance between the epiglottis and the arytenoid cartilages is reduced. Morrison and Rammage (1994) attribute this pattern of hyperfunction to poor vocal technique, 'tense pharyngolaryngeal postures', and/or an attempt to produce a particular resonance quality (e.g. the 'Bogart–Bacall' syndrome described by Koufman and Blalock, 1982). They also state that MTD Type 3 involves phonation in the low part of the speaker's dynamic range and is associated with vocal fatigue, particularly at low pitches.

This classification of muscular tension dysphonias developed by Morrison and Rammage (1994) has received some support from clinical investigations of subjects with hyperfunctionally related voice disorders, empirical studies of subjects simulating muscular tension in the larynx and experiments on human cadaver larynges (e.g. Belisle and Morrison, 1983; Morrison et al., 1983; Rammage, 1992). Because they describe the physiology underlying each of the three types of MTD, Morrison and Rammage's work also provides a possible framework for objective physiological assessment of vocal hyperfunction using techniques such as laryngeal videoendoscopy. Unfortunately, empirical evidence for the validity of their classification scheme is not complete and further research will be required to test the many proposals made by Morrison and Rammage concerning causality and the physiological and perceptual correlates of muscular tension dysphonia.

The notion that vocal hyperfunction may be reflected in either hyperadduction of the vocal folds or incomplete adduction has also been incorporated in a theoretical framework proposed by Hillman et al. (1989). Hillman et al. have postulated that vocal hyperfunction which leads to vocal fatigue and then to pathological changes on the vocal folds such as nodules and polyps is of an 'adducted' type; that is, increased muscle tension and collision forces in combination with tightly adducted vocal folds are responsible for injury to the vocal fold cover. In contrast, a 'non-adducted' type of hyperfunction, where there is increased muscle tension but incomplete approximation of the vocal folds, will result in dysphonia in the absence of pathological tissue changes. In this case, a further increase of hyperfunction would lead to aphonia where the vocal folds no longer vibrate.

Although Hillman et al. have not provided unequivocal evidence for this theoretical framework, they have begun to examine its validity and reliability by making objective acoustic and aerodynamic measures of the voices of speakers with normal voices, speakers with pathologies such as nodules, polyps and contact ulcers and those with dysphonia in the absence of secondary organic changes. Their initial research results have supported their propositions and have suggested that particular objective measures may have clinical applications for the evaluation of vocal hyperfunction. Adductive hyperfunction, for example, was associated with abnormally high levels of the glottal airflow waveform parameters of AC flow (assumed to indirectly reflect amplitude of vocal fold vibration) and maximum flow declination rate (an indirect measure of the velocity of vocal fold closure). On the other hand, non-adductive hyperfunction was correlated with the glottal airflow waveform parameter of unmodulated DC flow (an indirect measure of degree of glottal closure).

The work of Hillman et al. (1989) and Morrison and Rammage (1994), although incomplete, provides clinicians with some information on which to base their clinical evaluation of vocal hyperfunction. Laryngeal videoendoscopy with continuous and stroboscopic light can be used to assess parameters, which these authors have associated with hyperfunction (e.g. ventricular fold compression, anteroposterior supraglottic contraction, degree of glottal closure, glottal configuration, amplitude of vocal fold vibration, adequacy of the mucosal wave and vocal fold hyperadduction). Similarly, Hillman et al. have shown that inverse filtering of the oral airflow waveform to estimate the glottal flow waveform may provide useful indicators of hyperfunction (e.g. AC flow, DC flow, maximum flow declination rate). Other acoustic, aerodynamic and physiological parameters such as fundamental frequency, intensity, harmonic-to-noise ratio, mean airflow rate, subglottal pressure, and various electroglottographic measures may also prove to be useful measures of vocal hyperfunction, although clear research evidence for such relationships is not yet available. Further details on objective evaluation of voice can be found in Chapter 5 of this volume (see also Baken, 1987; Hirano and Bless, 1993; Colton and Casper, 1996).

There is reasonable face validity in the notion that certain perceptual and observational parameters (e.g. strain, breathiness, glottal fry, aphonia, larynx height) are likely to be good indicators of hyperfunction (Morrison and Rammage, 1994; Colton and Casper, 1996), so that perceptual rating of the client's voice is likely to be a valuable component of the evaluation process. Carding, in Chapter 5 of this book, outlines current approaches to the perceptual and observational assessment of voice.

Finally, assessment of vocal hyperfunction will, at the very least, require careful documentation of the hyperfunctional behaviours listed earlier in this chapter (e.g. yelling and screaming, speaking with hard glottal attack, excessive coughing and throat clearing). Documentation of the nature, frequency and severity of such behaviours is most effectively conducted using the self-report of the client, reports of significant others such as parents and teachers and direct observation of the client in the clinic and in naturalistic speaking and/or singing environments. Observation of vocal behaviours in naturalistic situations such as playgrounds, theatres, sports fields and classrooms is particularly important as the client's voice use in the clinical environment will often be unrepresentative of their everyday vocal patterns (Boone and McFarlane, 1994).

Management of voice disorders associated with vocal hyperfunction

Successful management of voice disorders related to vocal hyperfunction requires that clinicians address three major factors; the underlying causes and contributing factors of hyperfunctional voicing, the specific hyperfunctional behaviours themselves, and the client's general hyperfunctional vocal technique. The effects of underlying medical and psychological factors as well as laryngeal irritants and faulty learning patterns need to be minimized, specific hyperfunctional behaviours such as yelling and throat clearing need to be reduced or eliminated, and the client needs to learn to use vocal techniques which promote optimum levels of laryngeal muscle tension and normal voice quality, pitch and loudness.

Minimization of the effects of the underlying causes of vocal hyperfunction

For many clients with hyperfunctional voice problems, a symptomatic approach which focuses only on changing vocal behaviours is likely to be less effective than an approach which also addresses the causes of the hyperfunctional patterns (Aronson, 1990; Stemple et al., 1995a; Colton and Casper, 1996). Causal and contributing factors will vary depending on the client, so that the diagnostic process of searching for individual aetiological factors will be critical for the design of the management programme.

Where there are medical conditions such as laryngopharyngeal reflux, chronic sinusitis, allergic reactions of the vocal tract and chronic airways disease which predispose the client to vocal hyperfunction and coughing or throat clearing, referral for medical and, possibly, surgical management is warranted (Sataloff, 1987c). Laryngopharyngeal reflux, for example, may be controlled with high doses of H_2-receptor agonists such as omeprazole and lifestyle modifications (e.g. avoidance of foods which trigger reflux, avoidance of eating close to bedtime, elevation of the head of the bed by 12 cm during sleep, use of antacids) (Morrison and Rammage, 1994; Koufman et al., 1996). It should be remembered, however, that many medications used to treat other conditions such as allergies and sinusitis may have a negative effect on the vocal fold cover and that these conditions are also notoriously difficult to resolve (Reed Thompson, 1995; Colton and Casper, 1996).

In cases where laryngeal irritants are likely to underlie vocal hyperfunction, the client will work with the clinician to either remove those irritants or to reduce their effects on vocal behaviour. Tobacco and marijuana smoking and the use of other recreational drugs such as cocaine will be discouraged, but referral to a formal programme for elimination of such drug use may be necessary because many clients need considerable support and counselling in order to abandon the habit. Similarly, clients who have a high caffeine intake will be advised to reduce the number of drinks containing caffeine and to increase water intake to compensate for the dehydration which can be associated with caffeine. The client will also be advised to avoid environments which are excessively dry, dusty or polluted or to minimize their potential harm by increasing oral hydration and environmental humidity levels. Although cessation of medications for medical conditions such as asthma, hypertension and depression will be contraindicated, consultation with the client's medical practitioner may allow for changes in medication and modification of dose levels which will reduce the negative effects of the medication on vocal functioning.

When hyperfunctional voicing appears to result from faulty learning mechanisms, an aetiological approach will also be required. A common example is the person who adopts a low pitch and glottal fry in an effort to convey authority (Stemple et al., 1995a). This pattern was once almost exclusive to men, but with recent sociocultural changes (Pemberton et al., 1998), women may also demonstrate such learned hyperfunction. In this case, effective intervention will involve counselling which focuses on the client's vocal image and the vocal damage which may result, as well as teaching the client to use alternative means of conveying the desired image (e.g. altering prosodic patterns and non-verbal behaviour).

Although psychogenic factors can underlie vocal hyperfunction (Rollin, 1987; Aronson, 1990; Goldman et al., 1996), there is considerable controversy as to whether effective management of hyperfunctionally related voice problems requires approaches such as affective counselling or psychotherapy. It is widely accepted that a therapeutic relationship characterized by empathy, active listening, and encouragement on the part of the clinician is associated with effective intervention (Rollin, 1987; Wilson, 1987; Aronson, 1990; Stemple et al., 1995a), but whether or not successful intervention requires a psychological approach is not clear. Research evidence which demonstrates the efficacy of counselling and psychotherapy for clients with hyperfunctional voice disorders is scarce (see for example, Mosby, 1970, 1972) and the majority of authors focus on voice therapy techniques rather than psychological interventions in their recommendations for management of clients with these voice disorders (e.g. Boone and McFarlane, 1994; Stemple et al., 1995a; Colton and Casper, 1996). Nevertheless, clinicians are advised to be alert to the possibility that personality characteristics, emotional reactions to life stressors, dysfunctional interpersonal relationships and emotional disturbances may prevent the client from being able to change their vocal behaviours (Brodnitz, 1981; Rollin, 1987; Roy et al., 1997a). This may occur, for example, when a child's vocal hyperfunction is a response to disturbed family relationships (Wilson, 1987; Andrews, 1991; Morrison and Rammage, 1994). In such cases, the clinician will need to address the psychological contributors underlying vocal hyperfunction and referral to mental health professionals may be required. A more extensive discussion of the role of the psychological approach to voice therapy is provided in Chapter 8 of this book.

Reduction or elimination of specific hyperfunctional vocal behaviours

A traditional intervention approach for voice disorders related to vocal hyperfunction has been to employ a behaviour modification programme to eliminate specific hyperfunctional behaviours such as yelling, loud talking and speaking with hard glottal attack. Such programmes typically involve identification of hyperfunctional behaviours and the situations in which those behaviours occur, educating the client about the rationale for reduction of hyperfunction, teaching the client to recognize when they are using hyperfunctional voicing, collecting baseline data on the frequency of each behaviour, self-monitoring and regular charting or graphing of the incidence of hyperfunctional behaviours, and providing positive reinforcement or rewards for reductions in those behaviours. Examples of such behavioural programmes include Boone's 'Voice Program for Children' (Boone, 1993), Johnson's 'Vocal Abuse Reduction Program' (Johnson, 1985a) and Wilson's '10-step Outline for Voice Abuse' (Wilson, 1987).

Most of the major texts in the voice field also outline similar procedures to assist clients in reducing hyperfunctional behaviours (e.g. Boone and McFarlane, 1994; Colton and Casper, 1996).

While there is some research evidence which demonstrates that behavioural programmes for reduction of hyperfunctional behaviours can be effective (e.g. Johnson, 1985b), there are several limitations to this approach which may reduce its value for many clients. First, without also addressing the many situational factors which are conducive to vocal hyperfunction, behaviour modification will often be inadequate (Stemple et al., 1995a). Poor environmental acoustics or air quality, high levels of background noise, communicating with people with attentional or hearing impairments, participating in or observing sporting events, working in jobs which necessitate extensive speaking or singing and being required to sing or act using a voice outside of a comfortable range may all lead to hyperfunctional voice use. Instructing clients to tally the number of times they yell or use a loud voice will be of little value unless they are also assisted to alter these situational factors or to develop strategies to compensate for the environmental conditions. Improving room acoustics and air quality, turning down background noise, planning the working day to incorporate voice rest periods, allowing time for vocal recuperation after extensive voice use, refusing to perform roles that ask for potentially harmful vocalization, and using fold-back speakers when singing with bands are likely to be more effective than behaviour modification of specific hyperfunctional voicing patterns.

Planning recuperation time is particularly important because the extraordinary vibration and collision rates of the vocal folds in phonation mean that the cover of the vocal folds is susceptible to damage and needs recovery time after use (Titze, 1994). In addition, compensatory strategies including moving close to other people when speaking, moving away from the source of background noise, using voice amplification devices, arranging the communicative environment to facilitate lip reading on the part of the hearing impaired conversational partner, swallowing hard instead of clearing the throat, and using gesture and non-vocal sounds such as whistles and hand-clapping to gain attention will also be required if hyperfunctional behaviours are to be successfully reduced.

A second limitation of behavioural programmes for reduction of vocal hyperfunction is that it is often unrealistic to expect clients to eliminate or reduce a particular vocal behaviour. Consider the six-year-old child whose peers all yell and scream in the school playground, the musical theatre actor whose role requires screaming, the auctioneer whose voice must penetrate over large distances in the open air, the swimming instructor who must teach groups of noisy children in an outdoor pool. These people cannot easily relinquish their vocal hyperfunction without risking adverse effects such as social isolation and loss of employment.

The recognition of this important limitation of vocal abuse reduction programmes has led to a shift in approaches to vocal hyperfunction whereby clients are taught, not to stop shouting and loud talking, but to do so in a more effective and less vocally harmful manner (Bagnall, 1995; Stemple et al., 1995a; Wilson, 1987). Stemple et al. (1995a) recommend, for example, that children with voice disorders who shout frequently be taught how to shout in a better way, that is, by using a lower pitched voice and improved breath support. Other authors and clinicians recommend that the client is taught to shout by initiating voicing at a high lung volume and using a more resonant or better projected voice along with adopting a diaphragmatic-abdominal focus for speech breathing and cupping the hands around the mouth to simulate a megaphone effect (e.g. Wilson, 1987; Martin and Darnley, 1992). Improved projection may be achieved using more oral openness and techniques such as resonant voice therapy or improving the tone focus of the voice (Lessac, 1967; Boone and McFarlane, 1994; Morrison and Rammage, 1994; Stemple et al., 1995a; Colton and Casper, 1996).

Bagnall (1995) has also developed an approach to modifying vocal hyperfunction which teaches clients to 'yell well'. This approach derives from the 'Compulsory Figures for Voice' (Estill, 1997), a model proposed by Jo Estill to train singers and other voice users in the independent control of the structures of the vocal tract and in the production of a range of voice qualities (speech, falsetto, sob, twang, opera and belt). Bagnall (1995) suggests that children or adults with hyperfunctional voice disorders who need a very loud voice in speaking or singing be taught to use belting. Belting, or high-intensity voicing, involves release of laryngeal constriction using a silent 'giggle' posture in the vocal tract, anchoring (strong muscle contraction) of the large muscles of the head, neck and torso, a glottal stroke onset (i.e. complete glottal adduction without constriction), narrowing of the aryepiglottic area in the larynx, a high larynx and tongue position and high levels of vocal energy. No specific attention to breathing patterns is required to achieve this high intensity voice. Because there are several potential risks of using belting incorrectly (e.g. back and neck discomfort, laryngeal constriction, vocal fold pathology), it is recommended that clinicians who wish to teach this technique to their clients obtain specialist training (Bagnall, 1995; Estill, 1997).

In cases where the client requires a voice which carries well over distance and above background noise, but where belting would be too loud, Yanagisawa et al. (1989), Bagnall (1995) and Estill (1997) recommend the use of the 'twang' voice quality. To produce the 'bright, penetrating' twang quality, the client is taught to release laryngeal constriction with a silent 'giggle' posture, use the glottal stroke onset, narrow the aryepiglottic area of the larynx, raise the larynx and keep the back of the tongue high in the mouth. Imitation of the 'witch's cackle', 'child's taunt' ('nya, nya, nya nya, nya'), horse's whinny and similar vocal sounds will also assist the client to learn to produce the twang quality. Again, because laryngeal constriction can easily occur if this technique is applied poorly in speech or singing, the clinician should develop considerable expertise before teaching twang quality to clients with hyperfunctional voice disorders (Bagnall, 1995). Twang quality may, however, be particularly useful for clients who lecture, teach or socialize in large spaces or in noisy environments (Colton and Casper, 1996).

Modification of hyperfunctional vocal technique

In addition to addressing the underlying reasons for vocal hyperfunction and reducing specific hyperfunctional behaviours, the clinical literature recommends that clients with voice disorders related to vocal hyperfunction be taught to alter their general voice production technique for all voice contexts. The general aim is to teach the client to use vocal techniques which are incompatible with hyperfunction and which can be used by the client in everyday speaking and singing activities. All of the major texts on voice disorders describe a large number of voice therapy procedures designed to achieve this aim (e.g. Wilson, 1987; Aronson, 1990; Boone and McFarlane, 1994; Andrews, 1995; Stemple et al., 1995a; Colton and Casper, 1996; Dworkin and Melecca, 1997). A number of voice therapy manuals and texts which describe specific therapy approaches are also available (e.g. Lessac, 1967; Martin and Darnley, 1992; Kotby, 1995). Rather than reiterate the material provided in these resources on the procedural details for therapy techniques, the remainder of this chapter outlines the rationales for those therapy techniques purported to reduce hyperfunctional voicing, discusses any limitations of those approaches and comments on treatment efficacy.

An underlying principle of voice therapy to reduce hyperfunctional voicing is that clients' responses to intervention and the efficiency of their learning will be maximized if they are educated to monitor their own vocal performance (Aronson, 1990; Boone and McFarlane, 1994; Colton and Casper, 1996; Hicks and Bless, 1996). Self-monitoring is considered to be an essential prerequisite for changing vocal technique; unless clients can identify the faulty aspects of their voices and can tell whether or not their voice production meets the desired vocal performance, vocal improvement will be difficult to achieve.

Enhancing self-monitoring of vocal performance is most commonly approached through auditory training, although tactile, proprioceptive, and visual monitoring can be valuable adjuncts to working through the auditory channel. Vocal self-monitoring can be facilitated, for example, by providing clients with biofeedback from devices such as audio- and video-tape recorders, laryngeal videoendoscopy systems, electromyographic biofeedback units, and acoustic and respiratory analysis systems (Boone and

McFarlane, 1994; Stemple et al., 1995). While vocal self-monitoring is accepted as fundamental to successful voice therapy, few studies have investigated the efficacy of this approach for clients with hyperfunctional disorders. The small amount of research evidence available, however, indicates that the use of biofeedback can enhance treatment efficacy (e.g. Prosek et al., 1978; Stemple et al., 1980; Andrews et al., 1986; Bastian and Nagorsky, 1987).

Therapy techniques designed to reduce hyperfunctional voicing can be broadly categorized as those which focus on the support functions for vocalization, those which aim to directly reduce laryngeal muscle tension and constriction, and those that are holistic. There is no particular technique which is best for specific disorders. Rather, the clinician is advised to select therapy approaches on the basis of their knowledge of the physiological basis of the client's impaired vocal functioning (Stemple et al., 1995a; Colton and Casper, 1996). That is, a physiological approach to voice therapy is recommended; inappropriate physiologic activity in the laryngeal and respiratory musculature is modified directly through exercise and/or manipulation (Stemple et al., 1995a). It is also important, however, to employ therapy techniques which are appropriate for the client's personality and emotional and vocal needs as well as techniques with which the clinician is experienced and confident.

Therapy techniques which focus on the 'support' functions for vocalization

This category of therapy technique includes efforts to improve the client's postural alignment, general muscle tension levels and respiratory patterns. If the evaluation of the client has demonstrated that faulty posture, excess general body tension levels or inefficient or faulty breathing patterns are likely to be contributing to their hyperfunctional vocal behaviours, then such intervention is warranted. Methods for improving postural misalignments are comprehensively described by Martin and Darnley (1992) and Morrison and Rammage (1994). The clinician may also consider referring the client to other professionals for specific postural education (e.g. Alexander and Feldenkrais practitioners, exercise physiologists). General body and head and neck relaxation methods are also outlined in many voice texts (e.g. Martin and Darnley, 1992; Boone and McFarlane, 1994) as well as in specific relaxation manuals (e.g. Bernstein and Borkovec, 1973). A cautionary note is required here, however, as the role of general muscle tension (other than that within the vocal tract) in hyperfunctional voice disorders has not been established and long periods of time devoted to general body and head and neck relaxation training may have no significant effect on vocal hyperfunction (Boone and McFarlane, 1994). Indeed, Estill (1997) has suggested that increased tension of the large muscles of the neck, face and torso can reduce the need for constriction within the larynx by dispersing effort to those other parts of the body. General body relaxation would then be counterproductive if Estill's proposal is correct.

The role of respiratory dysfunction in hyperfunctional voice problems is also controversial (Reed, 1980; Colton and Casper, 1996) and there is almost no evidence to support the efficacy of respiratory training for clients with vocal hyperfunction (Hillman et al., 1990). Nevertheless, the voice literature abounds with recommendations that clients with hyper-functional voice disorders will benefit from training which aims to improve breathing technique (e.g. Wilson, 1987; Martin and Darnley, 1992; Boone and McFarlane, 1994).

There is little argument with the proposition that signs of poor coordi-nation between breathing and phonation such as speaking on reserve air, initiating everyday speech at very low or excessively high lung volumes, holding the breath before speaking, or attempting to speak for too long on one breath require direct modification if they are evident in clients with hyperfunctional voice disorders (Colton and Casper, 1996; Hicks and Bless, 1996; Wilson, 1987; Martin and Darnley, 1992; Boone and McFarlane, 1994). Similarly, there is general agreement that assisting clients to use relaxed and coordinated breathing can reduce hyperfunction of the laryn-geal muscles, even if only by distracting the client from their laryngeal focus (Colton and Casper, 1996; Wilson, 1987). When ineffective breathing patterns are seen, however, it is important to recognize that those patterns may simply result from the disrupted phonation and, sometimes, from postural misalignment. In such cases, breathing exercises are likely to be unhelpful and vocal and postural re-education will be more effective.

The admonition that clients with hyperfunctional voice disorders will benefit from learning to use diaphragmatic-abdominal breathing patterns and extensive training in respiratory control (e.g. Wilson, 1987; Greene and Mathieson, 1989) has recently been questioned (Aronson, 1990; Boone and McFarlane, 1994; Colton and Casper, 1996; Hicks and Bless, 1996). The underlying tenet here is that most clients with hyperfunctional voice problems do not exhibit faulty breathing *per se*; instead, it is more likely to be the coordination between breathing and phonation that is deficient (Boone and McFarlane, 1994; Hicks and Bless, 1996). Colton and Casper (1996), for example, propose that speakers who are not profes-sional voice users do not need to learn diaphragmatic-abdominal breathing and that only those clients who need to speak or sing with very low or high lung volumes will benefit from specific respiratory training. Colton and Casper (1996) indicate that the latter group of clients may require training in using diaphragmatic-abdominal breathing and in learning to support very high or low lung volumes with appropriate control of inspiratory and expiratory musculature. Estill (1997), however, takes this point further and suggests that even professional voice users such as singers do not require specific respiratory training as long as they learn effective control of laryngeal and supraglottic functioning and control of the large muscles of the back, neck and face for high-intensity voicing.

In cases where the clinician's evaluation of the client indicates that respiratory training is likely to reduce vocal hyperfunction, most voice texts and manuals describe therapeutic procedures which can be used (e.g. Wilson, 1987; Martin and Darnley, 1992; Boone and McFarlane, 1994; Hicks and Bless, 1996). Clinicians should remember, however, that many of the techniques outlined in these texts were derived from early speech and drama and singing pedagogy and have not always been supported by physiological evidence. Clinicians are therefore advised to ensure that they select respiratory training techniques which are consistent with current understanding of respiratory function for speech and singing (e.g. Hixon et al., 1976; Sundberg, 1987; Watson et al., 1990; Titze, 1994; Hixon and Weismer, 1995; Hoit, 1995). It is also important to recognize that there are individual differences in the respiratory patterns which are most appropriate; 'what is efficient for one individual may be less efficient for another' (Titze, 1994).

Therapy techniques which aim to directly reduce laryngeal muscle tension and constriction

Many therapeutic techniques designed to reduce the hallmark of vocal hyperfunction, excess laryngeal muscle tension, are described in the voice literature. These include the breathy or 'confidential' voice, the sigh, aspirate or easy initiation of voicing (e.g. initiation of words with /h/ or a silent /h/), and the yawn-sigh (see Wilson, 1987; Boone and McFarlane, 1994; Colton and Casper, 1996). Each of these techniques aims to counteract the medial compression and force of contact between the vocal folds, minimize ventricular fold compression and anteroposterior supraglottic constriction, eliminate hard glottal attack, reduce loudness and restore the position of the larynx to its resting position in the neck. The sigh, aspirate initiation of voicing and yawn-sigh also aim to assist clients to develop easy coordination between airflow and voicing. The rationale for these therapy approaches is supported by a small amount of research data and is in accord with current understanding of laryngeal function in healthy and impaired voices (Belisle and Morrison, 1983; Casper et al., 1989; Hillman et al., 1989; Titze, 1994). Although the efficacy of these techniques has rarely been investigated through experimental studies using objective measures of vocal functioning, a small number of published reports have shown that at least the breathy or confidential voice and the yawn-sigh can be effective for clients with hyperfunctional voice disorders (Boone and McFarlane, 1993; Verdolini-Marston et al., 1995).

While therapy techniques such as yawn-sigh, sigh, aspirate initiation and the breathy or confidential voice can have positive effects on vocal functioning, a number of caveats should be recognized. First, because each of these techniques promotes suboptimal voicing with incomplete glottal closure, breathiness and low loudness levels, they are normally not appropriate as the client's permanent vocal technique. Rather, these procedures are useful for a circumscribed period in the early stages of vocal rehabilitation to break the hyperfunctional pattern. Secondly, because these therapy approaches are associated with decreased glottal closure and increased airflow through the glottis, it is possible that drying of the vocal fold mucosa will result (Colton and Casper, 1996). For this reason, these techniques are suitable only in the short term and clients may need to be advised to increase oral hydration during this period of rehabilitation. Thirdly, the yawning component of the yawn-sigh technique is not always associated with the desirable effects of reduced laryngeal muscle tension and a lowering of the height of the larynx in the neck. Although the initial stages of a yawn lead to these outcomes, the final stages of the yawn often lead to raising of the larynx and increased supraglottic muscle tension. The positive result of the early part of the yawn is therefore compromised. Fourthly, while these therapy techniques are designed to minimize antero-posterior supraglottic constriction, Yanagisawa et al. (1989) have suggested that there are some circumstances in which such constriction is desirable. These authors have demonstrated that the use of aryepiglottic narrowing is a normal correlate of efficient loud voicing and suggest that clients may benefit from learning to use this type of constriction to produce a loud voice in a 'safe' manner (i.e. the 'twang' technique outlined earlier in this chapter). Finally, whether the breathy voicing and incomplete glottal closure promoted by these techniques is beneficial for clients with the form of hyperfunction labelled as non-adductive by Hillman et al. (1989) or as Muscular Tension Dysphonia Type 3 by Morrison and Rammage (1994) is unclear. Casper et al. (1989) indicate that these techniques may in fact encourage this type of hyperfunction and Titze (1994) suggests that such procedures would not benefit clients who already have the breathy voice associated with non-adductive hyperfunction.

Estill (1997) has proposed an alternative approach for reducing laryngeal muscle tension and constriction. Her approach involves teaching clients to reduce medial compression of the vocal folds and to retract the ventricular folds by consciously adopting a silent 'giggle' or laughing posture in the larynx during speech and singing. Estill and Yanagisawa (1991) have shown empirically that this manoeuvre can indeed achieve these aims and it may be that this approach is more viable for long-term use than the group of breathy, sigh, yawn-sigh, and aspirate initiation techniques outlined above. Experimental studies of the efficacy of Estill's deconstriction techniques for clients with hyperfunctional voice disorders, however, have yet to be conducted.

Aronson (1990) describes a further technique for modifying extrinsic and intrinsic laryngeal muscle tension and lowering the larynx to a position which is incompatible with vocal hyperfunction. His technique involves direct massage and manipulation of the laryngeal area to reduce musculoskeletal tension and muscle 'cramping' and to reduce the laryngeal pain and other signs of throat discomfort which may be associated with hyperfunction. Aronson suggests that this technique, known as 'manual laryngeal musculoskeletal tension reduction' or 'manual circumlaryngeal therapy' (Roy et al., 1997), should be used as the primary approach for clients who show signs of excess musculoskeletal tension of the larynx. Although Aronson has not provided any research data to support his contentions, his approach has been evaluated in a series of experimental studies by Nelson Roy and his colleagues (e.g. Roy and Leeper, 1993; Roy et al., 1997). These investigations have demonstrated consistent short-term voice improvement and reduction in laryngeal pain and tenderness in clients with functional voice disorders in the absence of laryngeal pathology. Long-term outcomes for some clients were impressive, but partial and infrequent recurrences of the vocal problems were seen in the majority of clients. Further research is required to determine the physiological and psychological basis of voice improvement associated with Aronson's approach and to compare its efficacy with that of alternative techniques for laryngeal hyperfunction. In the meantime, there is sufficient evidence for clinicians to consider this approach for clients with hyperfunctional voice disorders. Again, there are some limitations of Aronson's approach that should be kept in mind. Manual circumlaryngeal therapy can induce temporary pain in some clients (Aronson, 1990), the technique can be counterproductive for clients who do not speak with an elevated larynx (Colton and Casper, 1996), and the procedures will be difficult to use in young children with immature laryngeal structures (Wilson, 1987).

Holistic therapy techniques

The final category of therapy techniques which may be effective for clients with vocal hyperfunction includes techniques which take a more holistic approach and aim to improve several aspects of voice production simultaneously. The goal is to assist clients to integrate the various respiratory, phonatory and resonance components of voicing in a balanced and non-hyperfunctional manner. Examples of such holistic approaches are the accent method, the chewing technique, resonant voice therapy and vocal function exercises.

The accent method was developed by Svend Smith, a Danish speech therapist and speech scientist (Smith and Thyme, 1978; Kotby, 1995). This method incorporates teaching of diaphragmatic-abdominal breath support, rhythmic vowel play with systematic variation of intensity, rate and duration, and then progressive carryover to connected speech. Rhythmic body and arm movements accompany the phonatory exercises and general body, pharyngeal and laryngeal posture and glottal onsets are also addressed. The aims of the accent method are to eliminate hyperadduction of the vocal folds, reduce any glottal chink, improve the coordination of breathing with voice and speech, optimize pitch and pitch range, enhance projection and loudness range, and normalize voice quality. Although the underlying rationale for the accent method has not been described in detail, Smith hypothesized that diaphragmatic-abdominal support is the main mechanism for vocal improvement. Titze (1994) has proposed that the procedure of varying intensity systematically and repeatedly with diaphragmatic-abdominal muscular effort is indeed likely to reduce the adductory force required at the vocal fold level for the production of syllabic stress. Kotby (1995) also postulates that vocal intensity is increased because the accent method increases glottal airflow and subglottal pressure, that the average and range of fundamental frequency is increased because the technique promotes cricothyroid muscle activity, and that improved coordination between exhalation and initiation of voicing reduces laryngeal hyperfunction. The efficacy of the accent method has been examined by Nasser Kotby and his colleagues in a series of investigations (e.g. Kotby et al., 1991) and by Fex et al. (1994). The general conclusion of these studies has been that the method results in significant vocal improvements in most clients with hyperfunctional voice disorders without vocal fold pathology as well as clients with vocal nodules. It should be noted, however, that not all clients who participated in these studies demonstrated vocal improvement, that control groups were not included in any of these investigations and that comparisons with other therapy techniques have not been conducted.

The chewing technique originated from the work of Froeschels who proposed that because chewing is a natural vegetative act, if a person was taught to chew and speak simultaneously, then vocal hyperfunction would be reduced, resonance would be enhanced through reduced oral and mandibular muscle tension, and pitch would become normal (Froeschels, 1952). This therapy technique is strongly recommended by Wilson (1987) for children with hyperfunctional voice disorders, but is no longer listed by Boone and McFarlane (1994) among their facilitating techniques because their surveys have shown that chewing is rarely used by practising clinicians. There are no published experimental studies of the utility of the chewing method, but clinical case studies and anecdotal reports indicate that the approach can release excess laryngeal and jaw tension (Wilson, 1987; Colton and Casper, 1996). It is clear that some clients who have been socialized to chew unobtrusively will experience difficulty in learning this technique because of the embarrassment associated with exaggerated chewing. The clinician must therefore be skilled in using the method and comfortable in demonstrating chewing to the client (Colton and Casper, 1996).

Resonant voice therapy (Verdolini-Marston et al., 1995) and a host of related techniques such as humming and nasal consonants (Colton and Casper, 1996), the *um-hum* procedure (Cooper, 1973), altering tone focus (Perkins, 1983; Wilson, 1987; Boone and McFarlane, 1994; Stemple et al., 1995) and the Ybuzz (Lessac, 1967) are holistic approaches that promote a vocal technique that purported to be incompatible with hyperfunction of the laryngeal muscles and that can be used as a long-term vocal technique. These resonance approaches entail teaching the client to use particular speech sounds (mainly nasal consonants, /j/ and /i/) to increase propriocep-tive sensations of skull vibration during voicing. The client is encouraged to use imagery (e.g. the 'inverted megaphone' described by Lessac, 1967) and tactile and/or kinaesthetic self-monitoring to 'focus the tone forward' in the skull (i.e. to feel for vibration in the regions of the lips, hard palate and teeth, the nose and cheek bones, and the forehead). Use of chanting may also be incorporated with these techniques to enhance the forward focus and to make it easier for the client to alter voice production than it would be in normal speech (Colton and Casper, 1996). Once the client has learnt to alter the tone or resonance focus in this way, the dependence on partic-ular speech sounds and chanting is gradually reduced.

The rationale for these resonance techniques is not easy to discern from the literature. Most of these techniques developed from speech and drama and singing pedagogy and much remains to be learnt about the physiological and acoustic mechanisms underlying their effects (Titze, 1994; Verdolini-Marston et al., 1995). The general assumption is, however, that the voices of clients with hyperfunctional disorders are focused mainly in the larynx rather than being balanced between the larynx and the supraglottic resonators. The voices of these clients therefore sound and feel as if they are being squeezed or pushed out of the throat with excess laryngeal muscle tension. Resonance techniques aim to restore a more normal tone focus, with vocal effort in the laryngeal area becoming more evenly distributed throughout the vocal tract. In this way, the proponents of these techniques claim that vocal fold hyperad-duction and ventricular fold compression are reduced, that glottal closure is improved and that pitch becomes normalized (Lessac, 1967; Perkins, 1983; Wilson, 1987; Boone and McFarlane, 1994; Stemple et al., 1995a; Verdolini-Marston et al., 1995; Colton and Casper, 1996). It is also suggested that these approaches improve voice projection and therefore reduce the need for the client to use hyperfunctional mechanisms to produce a loud voice. Although this rationale for resonance approaches has some face validity, it may be that these techniques reduce laryngeal muscle tension and constriction by simply distracting clients from their preoccupation with the larynx and throat areas.

Whatever the case, further exploration of the mechanism of action of resonance techniques is required.

As with most voice therapy techniques, very little experimental research on the efficacy of these resonance approaches has been reported. A notable exception is the report of Verdolini-Marston et al. (1995a) who conducted a preliminary study of the efficacy of resonant voice therapy for women with vocal nodules as compared with confidential voice therapy and a vocal hygiene control condition. Although therapy was provided for only two weeks (9 sessions in total) and the follow-up period was only two weeks, the results demonstrated that both therapy techniques were associated with greater improvements in self-ratings of vocal effort, perceptual judgements of the voice and visual judgements of the health of the vocal folds than was the control condition. There was, however, no difference in the likelihood of vocal improvement between resonant voice therapy and confidential voice therapy.

Stemple, Glaze and Gerdeman (1995) have outlined a programme of vocal function exercises that are also holistic in that the programme is designed to balance and co-ordinate the respiratory, phonatory and resonatory subsystems of voice production. The client is taught a series of four exercises (sustaining /i/ for as long as possible on the note F above middle C for females and below middle C for males, gliding from high to low on the word 'knoll', gliding from low to high on 'knoll', and sustaining /o/ on the notes C, D, E, F, and G starting from middle C for females and an octave lower for males) which are then practised twice each, twice each day. Each exercise is practised as softly as possible with easy voice onsets (but no breathiness) and with a forward resonance focus. Stemple et al. (1995) propose that this exercise regime is akin to physiotherapy and that it is likely to improve laryngeal muscle control and flexibility, minimize laryngeal muscle hyperfunction, reduce vocal fatigue and create an optimal balance between airflow, laryngeal activity and supraglottic control. Whether such physiologic changes do result from the vocal function exercises and whether these exercises are effective for clients with hyperfunctional voice disorders has yet to be empirically demonstrated. Some early support for Stemple et al.'s contentions, however, has been provided in a study of the effects of the programme on the normal voices of adult women (Stemple et al., 1994). Acoustic, aerodynamic and videostroboscopic measures demonstrated significant positive changes in the voices of the women who underwent four weeks of vocal function exercising, whereas no significant changes occurred for control and placebo groups.

Modification of pitch, loudness and glottal fry

Although many of the therapy techniques outlined earlier are likely to have indirect effects on pitch, loudness and glottal fry, brief comment is required here as to whether direct modification of these vocal parameters is also beneficial for clients with hyperfunctional voice disorders. Because speaking or singing with excess loudness levels can be a possible cause of vocal dysfunction, it may be necessary to assist the client in learning to self-monitor loudness (e.g. using biofeedback devices such as audio-tape recorders and acoustic analysis systems) and to readjust their habitual loudness levels to be more situationally appropriate (Stemple et al., 1995; Wilson, 1987). For clients who have mucosal changes such as oedema, inflammation and vocal nodules, short-term restrictions on loud voice use will often be necessary; the client may, for example, be instructed to speak only in a soft, slightly breathy voice and to eliminate any voice use in noisy environments (Colton and Casper, 1996). Such extreme restrictions should, however, be temporary with a more appropriate long-term aim being for the client to develop vocal techniques which allow them to produce a well projected or loud voice in a 'safe' manner.

The need for direct modification of pitch in hyperfunctional voice disorders is particularly controversial. This controversy arises from disagreements surrounding the validity of the concept of optimal pitch, the role of inappropriate pitch as a cause of hyperfunctional voice problems and whether or not direct pitch modification is effective. The voice literature and available research data has generally rejected the concept of optimal pitch, is inconclusive as to whether inappropriate pitch can be a cause of hyperfunctional disorders, and indicates that direct pitch modification is difficult and often unnecessary for clients with these vocal disorders (see, for example, Wilson, 1987; Aronson, 1990; Roy and Tasko, 1994; Stemple et al., 1995a; Colton and Casper, 1996). In the majority of cases, therapy which focuses on reducing laryngeal muscle tension and constriction, either directly or holistically, is likely to result in an appropriate pitch level without the need for specific attention to pitch (Aronson, 1990; Colton and Casper, 1996). A notable exception to this generalization is the client whose hyperfunctional disorder appears to be due to the use of the 'pseudoauthoritative' voice; that is, an habitual low-pitched voice which is often accompanied by excessive use of glottal fry (Stemple et al., 1995). In this case, if an indirect approach focusing on the client's vocal image and modification of laryngeal muscle tension is not effective, direct alteration of pitch may be required. Aronson (1990) and Stemple et al. (1995) outline useful therapy techniques which involve establishing a comfortable target pitch using Cooper's (1973) *um-hum* procedure as well as self-monitoring and biofeedback. Specific attention to glottal fry may also be necessary for such clients; auditory, visual and proprioceptive self-monitoring and increasing subglottal pressure and airflow are likely to be effective methods.

Conclusion

Hyperfunctional vocal behaviours are considered to be a primary cause of the most common voice disorders; throat discomfort, vocal fatigue, nodules, polyps, oedema, inflammation and haemorrhage. Such vocal behaviours will therefore be the primary focus of evaluation and treatment programmes for clients with these disorders. There is little disagreement as to the types of vocal behaviours which are hyperfunctional, but further research is necessary to determine the underlying physiology of these behaviours and the precise aetiological role of vocal hyperfunction. Clinical evaluation of vocal hyperfunction aims to determine the medical, situational, psychological, laryngeal irritant, compensatory and learning factors that are at the basis of that hyperfunction and to measure hyperfunction in a valid and reliable manner. Our understanding of the classification of vocal hyperfunction and our ability to measure it has advanced considerably in the last decade so that clinicians can now more confidently operationalize and assess mechanical stress on the vocal mechanism. Scientific research must continue, however, to delineate more clearly the physiological, acoustic and perceptual features of hyperfunctional voicing and to establish which are the most useful measurement techniques.

The treatment of clients with voice disorders related to hyperfunction addresses the underlying causal and contributing factors of the hyperfunction, specific hyperfunctional behaviours, and the client's general vocal technique. Management which focuses on only one or two of these three considerations is unlikely to be maximally effective. Behavioural programmes for eliminating or reducing specific hyperfunctional behaviours have altered in recent years so that we now have more realistic expectations of our clients and, rather than severely restricting their voice use, assist them to be able to use their voices to the full, but in a manner which is less harmful to the vocal mechanism. Approaches to the modification of our clients' general vocal technique continue to rely on traditional therapy techniques, but we have seen a shift towards a more physiologic approach to voice therapy with less importance placed on techniques which promote suboptimal voice production. Although voice therapy is now based more clearly on physiological principles, further research needs to be conducted to develop a better scientific understanding of the mechanism of action of particular intervention methods and to establish the efficacy of therapy techniques. Experimental designs that use control groups or no-treatment baseline conditions, provide operational definitions of the voice outcomes targeted in therapy and clear details of therapy procedures, and that examine the role of factors unrelated to the therapy technique (e.g. client motivation and expectancies) will be required if voice therapy for hyperfunctional disorders is to advance to the stage where it can be considered to be an effective science as well as an art.

CHAPTER 8

Psychogenic, psychological and psychosocial issues in diagnosis and therapy

MARGARET FREEMAN

Introduction

This chapter aims to explore some of the issues raised by the terms 'functional' and 'psychogenic'. It is well recognized that both of these terms are used in a number of different ways in the literature. In the medical sense, for example, 'functional' is a general classification used by laryngologists for any voice disorders that are not caused by organic conditions such as disease or structural abnormalities (Groves and Gray, 1985). This classification covers many different patterns of vocal dysfunction, which are all associated with tension in the muscles involved in phonation (Morrison and Rammage, 1994). Because of the absence of an adequate physical explanation, it has been assumed that these problems were caused or strongly influenced by underlying psychological or 'psychogenic' processes (House and Andrews, 1987; Morrison and Rammage, 1994).

The history of voice therapy shows us that there has been a long-standing debate about the way to explain and categorize the different clusters of clinical signs and symptoms which come into the general classification of 'functional voice disorders'. As Butcher et al. (1993) have observed, this has produced an abundance of different terms and definitions. In general, however, it seems that most clinicians would agree that 'functional' and 'non-organic' refer to voice disorders not associated with specific organic aetiology (Morrison and Rammage, 1994), whereas the term 'psychogenic' implies that the problem has been caused or maintained by psychological factors (Brodnitz, 1959) or underlying 'psychologic disequilibrium' (Aronson, 1980, p.131).

In this chapter, it is suggested that the debate about 'psychogenic' and 'functional' voice disorders has combined two main concerns. The first is the question of how we can explain voice disorders that occur in an apparently healthy larynx (Roy et al., 1997). The second reflects broader concerns about the psychological processes that play their part in all of our work with clients who have voice disorders (Butcher et al., 1993). In the past, many clinicians firmly believed that these two elements were part of the same process. All non-organic voice disorders, including vocal abuse and misuse, were considered to reflect underlying unconscious psycho-emotional causes (Morrison and Rammage, 1994; Butcher, 1995). As House and Andrews (1987) have observed, however, these theories of psychological causality developed as a result of clinical opinion and anecdotal evidence, rather than research into the psychological characteristics of clients with different types of voice disorders.

Some of the traditional theories about psychological causes have been challenged as a result of clinical research and developments. A specific example of this is spasmodic dysphonia, which was traditionally described as 'spastic dysphonia' and attributed to personality disorder (Greene, 1964). Clinical research has shown us, however, that there are several different sub-types of spasmodic dysphonia, some of which are associated with neurogenic changes (see Whurr, Chapter 11, this volume). Other clinical research has shown us that various physiological factors can impinge on vocal function, so that there is no clear distinction between 'functional' and 'organic' (Morrison, 1997).

At the same time, however, many clinicians recognize that many psychological issues can be raised in our work with people who have voice disorders. This includes the growing awareness that most voice problems, whether they are permanent or potentially reversible, can have quite severe psychosocial consequences (Andrews, 1995; Ritchie, 1996; Smith et al., 1996; Ramig and Verdolini, 1998).

All of these factors have led expert clinicians to suggest that we need to review the way we consider voice disorders (Morrison, 1997) and, in particular, the way we think about the psychological and psychosocial factors which influence our work with voice disordered people (Butcher, 1995; Ritchie, 1996; Morrison, 1997). Because the history of voice therapy shows that theories of causality have evolved over time, the first section of this chapter reviews some of the key influences. The later sections review some recent developments and consider their implications for management and therapy.

Theories, definitions and classifications

The first priority for all patients with voice disorder is to ensure that conditions that require primary medical or surgical treatment are identified and managed appropriately. As we have seen, when all possible organic factors have been excluded, the laryngologist may describe the disorder as 'functional'. Probably the most objective definition of this term is that it describes transient or chronic disturbances in normal function that are not attributable to organic disease (Mayer, 1996; Roy et al., 1997b). Technically, therefore, this covers changes to the mucosa because of abuse/misuse, as well as problems where there are no visible laryngeal signs.

The functional-organic dichotomy

Speech and language therapists, along with many other health care workers, have recognized that there are problems with the 'functional-organic dichotomy' (Van Riper and Irwin, 1958, cited by Fawcus, Chapter 4, in this volume). It has been suggested that this classification system – which tends to imply that ill-health can be caused by *either* the mind *or* the body – originated in the seventeenth century (Descartes, 1664, cited by Posner and Raichle, 1997, p. 2). Descartes' view was that the mind and body were two separate systems that had little interaction. He advised that doctors should concentrate on the scientific investigation of the physical processes, whereas the mind was the province of religion and philosophy (Bakal, 1979; Damasio, 1994; Mayer, 1996; Ogden, 1996; Posner and Raichle, 1997; White and Moorey, 1997). This way of thinking was still dominant when voice disorders were first described in the medical literature; Russell (1864, p. 618) stated, for example, that functional disorders were 'mental or moral problems, requiring moral treatments'.

Psychodynamic theory

The most influential explanation of psychological aetiology has come from psychodynamic theory, particularly Freud's (1905) description of a case of aphonia as a conversion disorder. It is of note that aphonia has been consistently described as a conversion disorder, hysteria or emotional distress in most ENT textbooks and much of the voice therapy literature, without modification, until quite recently (Boone, 1983; Butcher et al., 1987; House and Andrews, 1987; Morrison and Rammage, 1994; Rosen and Sataloff, 1997b). The concept of aphonia as a conversion disorder is reviewed in more detail in a later section.

Although the symptoms of aphonia and spastic (now 'spasmodic') dysphonia were identified as indications of separate and more severe psychopathology, it seems that many clinicians considered that all functional voice disorders, including 'habitual dysphonia' and 'vocal strain' were manifestations of other, less severe psychological processes, such as personality disturbance, anxiety and neurosis. Brodnitz (1959), for example, described functional voice disorders as two sides of a coin, with the physical symptoms on one side and the psychological factors on the other. Therapy for these disorders therefore combined 'technical voice training' and psychotherapy or counselling (Wyatt, 1941; Brodnitz, 1958; Heaver, 1958).

The balance of physical and psychological factors

Discussions about the psychological and physical mechanisms involved in functional voice disorders began in earnest in the 1960s. Perello (1962) suggested that there were identifiable clusters of problems, some of which were predominantly 'mechanical' problems such as vocal abuse, whereas other voice disorders may have predominantly psychological aetiologies. Murphy (1964) described a slightly different concept; he suggested that aetiologies of voice disorders existed on a continuum, with physical/organic factors at one end and psychological/functional influences at the other. Included in his model was the recognition that some people may simply have faulty vocal habits; because they did not understand how their vocal mechanism worked, they were more prone to developing dysphonia. Luchsinger and Arnold (1965) proposed a different model, based on the stress response. They suggested that the muscular tension associated with voice disorders could be the result of two different types of stressors: *exogenous* sources, which were those related to external demands such as overwork or unhappy relationships and *endogenous sources* such personality characteristics and other personal attributes.

It seems that each different explanation of functional voice disorders has produced new definitions and descriptions. The successive editions of Margaret Greene's (1957, 1964, 1972, 1980) book provide excellent documentation of the ways theories developed and changed. Unfortunately, this has also led to more variations in the terminology (the chapter by Margaret Fawcus discusses this in more detail).

Behavioural descriptions: abuse and misuse

During the 1970s, when there was a general movement towards a more scientific approach, the emphasis shifted towards behavioural descriptions of voice disorders and greater emphasis on the techniques of voice therapy (Boone, 1971; Moncur and Brackett, 1974; Perkins, 1983). Most of the focus moved to symptom-based therapy to reduce vocal abuse and misuse, with a corresponding swing away from psychodynamic interpretations. Boone and MacFarlane (1994) make the point that the original cause of the problem is often lost in the mists of time, and is therefore irrelevant, by the time most clients attend for voice therapy.

Recent studies have certainly confirmed that symptomatic voice therapy – especially when combined with explanation of the problem and therapeutic support – can be beneficial to the majority of clients with non-organic voice disorder (Carding and Horsley, 1992; Ramig and Verdolini, 1998). This change in approach was not with universal approval, however. Moore (1977) observed that improvements in techniques were only useful if the patient wanted to change. Brodnitz (1981, p. 24), who had always advocated a holistic approach which took account of the psychogenic or 'emotional dynamics' of voice, rejected the notion that therapy should be simply a routine. He described this approach as 'vocal gymnastics', which treated the symptoms, rather than the cause.

Psychogenic

The debate about the differences in the concepts underlying 'functional' and 'psychogenic' began again in earnest after Aronson (1980, p. 131) reasserted the view that all non-organic voice disorders were 'a manifestation of one or more types of psychologic disequilibrium, such as anxiety, depression, conversion reaction, or personality disorder, that interfere with normal volitional control'. Aronson suggested different personalities respond to stress in different ways, which can include an innate predisposition towards laryngeal tension. He therefore considered that personality characteristics influenced the type of non-organic voice disorder an individual would develop (Aronson, 1990).

A number of clinicians have challenged Aronson's conceptualization, because, they argue, predictions about personality cannot be made on the basis of the vocal and laryngeal symptoms alone (Boone and McFarlane, 1994; Morrison and Rammage, 1994; Colton and Casper, 1996; Rosen and Sataloff, 1997b). Aronson's (1990) views have, however, stimulated debate about the processes involved in the development of vocal tract tension. Whereas Aronson (1990) identifies this as a stress response, others have suggested that at least some of the tension observed in voice disordered clients may be an attempt to compensate for, or adapt to, other changes in the vocal tract (Freeman and Schaeffer, 1988; Boone and McFarlane, 1994). In reality, as Butcher (1995, p.468) has observed, it can be difficult, by the time the client reaches voice therapy, to identify whether processes such as 'psychological causes', habitual tension and adaptive vocal abuse are a cause or a result of the voice disorder.

The current debate about 'psychogenic' voice disorder

The term 'psychogenic' has been adopted by many clinicians, but, unfortunately, there are two quite different interpretations in common usage. Some clinicians use this term specifically for the small group of clients who have aphonia or dysphonia without any change to the vocal fold mucosa (Schalen et al., 1992; White et al., 1997), while others use 'psychogenic' specifically to imply that 'there is an observable voice problem and that the causative and perpetuating factors are largely psychological' (Butcher et al., 1993, p. 2; Morrison and Rammage, 1994).

Many clinicians tend to identify voice disorders associated with overt laryngeal signs of abuse or 'wear and tear' (Sapir et al., 1990) as characteristically different from symptoms of aphonia or transient dysphonia which show no signs of mucosal damage. This latter group are either described as 'functional' (Roy et al., 1997) or 'psychogenic' (Schalen et al., 1992). As we shall see below, one of the major developments in the past few years is that research has begun into the psychological characteristics of people with these voice disorders.

Voice disorders as an interactive process

The 'explosion of interest in voice' during the 1980s (Colton and Casper, 1996, p. v) with the strong emphasis on integrated, multi-disciplinary approaches has led to many changes, including the establishment of specialist voice teams who have adopted a collaborative, problem-solving approach to voice disorder. This in turn has led to the recognition that many voice problems develop from a combination of factors, rather than a single cause. Some experts in voice now consider that the traditional functional-organic classification system is an inappropriate model for diagnosis of voice disorders (Morrison, 1997).

Clinical research has demonstrated, for example, that some people's voice disorders may be triggered by chronic or acute conditions such as colds, upper respiratory tract infections, allergies, asthma or gastro-oesophageal reflux, as well as by emotional or other stress responses (Freeman and Schaefer, 1988; Morrison and Rammage, 1994). The effect of many of these conditions may be insidious, rather than sudden. We also know that many people do not recognize the relevance of the early symptoms, which explains why clients often cannot pinpoint the exact time of the onset (Haynes and Pindzola, 1998). It is hypothesized that once the process of voice deterioration has started, it requires only a small amount of tension, misuse or abuse to perpetuate the problem (Morrison and Rammage, 1994; Haynes and Pindzola, 1998). Even in the early stages of voice change, however, the problem may be compounded by psychosocial factors. Andrews (1995) suggests that any vocal limitations can have an effect on an individual's interactions with others, either through the listener's reactions or because of the difficulties faced by the voice-impaired person as he or she attempts to communicate in all activities of daily life.

A picture is therefore emerging of voice disorders which develop from a self-perpetuating spiral of causes and effects which can include changes in voice and reduction of the sense of well-being, exacerbated by the person's lack of understanding of the processes involved in voice production. If this is the case, it may explain why the majority of clients respond so well to symptomatic voice therapy (Carding and Horsley, 1992; Ramig and Verdolini, 1998). We also know that some people seem to tolerate their vocal symptoms for a considerable time whereas others seek medical attention quite rapidly (Smith et al., 1996). There are two questions raised by this. First, do factors such as personality account for the differences in seeking help? Secondly, does the duration of the symptoms relate to the differences in the pattern of laryngeal signs (Kotby, 1995)?

Psychological and psychosocial characteristics

In parallel with research from voice clinics, studies of the psychological characteristics of clinical populations have been undertaken. House and Andrews (1987, 1988) used structured psychiatric interviews and assessment of recent life events with a group of people referred for voice therapy with functional disorder, defined as 'voice disorder for which there was no adequate physical explanation' (House and Andrews, 1987, p. 484). The findings were that only two out of 71 patients met the criteria for personality disorder, both of which were of the histrionic type. Of the five patients with 'whispering aphonia', two patients had clinically diagnosable anxiety disorders. Overall, no direct association between the type of voice disorder and psychiatric pathology was found. However, around a third of the patients showed what House and Andrews (1988) described as 'conflict over speaking out' (CSO) in demanding situations that the patients had experienced during the year preceding the voice disorder and that created a sense of futility and vulnerability.

The same theme of difficulty with expression of feelings and/or a sense of being stuck in relationships or situations that are unfulfilling was also identified by Butcher et al. (1987) in clients who were unable to respond to traditional voice therapy. Butcher (1995) has noted that this sense of feeling helpless and unable to change is one of the responses to long-term stress, which Seligman (1975) suggested could eventually lead to depression and anxiety.

Studies of Functional or Psychogenic Aphonia and Dysphonia

Several studies have specifically evaluated groups of clients with aphonia or intermittent dysphonia. These impairments are identified as either 'functional' (Kinzl et al., 1988; Roy et al., 1997) or 'psychogenic'

(Gerritsima, 1991; Schalen et al., 1992; Friedl et al., 1993; White et al., 1997). Schalen et al. (1992) and Roy et al. (1997) report that clients with these symptoms generally represent just over 10% of cases referred for voice therapy. Their vocal symptoms include intermittent or ongoing aphonia, dysphonia or 'whispering dysphonia' (White et al., 1997) despite competent vocal fold closure during non-phonatory activity such as coughing. Typically, the descriptions of this group of voice disorders indicate that they are far more frequently found in women. The voice problems may be transient or have a tendency to recur (House and Andrews, 1988; Schalen et al., 1992; White et al., 1997).

These studies have explored factors such as personality characteristics, emotional status and responses to life stress in clients with non-organic voice disorders (House and Andrews, 1987, 1988; Kinzl et al., 1988; Gerritsima, 1991; Roy et al., 1997; White et al., 1997). Taken together, the results show that although each of these factors may play a part, there are wide variations among clients with apparently similar vocal signs and symptoms. Although some clients in each study showed some degree of anxiety, depression or introversion, a significant proportion of the clients were found to have psychological profiles within the 'normal' range. Overall, these studies confirm Kinzl et al.'s (1988) finding that clients with the vocal symptoms of aphonia and intermittent dysphonia do not have homogenous psychological profiles.

Cause or effect?

Significantly, the group psychological profiles of clients with aphonia and non-organic dysphonia are similar to those reported for groups of people with organic voice disorders (White et al., 1997) and with vocal nodules and related conditions (Goldman et al., 1996). In each of these studies, there is a general tendency for patients with voice disorder to show slightly higher levels of anxiety-related scores in comparison with other, non-voice disordered outpatients (House and Andrews, 1987; White et al., 1997) or with healthy controls.

This seems to confirm the clinical observations that having any type of voice disorder may, in itself, be a source of stress and distress (Aronson, 1990; Andrews, 1995). We noted above that Andrews (1995) has emphasized the psychosocial aspects of voice disorder. This has been further underlined in a recent study (Smith et al., 1996) that explored the quality of life experienced by clients with voice disorders of many different aetiologies. The findings show that clients with voice disorder reported significantly more adverse quality of life effects than a matched, healthy control group. A larger proportion of the group with voice disorders also reported psychological problems, including depression and reduced professional self-esteem. Physical discomfort and phonatory effort were also identified as problems among the client group.

Social and psychosocial issues in voice disorder

The information from both physiological and psychological studies shows that we need to revise our concepts about the psychology of voice disorder (Butcher, 1995; Ritchie, 1996; Smith et al., 1996; Rosen and Sataloff, 1997b). We also need to obtain more information about the processes that influence the onset of voice disorder (Enderby and Emerson, 1995). It is generally accepted, for example, that few lay people understand how voice is produced. There is also evidence that there may be a fairly long delay between the onset of the symptoms and the presentation for voice evaluation, for some of our potential clients. According to Smith et al. (1996), for example, many patients reported that they had had their voice disorder for two years before attending voice therapy, although some reported up to twelve years' experience of vocal symptoms. The patients with vocal nodules studied by Goldman et al. (1996) reported vocal symptoms of between 9 weeks and 9 years duration; eight out of the 27 patients had previously received voice therapy.

There may be many different reasons for this, but one startling fact is reported by Schalen et al. (1992), who found that 16 out of 34 consecutive patients with non-organic voice disorders had received antibiotics on 1–7 different occasions, while others had undergone testing for allergy or had been diagnosed as asthmatic, prior to referral to the ENT clinic. It seems probable that the process of medical diagnosis may be an influential factor in some voice disorders. Occupational use of voice may be an influential variable (Koufman and Blalock, 1991).

Another issue which has been raised by many clinicians is that women make up a sizeable proportion of all referrals with so-called functional voice disorder (House and Andrews, 1987; Butcher et al., 1993; Wilson et al., 1995; Smith et al; 1996; White et al., 1997) and other non-organic conditions such as nodules, polyps and Reinke's oedema (Colton and Casper, 1996). Because it is recognized that women tend to seek medical consultations more frequently than men (Jones, 1994) and are more frequently diagnosed with mental health problems (Gravell and France, 1991), it has been assumed that women's voice problems reflect a general susceptibility to psychological difficulties (Butcher, 1995). We have noted above that women's social roles and responses have been considered to play their part (House and Andrews, 1988; Butcher, 1995), but it has also been suggested that hormonal variations (Butcher, 1995; Sataloff et al., 1997a) and other biophysiological differences may be influential (Sodersten and Lindestadt, 1987).

Concepts from health psychology

Health psychology has evolved from the need to develop an integrated understanding of the ways that medical, social and psychological factors combine to influence health and illness (Engel, 1977; Ogden, 1996). The emphasis is on drawing together information from research on stress, emotions, beliefs, learning and social psychology into a cohesive framework. Health psychologists aim to explain changes in health from a psychological perspective and, in turn, to promote better understanding of the psychological issues involved in health care (Ogden, 1996). Many of the issues raised in voice diagnosis and therapy have been explored by health psychologists (Butcher, 1995; Ritchie, 1996; Rosen and Sataloff, 1997). The following section summarizes some of the most obvious examples.

Stress

References to stress in the voice literature are often based on the 'fight or flight response' (Cannon, 1932), which described the rapid physiological changes, such as increases in blood flow, respiratory rate and muscle tone, which enable the individual to respond to an acutely demanding situation. The flight and fight reaction provides a useful explanation of immediate, short-term reactions to an emergency, but it does not fully explain how longer term, habituated musculoskeletal tension develops.

Selye (1956) proposed a model (the General Adaptation Syndrome), to explain the long-term effects of stress. *The alarm phase* is similar to the fight and flight response. If the demand continues, the individual responds by *adaptation*, when the physiological responses tend to be less extreme. In the final phase, *exhaustion*, the individual begins to show physical reactions (Ogden, 1996; Rosen and Sataloff, 1997b).

Life events theory and ongoing stress

Selye's model prompted much of the work about the relationship between stressors such as life events, including bereavements, divorce or changes of work or home life and the onset of illness (Holmes and Rahe, 1967). This led to recognition that some stressors are insidious, rather than specific. Chronic demands such as overwork, professional, family or personal worries can lead to stress responses such as anxiety and depression or physical symptoms (Moos and Swindle, 1990). Once the stress response has been triggered, the situation tends to become self-perpetuating, as the physiological responses and psychological effects interact (White and Moorey, 1997). These descriptions are very similar to the processes identified in some of the work with voice disordered clients (House and Andrews, 1988; Butcher et al., 1993; Morrison and Rammage, 1994; House and Andrews, 1997).

Coping styles in response to stress

People can react very differently to similar experiences. While one person may perceive a situation as a threat, for example, another person may perceive the same situation as a challenge. Lazarus (1975) suggested that our appraisal of the situation is influenced by our previous experiences and coping styles. Some typical coping strategies are direct action, seeking more information, doing nothing or developing alternative ways of coping with the stress by, for example, relaxation or invoking defence mechanisms (Ogden, 1996). If we already have an effective coping strategy, we show less physiological arousal; when we perceive a situation as new or threatening, the impact is far greater (Wiedenfeld et al., 1990). Three different types of changes can be evoked as a stress response. These include sympathetic arousal, including increases in the release of stress hormones; increases in heart rate, blood pressure and muscle potential (the fight or flight response) and changes in psychological factors such as increases in fear and anxiety and/or reduction in cognitive ability and sensitivity towards others (Ogden, 1996).

We need to keep in mind that situations that seem stressful to us may not have been perceived as stressful by the individual concerned. For example, some people may cope successfully with demands because they can draw on previous experience, whereas others might respond to a similar situation by repressing their feelings. Ogden (1996) also points out that patients' recall of events may be coloured by their current experiences. If someone believes that there is stigma attached to being unable to cope with stress, they may be unable to consider this as part of their problem. Others, however, may have recognized that their lifestyles have influenced the onset of their symptoms and are keen to make some changes.

Coping styles, coping strategies and personality in voice disorder

The concept of coping styles and strategies can help us to think about the variables that influence the onset of voice disorder, and also about clients' responses to therapy. In their exploration of the coping styles and personality traits of people with vocal nodules and vocal polyps, McHugh-Munier et al. (1997) identified patterns of thinking that are very similar to factors reported by others (Butcher et al., 1987; House and Andrews, 1988; Roy et al., 1997). These included the need to respond to others, internalization of responsibility and introspection. Like Butcher and his colleagues, McHugh-Munier et al. (1997) identify two different patterns of coping strategies. McHugh-Munier and colleagues identify these as 'emotional coping strategies' and 'cognitive coping strategies', while Butcher and Elias (1995) have suggested that some clients use repression as a coping mechanism, whereas other use suppression: 'in other words, these individuals consciously inhibit expressing their feelings' (Butcher and Cavalli, 1998, pp. 62–3). Baker (1997) has also described two different patterns of responses in voice-disordered clients.

Butcher and Cavalli (1998) have suggested that these different types of coping strategy can influence our clients' ability to respond to therapy. Because people who cope by suppression use more cognitive processes of repression, their problems are 'nearer the surface' and are therefore more easily accessible to patient and therapist. By contrast, the very small proportion of our clients who cope by emotional repression and denial tend to be more locked in by their problems. It is this group who fit the criteria for conversion disorder (Butcher, 1995; Baker, 1997). In her account of a psychotherapeutic approach, Baker reports on two clients who were unable to respond to voice therapy alone. She describes the lengthy and difficult process of psychotherapy with these clients as like peeling the layers of an onion. Each layer has to be peeled off slowly 'with many weeks, or even months of pungent odours and weeping eyes before reaching the true centre' (Baker, 1997, p. 528).

Beliefs and cognitions about health and illness

Health psychologists suggest that the process of seeking and responding to medical advice can be strongly influenced by 'a patient's own implicit common sense beliefs about their illness' or 'illness cognitions' (Leventhal et al., 1985, cited by Ogden, 1996, p. 38). These are the beliefs and knowledge which help us to recognize symptoms and decide on the appropriate 'illness action', such as taking a tablet, staying in bed or consulting the doctor. The consultation option is more likely to happen if the symptoms are severe or unfamiliar or if they do not follow the predicted time course.

Other factors can influence the decision to seek a medical consultation. Some people avoid going to the doctor because they believe their symptoms are insignificant or 'not real' health problems (Ogden, 1996). This may change if the individual learns new information which raises anxieties about the cause, or if others begin to comment on the problem (Ogden, 1996). In some cases, people can apparently tolerate certain types of symptoms until other factors, such as increased stress, reduce their ability to cope (Cooper et al., 1988).

Health and illness beliefs also influence the way people respond to medical advice and information. This includes beliefs about how much control and responsibility we have over our health and our susceptibility to illness. People who believe that their actions and behaviours influence their health are described as having an internal health locus of control. By contrast, someone with an external locus of control may attribute their problems to fate or chance and therefore be unable to accept that their actions may be influential (Wallston and Wallston, 1982).

Implications for diagnosis and therapy

By the time clients reach voice therapy, it is highly probable that they will have had a range of thoughts and feelings because of the voice disorder. Once people realize that a problem exists, they also formulate theories about the cause (Ogden, 1996). Most clients report they have had fears about the possibility of cancer or other serious illness, many have also considered that the problem may be a stress response (or 'psycho-logical'). The process of medical diagnosis, including being referred to a specialist clinic, can also raise anxieties. Throughout this time, clients will also be experiencing the frustrations of attempting to carry out their everyday lives with a problem which is apparent in every communicative act. Clearly, there are many different psychological and psychosocial factors which can undermine our clients' coping skills (Andrews, 1995; Smith et al., 1996).

The diagnostic interview

There are some excellent descriptions of voice history interviews in the voice therapy literature (Aronson, 1990; Butcher et al., 1993; Colton and Casper, 1996; Harris, 1998), each of which emphasizes slightly different perspectives. The following sections focus on some of the psychological factors, in particular.

All clinicians emphasize the importance of listening skills during the diagnostic interview. Listening serves two key functions. First, clients tend to value and respond more readily to an empathic listener who shows interest in their views and who is willing to provide information (Ley, 1989). Secondly, the clinician can gain valuable information about the client's health beliefs, their attributions about the cause and their attitude to the referral to voice therapy.

Clients can arrive for voice evaluation and therapy with very different expectations, attitudes and health/illness cognitions. They also tend to have questions about the laryngologist's diagnosis. As Brodnitz (1965) has observed, the busy ENT clinic is not an appropriate setting for a detailed exploration of causes. This means that the voice history interview may be the first opportunity for the client to discuss his or her voice problem in detail, with an informed person.

Many clients find that the chance to simply recount the story of how the voice problem has developed, to an empathic and informed listener, is therapeutic. In the same way, the information we can provide, either explicitly or implicitly through our questions, can be enabling. Some clients engage in the process of exploring their behaviour and related causes with enthusiasm, because it provides them with the explanation of how the problem developed. These clients seem to fit the profile of people with an internal locus of control (Wallston and Wallston, 1982).We could hypothesize that the diagnostic interview may enable these clients to change their illness cognitions about the voice disorder. When the action plan fits with the client's health beliefs, the chances are that they have a good prognosis.

Other clients may have a different type of agenda. Harris et al., (1998) points out, for example, that clients who had fears about the cause of the voice problem may have gained the reassurance they needed from the laryngologist's diagnosis. They may come to the voice therapy interview to comply with the laryngologist's recommendations, rather than because they want voice therapy. For these clients, it may be appropriate to simply provide written advice on vocal hygiene and information about how to seek re-referral.

Andrews and Summers (1991) suggest that people enter therapy at different levels of readiness. Some may 'test' the voice clinician to make sure that we can be trusted and have the ability to help before they disclose personal information. Others may have had strong convictions that the voice problem was the result of illness and were expecting that the doctor would provide a cure, such as medication (Colton and Casper, 1996). This means that we need to explain what therapy will involve and provide information to help the client to understand the symptoms and, perhaps, reformulate his or her cognitions. Again, however, people vary in their response. People with an external locus of control (Wallston and Wallston, 1982) may have great difficulty in accepting the responsibility for change. One example cited by Colton and Casper (1996) is clients who continue to smoke despite medical advice. If this is a key concern, it may be more appropriate to recommend that the client attends a smoking cessation clinic (DiClemente et al., 1991) rather than voice therapy.

Stress

Clients also vary in the way they are able to review stress factors in their lives. Even the slightest hint of associations between the voice problem and stress can be threatening to some people, who may initially react with a firm denial. This may be particularly true if the laryngologist's well-intentioned reassurance that 'there's nothing wrong physically' is interpreted by the client as 'it's all in the mind' (White and Moorey, 1997). Other clients may believe that to admit one is unable to cope is a sign of personal weakness, while a small minority may still be coping with their problems through denial and repression (Baker, 1997; Butcher and Cavalli, 1998).

Musculoskeletal tension

We need to consider these different perceptions and definitions of stress in relation to musculoskeletal tension, which is one of the most consistent presenting features of voice disorder. This tension has been attributed to different processes by clinicians. As we have seen, Aronson (1990) considers that musculoskeletal tension is predominantly a response to emotional reactions such as anxiety or other responses to stress (see also Butcher et al., 1993; Nichol et al., 1993; Stemple, 1993). Others have suggested that musculoskeletal tension can result from attempts to compensate for, or control, the changes in the voice (Boone and McFarlane, 1994). Morrison and Rammage (1994) also point out that some people simply have poor habitual posture, which reduces vocal efficiency.

Therapists need to take a pragmatic approach, especially if the reduction of the tension is a primary goal of therapy. The client who believes that this tension is the *result* of the voice problem, rather than the *cause*, may reject explanations which emphasize the stress–tension relationship and could perceive that the clinician is presenting an implicit challenge to his or her beliefs. For these clients, the introduction of relaxation techniques may be more acceptable if the emphasis is placed on reduction of mechanical strain, rather than stress: for example, 'stiff muscles' or 'putting in too much effort'. Often, as clients gain benefits from relaxation, they may be more able to reconsider the wider implications of stress in their lives and may spontaneously raise the topic again.

Personal and psychosocial factors

Most of our adult clients consider themselves relatively fit and well, apart from their voice disorder. Although they may be classed as patients and attend for treatment, clients also continue with their usual everyday activities. Finding time for voice therapy may be an additional stressor for some people; others may find the voice therapy makes them feel self-conscious and uncomfortable. The voice therapy interview itself raises new issues and focuses on aspects of behaviour, such as personal habits and communication style, which are not usually discussed with strangers. It can be useful to offer the opportunity to discuss these issues, including how the client will cope with the extra demands of therapy, as part of the first interview.

Sifting the information

By the end of the first interview in particular, clinicians can be left with feelings of uncertainty about the client's 'personality' or 'psychological' issues. This can be because we have raised issues that the client had not considered before, so he or she has difficulty in responding. In some instances, a client may be unwilling to disclose personal information or feelings to a new person, in a new and uncertain situation (Andrews and Summers, 1991). Typically, however, the information gained from the case history and evaluation of vocal function enables the clinician to explain the vocal symptoms to the client and to propose a course of action.

There are strong positive benefits from proposing an initial, short-term programme of therapy. This enables both clinician and client to identify some immediate objectives, which they can review together after two or three sessions. Mutual agreement about the times and dates of appointments and an action plan can enable the client to feel a sense of control and focus. It also gives the clinician more time to obtain a clearer picture of the client's needs and to consider whether voice therapy is the most appropriate form of intervention.

Reflection and supervision

As clinicians, we also should take time to reflect on the information gained during the interview. Action such as writing the case notes and reporting back to the referral source is part of this process. Clinical supervision or case discussion with more experienced peers or colleagues in related disciplines can also help us to clarify our thoughts and responses to our clients (Baker, 1997; Syder, 1998). This may be part of the routine activity of the Voice Clinic team (Morrison and Rammage, 1994; Harris et al., 1998), as a result of interdisciplinary collaboration (Butcher et al., 1993) or with another professional, as part of one's own professional development (Syder, 1998). However it is organized, many experienced clinicians value the opportunity to reflect upon and evaluate the dynamics of the client–clinician relationship.

In many cases, the client engages in active reflection as well. As the therapeutic relationship develops, clients often return to issues which were raised in the initial interview, and which they have reconsidered in some way.

The aphonic client

Aphonia in the absence of laryngeal pathology is a relatively rare problem, with an incidence of less than 5% in the average caseload (House and Andrews, 1987, Butcher, 1995). As we have seen, although it has traditionally been described as a conversion disorder, few aphonic clients fit the psychological criteria for this condition (House and Andrews, 1987; Kinzl et al., 1988). Because it is still often perceived as a psychological problem by many people, however, this can cause problems for the client, who may feel trapped by the symptoms and feel the problem is not being taken seriously. We need to remember that, whatever the cause of the symptoms, the psychosocial consequences of voice loss can be quite devastating (Ritchie, 1996).

The physical concomitants of aphonia are well described. Typically, there is visible tension, with a tendency for jaw-jutting, tightness or near immobility of the mandible, a retracted tongue and palpable supra-hyoid muscles. Changes in breathing patterns, with a tendency for breath-holding in speech contexts may also be present (Morrison and Rammage, 1994). There are also several useful descriptions of the therapy techniques which are successful for regaining the voice. Some clinicians suggest direct laryngeal manipulation, such as depression of the thyroid cartilage (Greene and Mathieson, 1989) or massage of the laryngeal structures (Aronson, 1990). Boone and McFarlane (1994) also report success with facilitating techniques such as inspiration phonation or yawn-sigh. All descriptions emphasize that the clinician should be reassuring but persistent. The primary aims are to release the laryngeal tension, to elicit laryngeal sound of any sort, and then to keep experimenting. Once sound is produced, full voice is regained quite rapidly in many cases (Greene and Mathieson, 1989; Baker, 1997).

The processes which produce aphonia are less clearly understood. There are reports of some cases of intermittent aphonia triggered by allergic reactions (Freeman et al., 1987; Tsunoda et al., 1998). Clinicians have also reported associations with upper respiratory infections or viral agents (Boone and McFarlane, 1994). Other aphonias may reflect a pre-existing muscle misuse which is compounded by tension, attempts to compensate and other known or unknown factors (Kinzl et al., 1988; Boone and McFarlane, 1994).

Baker (1997, p. 528) has reported that clients often respond to return of voice with a 'cathartic emotional response' and the need to discuss the frustrations and difficulties associated with the whole experience of being aphonic. Some clients describe a sense of being hopelessly trapped by symptoms which felt (and were, physically!) real, but were not taken seriously by others. Most clients need time and support as they try to work through these and related issues, which may include questions about how and why the problem was reversed so quickly. There is also a need for some ongoing therapy, to ensure that the client can maintain the voice.

The client with intermittent aphonia or dysphonia

Clients whose voice problems are mild or intermittent can cause the therapist to feel a sense of uncertainty about the nature of the problem. Kotby (1995) suggests that these symptoms can be early indicators of vocal misuse, sometimes described as phonaesthesia (Verdolini et al., 1998). The voice evaluation can show that the client has an inefficient vocal pattern, despite the apparent lack of signs of laryngeal change. There are indications in the literature that a substantial proportion of these clients may have a recurrence of the symptoms, even after a course of voice therapy. Although this has been attributed to psychogenic factors, an alternative explanation may be that they needed a different approach, aimed at optimizing their vocal efficiency. The vocal function exercises described by Sabol et al. (1993) and Verdolini-Marston et al. (1995) are reported to be very effective for phonaesthesia.

Clients who are unable to respond to voice therapy

Lack of response to therapy can take many different forms. Some clients, for example, may be unable to change the established patterns of behaviour in their daily lives, despite their apparent motivation for therapy (Colton and Casper, 1996). Some of the strategies used in cognitive-behavioural therapy can help clients to think about their responses (Butcher et al.,1993). As an example, clients may find it useful to list the potential positive and negative consequences of behaviour change and then identify goals which can be translated into action. This may, of course, include the decision to leave therapy, but it may also enable the client to redefine personal goals and identify how to reach them.

Learning styles

With some clients, poor response within the therapy session may be related to teaching and learning styles. The processes involved in acquiring and then transferring new voicing patterns into everyday speech are not simple and may not come easily to some clients. This is an aspect of our therapy which needs more attention (Verdolini-Marston et al., 1995). Another issue is that voice therapy may be the client's first experience of one-to-one learning; this can be stressful, especially when the learning requires the heightened self-awareness, self-monitoring and sometimes, relatively subtle changes in vocal behaviour which may be required in voice therapy.

Clients may also vary in their learning strategies. Voice therapy has traditionally emphasized auditory feedback for self-monitoring, for example, but this can be a problem for some clients. Filter (1980) suggested that therapy should focus on stronger use of proprioceptive, tactile and kinaesthetic awareness for posture, relaxation and awareness of laryngeal control. Clients who have difficulty with auditory monitoring of voice can sometimes benefit from the visual feedback from computer programs such as Visipitch, SpeechViewer or the electroglottograph (Carlson, 1993). Different approaches to therapy, such as the Accent

Method, may be more appropriate for the needs of some voice disordered clients (Kotby, 1995). Another alternative is to change the routine to intensive daily therapy, which has been shown to benefit clients with non-organic disorders (MacIntyre, 1980) and other conditions, most notably those associated Parkinson's disease (Ramig, Chapter 9, this volume).

The client with ongoing problems

Outcome studies indicate that most clients who receive a combination of information, focused therapy and empathic support will benefit from voice therapy (Carding and Horsley, 1992; Ramig and Verdolini, 1998). As we have seen, however, there is a fairly small proportion of clients who may be unable to respond to voice therapy alone, because of pre-existing or current problems such as depression, anxiety or other stress responses (Butcher, 1995; Baker, 1997). Some clients feel able to disclose their problems during therapy, as their relationship with the voice therapist develops. Others may be unable to respond to voice therapy and may need help to come to terms with the need for further support or treatment. Many voice therapists now respond to these problems by working in close collaboration with psychologists or psychotherapists, either in conjoint therapy or with a period of psychologically based therapy followed by voice therapy. Butcher et al. (1993), Baker (1997) and Butcher and Cavalli (1998) provide detailed descriptions of different therapeutic approaches in their case studies of clients with ongoing psychological problems.

Conclusion

At the start of the 1980s, some clinicians expressed concerns that the increasing focus on the science of voice disorder might lead to reduced emphasis on the psychology of voice. As the information reviewed in this chapter shows, there is still a strong interest in the psychological aspects of voice disorder. We have seen, however, that the emphasis is shifting away from a predominantly psychodynamic model of causality and towards a broader framework, which considers how psychological and other factors interact in each person's unique set of circumstances. Although there is still clearly a need for more information about the voice–psychology relationship, the current approaches from health psychology can help us to understand and respond to the many psychological issues raised in our work with people who have voice disorders.

CHAPTER 9

Voice problems of speakers with dysarthria

LORRAINE OLSON RAMIG

Introduction

Voice disorders accompanying damage or disease to the nervous system are called neurological voice disorders. A significant number of neurological disorders such as myasthenia gravis, Parkinson's disease, essential tremor, dystonia and multiple sclerosis are accompanied by disordered voice (Aronson, 1980). However, except for the more common problem of laryngeal nerve paralysis and the unusual, but disabling, entity of spasmodic dysphonia (laryngeal dystonia), neurologically based voice disorders until recently have been a neglected topic for both basic and clinical research in the fields of speech pathology, otolaryngology and neurology (Smith and Ramig, 1995). This chapter will provide a background and a framework for the study of neurological voice disorders, as well as clinical assessment and treatment suggestions for select neurological voice disorders from the perspective of speech pathology (Ramig et al., 1995a,b).

Background on voice problems in speakers with dysarthria

Because neurological voice disorders reflect a wide range of characteristics and aetiologies, a number of classification systems have been proposed to assist in their description, diagnosis and treatment planning. Historically, neurological voice disorders were viewed in the context of dysarthria or motor speech disorders. Aronson (1980) labelled them 'dysarthrophonias' and referred to them in relation to the classic dysarthria classification system of flaccid, spastic, ataxic, hypokinetic, hyperkinetic and mixed dysarthrias (Darley et al., 1969a,b). Ward et al.

(1981) proposed a similar framework for neurological voice disorders which included the efferent motor subcategories of upper motor neuron (cortex and pyramidal tracts), extrapyramidal (reticular substance), cerebellar and nuclear (lower motor neuron). Aronson (1980) proposed an additional classification system based upon the constancy or variability of the acoustic symptoms accompanying the neurological voice disorders. He proposed the following categories: relatively constant (flaccid, spastic (pseudobulbar), mixed flaccid-spastic and hypokinetic), arrhythmically fluctuating (ataxic, choreic, dystonic), rhythmically fluctuating (palatopharyngolaryngeal myoclonus and organic essential tremor), paroxysmal (Gilles de la Tourette's syndrome) and loss of volitional phonation (apraxia, akinetic mutism and dysprosody of pseudo-foreign dialect). These approaches are based upon an association between the voice disorder and the corresponding site of neurological damage and have made important contributions to the description and diagnosis of neurological voice disorders.

New developments in voice problems in speakers with dysarthria: diagnostic and treatment implications

More recently, Ramig and Scherer (1992) proposed a system for considering neurological voice disorders with specific application to *treatment*. Rather than relating the neurological disorder to the site of neural damage and aetiology, this classification system focused on the existing laryngeal physical pathology and resulting voice characteristics. They proposed a number of categories of neural laryngeal physical pathologies including: glottal closure problems (hypoadduction and hyperadduction) and vibratory stability problems (short-term, e.g. hoarseness and long-term, e.g. tremor). Ramig and Scherer (1992) used these categories to organize approaches to treatment of neurological voice disorders which focused on modification of laryngeal physical condition with corresponding changes in perceptual characteristics of voice. This classification system has been further developed (Ramig et al., 1995b; Smith and Ramig, 1995).

The work of Ramig and Scherer (1992), Smith and Ramig (1995) and Ramig et al. (1995a), has highlighted the role of voice as an initial and significant treatment target for individuals with dysarthria. In addition to disordered voice, individuals with dysarthria typically have articulation and rate problems. While these articulation and rate problems are frequently the focus of speech treatment, Ramig and colleagues suggest that initiating treatment with the focus on *phonation* may offer a single motor organizing theme that maximally impacts other aspects of speech production (Froeschels, 1952; Berry, 1983; Rosenbek and LaPointe, 1985; Yorkston et al., 1988; Duffy, 1995; Ramig et al., 1995). This *'phonation first'* focus was the basis for the development of the Lee Silverman Voice Treatment (LSVT(CM)) which has had extensive application and positive outcomes for the treatment of dysarthria in individuals with Parkinson's disease (Ramig et al., 1995a,b). Clinically and statistically significant improvements in articulation and reductions in rate together with increases in vocal loudness and improvements in voice quality have been reported in individuals with Parkinson's disease following the LSVT(CM) (Dromey et al., 1995; Ramig et al., 1995b).

Voice problems in speakers with dysarthria: description and diagnosis

Dysarthria may accompany various neurological disorders and diseases. It is important for the speech pathologist to have basic knowledge regarding significant aspects of these disorders, such as aetiology/pathogenesis, incidence/demographics as well as medical diagnostic and treatment information. Various neurology texts are available, including those that were helpful in preparing this review (Yahr and Bergman, 1986; Rowland, 1991; Asbury et al., 1992; Weiner and Lang, 1995; Fahn et al., 1998; Paty and Ebers, 1998).

Aetiology/pathogenesis

The aetiologies of neurological voice disorders are varied. Any damage or disease of the components of the peripheral or central nervous system which control laryngeal function can affect voice production. Most common aetiologies of neurological voice disorders include trauma, cerebral vascular accidents, tumours, and diseases of the nervous system.

Flaccid voice disorders involve damage or disease to one or more components of the motor unit (nucleus ambiguus, vagus nerve, myoneural junctions or laryngeal muscles). Viral infections, tumours, strokes, trauma or degeneration of the cell bodies in the nucleus ambiguus or a wound to the recurrent laryngeal nerve branch of the vagus (cranial nerve X) could result in laryngeal muscle paralysis. Myasthenia gravis is caused by autoimmune mechanisms that reduce available acetylcholine receptors at the neuromuscular junction and reduce laryngeal neuromuscular transmission. Muscular dystrophies or myopathies such as myotonic dystrophy, an autosomal dominant disorder with variable expression, may cause atrophy of laryngeal muscle fibres. Flaccid neural laryngeal disorders may also result from laryngeal nerve involvement.

Spastic (pseudobulbar) voice disorders are associated with bilateral upper motor neuron damage. Such damage may occur with multiple, bilateral cerebral vascular accidents, any lesion of the corticobulbar tracts bilaterally and vascular and degenerative diseases involving motor cortical areas bilaterally. In addition, vascular diseases and tumours of the internal capsule or brainstem, degenerative diseases involving the entire cortico-bulbar tract system, infectious diseases and the congenital disorder of spastic cerebral palsy may be aetiologies for spastic neural laryngeal disorders. Consequent release of inhibition of excitatory nerve impulses to vagal nuclei (Aronson, 1985b) may result in hyperadduction of the true and false vocal folds observed in these disorders. It is important to distinguish spastic neural laryngeal voice disorders resulting from bilateral upper motor neuron damage from adductor spasmodic dysphonia associated with the hyperkinetic disorder laryngeal dystonia.

Ataxic voice disorders may occur following cerebellar damage resulting from strokes, traumas, toxins, tumours or diseases such as Friedreich's ataxia.

Hypokinetic voice disorders have been most commonly related to the degenerative neurological disorder idiopathic Parkinson's disease. The aetiology of this basal ganglia disease is unknown, however it has been associated with both genetic and environmental factors. In Parkinson's disease, degenerative changes in the substantia nigra result in depletion of the neurotransmitter dopamine. Parkinsonism is an umbrella term for other disorders that have some of the characteristics of idiopathic Parkinson disease but may be the result of a virus, head-trauma, carbon monoxide poisoning, toxic build-up or the historic influenza epidemic (Darley et al., 1975). These disorders include the multi-system disorders of postencephalitic parkinsonism, progressive supranuclear palsy and Shy-Drager syndrome.

Hyperkinetic voice disorders are generally associated with diseases of the basal ganglia and include a range of diseases such as Huntington's disease, organic essential tremor, orofacial dyskinesia, dystonia, athetosis, palatopharyngolaryngeal myoclonus and Gilles de la Tourette's syndrome. The abnormal 'choreiform' movements accompanying the autosomal dominant disease of Huntington's disease are associated with loss of neurons in the caudate nucleus. Vocal tremor accompanies a number of neurological diseases including organic essential tremor, and has been associated with both a central and peripheral mechanism. Lesions in the caudate nucleus, putamen, cerebellum, dentate nucleus and oscillations occurring in the olivocerebellorubral loop system have been suggested as the cause of essential tremor. Sustained muscle contractions that may cause twisting or repetitive movements or abnormal postures characterize the basal ganglia disorder of dystonia which has a laryngeal manifestation in spasmodic dysphonia. Primary dystonias may be inherited (usually autosomal dominant) or sporadic. Secondary dystonias may be observed with other neurological disorders, environmental (e.g. drug induced, tardive dystonia), or psychogenic.

Mixed voice disorders occur from damage or disease to multiple neural subsystems. For example, both lower motor neurons and bilateral upper motor neurons may be affected in amyotrophic lateral sclerosis (ALS) which is considered a flaccid and spastic dysarthria. The aetiology of ALS is unknown; theories include viral infection and environmental factors. Demyelinization of both upper motor and cerebellar neurons occurs in multiple sclerosis (MS) which is considered a spastic and ataxic dysarthria. Aetiologies of MS include an environmental agent (e.g. unspecified viral infection) in a genetically susceptible population.

Incidence and Prevalence information

The incidence of neurological voice disorders varies according to the incidence of the neurological disorder or disease it accompanies. Not every individual with a neurological disorder will have a voice disorder; however, in some cases, voice disorders may be the first sign of a neurological disease.

For example, myasthenia gravis has a prevalence of 2–10 per 100,000 persons (Newsome-Davis, 1992) and at least 15% of these patients have a speech or voice disorder (Grob et al., 1981). There are twice as many females as males who have myasthenia gravis. Myotonic muscular dystrophy has a prevalence of 3–5 cases per 100,000 persons (Barchi and Furman, 1992) and speech and voice disorders are reported to occur commonly.

There are 500,000 new stroke cases per year; the frequency of co-occurring voice disorders has not been reported.

Ataxic involvement can result from neoplasms, trauma, infarct and neural degeneration. It has been reported that the prevalence of Friedreich's ataxia is 1 and 2 per 100,000 (Harding, 1983, 1984) with 63–93% of these patients having dysarthria (Heck, 1964; Joanette and Dudley, 1980).

The prevalence of Parkinson's disease is 1000 in 100,000 over age 60 and 100 in 100,000 under age 60. It has been reported that one and one half million Americans have idiopathic Parkinson's disease with 89% of these individuals having a voice disorder (Logemann et al., 1978).

The autosomal dominant disorder of Huntington's disease affects 4 to 8 per 100,000 individuals, with voice and speech disorders reported to occur frequently. The neurologic symptom of tremor occurs in a number of neurological disorders such as Parkinson's disease, cerebellar disorders and essential tremor. The neurological disorder of essential tremor is the most prevalent, occurring in 414.6 per 100,000 individuals and affecting 5 million people (Haerer et al., 1982; Hubble et al., 1989). Vocal tremor occurs in 11–30% of essential tremor patients (Findley and Gresty, 1988; Elble and Koller, 1990; Koller et al., 1994) and may be the first or only sign of the disorder. Dystonia has been reported to affect approximately 250,000 people with laryngeal involvement observed in 22% of 2,556 cases of dystonia (Blitzer and Brin, 1992; Brin et al., 1992).

The mixed dysarthria of ALS has an incidence of between 0.4 and 1.8 per 100,000 population. Its peak incidence is at the fifth to seventh decade of life. The male-to-female ratio is 1.5 to 1.0. Brain stem or bulbar involvement occurs in 30% of cases (Carpenter et al., 1979) and progresses more rapidly than spinal involvement. It has been reported that 28% of patients with ALS presented with symptoms in the head, neck, larynx or voice (Bonduelle, 1975; Carpenter et al., 1979; Dworkin and Hartman, 1979; Mulder, 1980; Tandan and Bradley, 1985). In the northern part of the United States, the prevalence of the mixed dysarthria of MS is 100 in 100,000. Below the 37th parallel, the prevalence is 35.5 in 100,000 and above the 37th parallel, the prevalence is 68.8 in 100,000. Approximately 40% of patients with MS have disordered speech and/or voice with the ratio of females to males being 1.5 to 1 (Darley et al., 1972).

Medical considerations: diagnosis and findings

Certain classic medical symptoms contribute to the diagnosis of the neurological disorder and consequently the accompanying voice disorder. It is important for the speech-language pathologist to be aware of general symptoms of neurological conditions.

For example, in myasthenia gravis, the common initial symptom is in the extraocular muscles. Other classic symptoms of myasthenia gravis include fatigability, fluctuation and restoration of function after rest. In myotonic muscular dystrophy the classic symptom of clinical myotonia is seen as the delayed relaxation of skeletal muscle after voluntary contraction.

In Friedreich's ataxia, the most frequent first symptom is ataxia of gait. Diagnostic criteria include progressive gait and limb ataxia. Hypotonia and incoordination of muscles may also be observed in ataxia.

In Parkinson's disease, the physical pathologies of rigidity, tremor, reduced range of movement and slowness of movement are observed together with the classic symptoms of mask-like face and micrographia. Diagnosis is made when two of these primary symptoms are observed, plus a positive response to the neuropharmacological treatment of L-dopa.

Abnormal involuntary movements characterize the hyperkinetic movement disorders. In Huntington's disease, the choreiform movements (abrupt, jerky, purposeless) and progressive mental deterioration (loss of memory and intellectual capacity) are classic symptoms. Tremor has been observed in varied neurological disorders as well as in normal individuals under stress. The tremor accompanying the disease essential tremor may appear at rest and is finer and less rhythmic than Parkinson tremor. It may occur first in the hand and progress to the face, arms, neck, face. It can be accentuated by voluntary movement of the extremities or by emotional or physical stress. The twisting or repetitive sustained muscle contractions accompanying dystonias may be focal (isolated to a small group of muscles in one body part), segmental (contiguous muscle groups) or generalized (widespread muscle involvement). Spasmodic dysphonia is considered in most cases as a focal primary, function-specific, action-induced laryngeal dystonia.

The initial manifestations of ALS include muscle weakness, cramps, fasciculations (Carpenter et al., 1979). Classic signs of MS are varied; optic neuritis and sensory or motor disturbance of the limbs may be common presentations. Approximately two-thirds of the patients have exacerbation and remission of symptoms and in the other third, the symptoms are progressive.

The voice evaluation: diagnosis and findings

Unlike many other voice disorders, neurological voice disorders may exist in the company of disorders of the speech subsystems of respiration, articulation and resonance. In addition, swallowing problems are common in these neurological disorders. Furthermore, patients may compensate laryngeally for disorders in another part of the speech mechanism. These co-occurring speech mechanism disorders must be considered in the assessment of the voice. The cognitive (Mayeux et al., 1986; Bamford et al., 1989; Rao, 1990), emotional (Darley et al., 1969a; Mayeux et al., 1986) or sensory changes (Lidsky et al., 1985; Hallet, 1995) accompanying the neurological disorder are important considerations in assessment as well as in planning treatment. In some cases, voice disorders have been reported as the earliest symptom of a neurological disorder and this should be considered in assessment as well.

Voice characteristics: perceptual findings

The primary perceptual descriptions of neurological voice disorders come from the work of Darley et al. (1969a,b; 1975) and Aronson et al. (1968b). Myasthenia gravis has been characterized perceptually by inhalatory stridor, breathy voice, hoarse, flutter or tremor. Loudness is reduced and there is a restriction of pitch range (Aronson, 1990). There is progressively increased dysphonia including breathiness and reduced loudness while speaking (Walton, 1977). Mild breathy dysphonia and hypernasality have been reported (Wolski, 1967; Aronson, 1971; Neiman et al., 1975). Myotonic muscular dystrophy is characterized by weak, hoarse and nasal voices (Ramig et al., 1988).

Spastic (pseudobulbar palsy) voice is characterized by harshness (97%), strained-strangled quality (67%), abnormally low pitch (87%), monopitch (97%), pitch breaks and voice tremor (30%) (Aronson et al., 1968a, b). Nasality, monotone and reduced intensity have also been reported (Aring, 1965). These characteristics occur typically in the presence of accompanying dysarthria.

The voice of the individual with an ataxic disorder is frequently within normal limits. When disordered, it may be characterized by hoarse-harsh voice quality, sudden bursts of loudness, irregular increases in pitch and loudness or coarse voice tremor. The voice also may be monopitch, too low, strain-strangled and have pitch breaks (Darley et al., 1969b) and typically occurs in the presence of accompanying dysarthria (Aronson, 1990). The voice disorder accompanying Friedreich's ataxia has been reported to be harsh, have pitch breaks, prosodic excess and phonatory-prosodic insufficiency (Joanette and Dudley, 1980).

The voice of the individual with Parkinson's disease has been described as reduced in loudness, monopitch, breathy, rough, hoarse and in some cases, tremorous. Reduced volume and breathy voice may be the first sign of Parkinson's disease (Aronson, 1990). Logemann et al. (1978) found that 89% of 200 patients with PD showed laryngeal dysfunction and that 45% had laryngeal dysfunction as the only symptom. They reported the following voice characteristics: breathiness (15%), roughness (29%), hoarseness (45%) and tremulousness (13.5%). These observations are consistent with those of Pawlas and Ramig (in review) who reported the following voice characteristics in addition to reduced loudness in a group of 45 patients with Parkinson's disease: hoarseness (71%), monotone (49%), reduced stress (49%), unnatural prosody (40%), breathiness (40%), vocal fry (36%), mucus crackle (24%) and tremor (20%).

The voice of the individual with Huntington's disease is characterized by irregular pitch fluctuations and voice arrests (Ramig, 1986). Darley et al. (1969) reported sudden forced inspiration or expiration, harsh voice quality, excess loudness variations, strained strangle phonation, monopitch, monoloudness, reduced stress, transient breathiness and voice arrests (Aronson et al., 1968b; Aronson, 1985b) in the voices of individuals with Huntington's disease. The tremorous voice accompanying essential tremor is characterized by 'quavering intonation' (Brown and Simonson, 1963; Aronson, 1990; Colton and Casper, 1990) or rhythmic fluctuations in loudness. The pitch, loudness and regularity of vocal tremor has been reported to vary and there may be arrests of phonation. Laryngeal dystonia or spasmodic dysphonia is characterized by effortful, strain-strangle voice quality with frequent voice breaks as well as interruptions of breathy or whispered segments upon a normal or hoarse voice (Aronson, 1990). The former is considered as adductor spasmodic dysphonia and the latter as abductor spasmodic dysphonia.

The voices of individuals with ALS have been described in a number of studies. Carrow et al. (1974) studied 79 patients with ALS and reported that 80% had harsh voice quality; 65% were breathy, 63% had tremor, 60% were strain strangled; 41% had audible inhalation, 38% had excessively high pitch and 8% had excessively low pitch. Aronson et al. (1968a) reported voices in ALS patients that were harsh (79.75%), strained-strangled (59.5%) with some breathiness (64.5%), reduced loudness, audible inhalation, 'wet hoarseness' and hypernasality (74.7%). Rapid tremor or flutter was reported in 63.3% of the ALS patients studied by Aronson et al. (1992) on vowel prolongation. It was suggested that the specific profile of voice characteristics in ALS (e.g. more flaccid or spastic) depended upon the site of lesion. Darley et al. (1972) studied 168 MS patients and reported that of the 59% that were vocally disordered, their voices were characterized by the following: impaired loudness control (77%), harsh voice (72%), impaired intonation, inappropriate pitch and breathiness. Farmakides and Boone (1960) reported impaired loudness, harshness and hypernasality in individuals with MS.

Voice characteristics: endoscopic findings

Comprehensive endoscopic descriptive data sets do not exist on the majority of neurological voice disorders. Myasthenia gravis or myotonic dystrophy may reveal bilateral weakness of intrinsic laryngeal muscles. Sluggish vocal fold adduction and increasing weakness of arytenoid and vocal fold motion have been suggested in myasthenia gravis (Colton and Casper, 1990). Velopharyngeal inadequacy has been observed frequently in both myasthenia gravis and myotonic dystrophy. Aronson (1980) suggests that the voice disorder accompanying spastic (pseudobulbar) dysarthria is caused by hyperadduction of the true and false vocal folds (i.e. glottal constriction and resistance to exhalatory flow). Aronson (1990) reports that the folds appear normal in structure.

Kitzing (1985) suggested that, when hyperadduction occurs, there would be reduced vocal fold amplitudes, diminished mucosal waves, and excessive glottal closure. Hanson et al. (1984) reported bowing and greater amplitude of vibration and laryngeal asymmetry in individuals with Parkinson's disease. Smith and Ramig (1995) reported that 12 of 21 individuals with Parkinson's disease had a form of glottal incompetence (bowing or anterior or posterior chink) on nasal fibreoptic views. Perez et al. (1996) reported visually-rated laryngeal tremor in 55% of the 29 individuals with Parkinson's disease they studied; the primary site of tremor was vertical laryngeal motion. The most striking stroboscopic findings for these individuals were abnormal phase closure and phase asymmetry. Amplitude and mucosal waveform were essentially within normal limits in the majority of these patients.

Endoscopic descriptions of one individual with Huntington's disease revealed adductory movements at rest and termination of phonation seemingly by adductory laryngospasm (Ramig and Wood, 1983). Endoscopic descriptions of vocal tremor have revealed multiple sites of tremor, including posterior tongue and/or the posterior pharyngeal wall as well as laryngeal structures (Ardran et al., 1966; Ludlow et al., 1986; Koda and Ludlow, 1992; Smith and Ramig, 1995).

Laryngeal endoscopic reports of ALS revealed that, if there is spastic involvement, patients may adduct normally or may hyperadduct with the false folds. If there is flaccid involvement, there is less abductory, adductory excursion (Aronson, 1990). Garfinkel and Kimmelman (1982) reported pooling of saliva.

Voice problems in speakers with dysarthria: treatment options

Course of treatment; options and outcomes

Treatment for neurological voice disorders must be considered in the context of treatment for the overriding neurological disorder. Frequently individuals with neurological voice disorders are receiving neuropharmacological treatment or may have had neurosurgical treatment. Either or both of these treatments may or may not influence their voice.

Surgical

Individuals with a neurological voice disorder may have systemic treatment (e.g. neurosurgical treatment such as pallidotomy for Parkinson's disease or thymectomy for myasthenia gravis) or laryngeal surgical or injection treatment which may directly treat the disordered larynx (thyroplasty for vocal fold paralysis or Botox for laryngeal dystonia).

Various neurosurgical procedures have been used to treat Parkinson's disease: adrenal cell transplant, fetal cell transplant (Freed et al., 1993) and pallidotomy (Iacono et al., 1994) as well as dystonia: pallidotomy (Vitek et al., 1998). Data on corresponding speech and voice changes following these procedures are accumulating. For example, Baker et al. (1997) reported that, while measures of limb movement improved following fetal cell transplant, measures of speech and voice did not show systematic changes.

Thalamectomy has been used for a number of years to successfully reduce limb tremor (Manen et al., 1984). However, reduced vocal volume, velopharyngeal incompetence and swallowing problems have been associated with bilateral thalamectomy (Allan et al., 1966). Recently, Countryman and Ramig (1993) reported pre-, post and follow-up data following an intensive voice treatment programme (Lee Silverman Voice Treatment; LSVT(CM)) administered to an individual with idiopathic Parkinson's disease who had had bilateral thalamotomies. While the patient demonstrated statistically significant improvements following treatment on various measures of phonatory stability, intensity and fundamental frequency variation, in contrast to other individuals with IPD, she was unable to maintain these changes at 6 and 12 month follow-up. While data are variable in terms of the effects of surgical treatment on speech and voice production in Parkinson's disease, it appears that the magnitude and consistency of these effects are not adequate to impact on functional communication.

Pharmacological

Neuropharmacological treatments can be very useful in treating general motor symptoms of the neurological condition.

For example, in myasthenia gravis, positive effects of tensilon/ pyridostigmine (Mestinon) have been documented on symptoms of myasthenia gravis including the voice (Rontal et al., 1978). Neuropharmacological treatment for Parkinson's disease supports amelioration of general motor symptoms with, for instance, dopamine precursors or agonists (e.g. bromocriptine, pergolide mesylate). It has been suggested that Deprenyl may slow progression of disability (Shoulson and Fahn,

1989). However the impact of these drugs on speech or voice production is not established. While there are papers to support positive effects of medication on voices of individuals with Parkinson's disease (Audelman et al., 1970; Mawdsley and Gamsu, 1971; Wolfe et al., 1975), the findings do not support consistent and significant effects of neuropharmacological treatment on voice production. For example, in a study of on–off effects of medication on acoustic and electroglottographic measures of vocal function in two individuals with Parkinson's disease, Larson et al. (1994) reported no systematic or consistent relationship between drug cycle fluctuations and these measures. The medical treatment of Huntington's disease involves pharmacological attempts to control the choreic movements with antidopaminergic agents, phenothiazines, benzodiazepines, or antiseizure medications (Brin et al., 1992). The effects of these on voice in Huntington's disease has not been documented. Smith (personal communication) reports improved voice quality and ease of phonation in an individual with hyperadductory voice arrests associated with Huntington's disease following Botox injections into the thyroarytenoid muscle. The neuropharmacological treatment of essential tremor has involved various drugs (e.g. propranolol, primidone, acetazolamide, alprazolam, phenobarbital) with mixed results (Koller et al., 1986). Recently, Stager and Ludlow (1994) reported positive findings on use of Botox for treatment of vocal tremor.

Since 1987 when Botox was first injected into laryngeal muscles of individuals with spasmodic dysphonia (laryngeal dystonia) (Brin et al., 1987; Miller et al., 1987), it has been considered an important medical treatment for this disorder. There is a large literature reviewing various aspects of Botox treatment (e.g. Ludlow, 1995; Brin et al., 1998).

Speech pathology

Behavioural treatment for neurological voice disorders has only recently been addressed systematically (Ramig and Scherer, 1992; Smith and Ramig, 1995; Ramig, 1995a). In contrast to previous approaches to speech treatment that have been directed to the aetiologic classification of disorders, the approach suggested by Ramig and colleagues presents a treatment framework in relation to the physical pathology in the laryngeal mechanism. Neurolaryngeal disorders have been classified as: disorders of glottal closure (hypoadduction and hyperadduction) and instability (short-term and long-term).

Hypoadduction

Certain neurological disorders are accompanied by inadequate vocal fold adduction or hypoadduction. The particular type and extent of hypoadduction may be associated with the site and extent of the related neurological damage. Hypoadduction may accompany a variety of neurological disorders, but is often associated with lower motor neuron (flaccid) involvement, which is characterized by paresis (weakness) or paralysis (immobility), atrophy and fatigue. Recently the hypoadduction accompanying Parkinson's disease has received attention (Smith and Ramig, 1995).

In treatment for individuals with reduced adduction, the primary treatment goal is to increase loudness and reduce breathy, hoarse voice quality by increasing vocal fold adduction. Procedures to accomplish this include pushing, pulling and lifting while phonating (Froeschels et al., 1955). The goal is to maximize adduction by 'reinforcing the sphincter action of the laryngeal muscles engaged in phonation' (Froeschels et al., 1955). Other techniques to increase adduction include hard glottal attack, digital manipulation of the thyroid cartilage and turning the head to one side or the other – to increase tension on the paralysed fold (Aronson, 1990).

To facilitate the goal of increased loudness and improved quality, the respiratory system is often a focus of treatment. The goal of respiratory treatment is to achieve a consistent subglottal pressure during speech that is produced with minimal fatigue and appropriate breath group lengths (Netsell and Daniel, 1979). Stabilization of posture may be considered first (Murphy, 1965; Collins et al., 1982; Rosenbek and LaPointe, 1985). This may be followed by training to increase subglottal air pressure to '5 cm. of water pressure for 5 sec' (Netsell and Hixon, 1978). Other techniques include exercises against a resistive load and controlled exhalation (Putnam, 1988). To improve coordination of respiration and phonation, various techniques such as maximum duration vowel phonation (Stemple et al., 1994; Ramig et al., 1995b) and phonation with simultaneous respiratory and vocal feedback have been suggested (Yorkstone al., 1988). The individual with hypoadduction may also be encouraged to maximize oral resonance in order to increase loudness and quality. Details of these approaches have been reported by Ramig and Scherer (1992), Smith and Ramig (1995), Ramig (1995a) and Ramig et al. (1995b).

Hyperadduction

Certain neurological diseases result in excess vocal fold adduction, or hyperadduction. In some cases, the ventricular (false) vocal folds may hyperadduct as well (Aronson, 1990). The particular type and extent of hyperadduction may be associated with the site and extent of the related neurological damage. Hyperadduction most frequently occurs in cases of upper motor neuron system disorders characterized by spasticity and hypertonicity and extrapyramidal system diseases accompanied by abnormal involuntary movements (e.g. tics, chorea, dystonia) that may be focal or generalized. In addition, hyperadduction may be compensatory. For example, a patient may have weak respiratory support or velopharyngeal closure and hyperadduct in order to manage the air stream for adequate loudness (Putnam, 1988).

The primary focus of voice therapy for patients with hyperadduction is to decrease the pressed, strained voice by reducing vocal fold hyperadduction. Procedures to accomplish this include those designed to relax laryngeal musculature and facilitate easy voice onset. These techniques may begin with whole body relaxation (Jacobson, 1976; McClosky, 1977) and then focus on laryngeal musculature. Other approaches include laryngeal massage, chewing approach, the yawn-sigh, chanting and delayed auditory feedback (Froeschels, 1952; Boone, 1983; Pershall and Boone, 1986). These techniques are based upon the hypothesis that when phonation is produced in the context of these reflex-like (Aronson, 1990) or continuous phonation responses, it will be more relaxed and less hyperadducted.

To facilitate the goal of improved voice quality, the respiratory system is often a focus of treatment in individuals with hyperadduction. The goal of respiratory treatment is to achieve consistent, steady airflow with relaxed respiratory musculature (Aten, 1983). Once the patient's posture is stabilized, relaxed abdominal breathing may be trained to provide the greatest respiratory support with the minimum muscle tension (Prater and Swift, 1984). These activities may be combined with progressive relaxation exercises. To encourage reduced hyperadduction and remove the laryngeal focus, some clinicians (Cooper and Cooper, 1977) encourage 'placement' of the vocal resonance in the frontal nasal area.

Instability

Certain neurological disorders are accompanied by increased phonatory instability. The particular type, extent and regularity of the instability may be associated with the site and extent of the related neurological damage. Long-term fluctuations and short-term changes can occur as well as random or continuous use of alternative modes of voicing such as ventricular phonation, glottal fry, or diplophonia (Ramig et al., 1988; Aronson, 1990). These forms of instability may occur singly or in combination and may be related to the problems of adduction discussed previously.

The main focus of therapy for individuals with phonatory instability is to reduce the unsteady, hoarse, rough voice quality by targeting steady, clear phonation. Patients are encouraged to maximize respiratory and laryngeal coordination, as discussed previously, in order to sustain steady voicing with consistent good quality. Treatments discussed earlier to promote more efficient vocal fold adduction have been reported to have positive effects on phonatory stability as well. For example, improved phonatory stability has been measured in individuals with Parkinson's disease after therapy designed to promote increased vocal fold adduction (Dromey et al., 1995).

Augmentative communication

In some cases the severity of the neurolaryngeal disorder in combination with breakdowns in other parts of the speech mechanism, as well as the neurological disorder, makes a form of augmentative communication the best choice to facilitate communication. These devices can range from a simple manual board up to sophisticated computer-based technology. The more advanced devices offer synthesized or digitized speech output which can be customized to the patient's needs.

Prognosis

Recently, data have been presented on the efficacy of intensive voice treatment for individuals with neurolaryngeal disorders. These data have been generated primarily around an intensive voice treatment programme (LSVT) designed for individuals with Parkinson's disease. Data from administration of this treatment (Ramig et al., 1995b; 1996) support improved sound pressure level, fundamental frequency variation, vocal fold adduction and subglottal air pressure as well as maintenance of these changes for 6–12 months. The rationale and techniques for this treatment have been summarized elsewhere (Ramig et al., 1995b). These data are consistent with data reported by others on the usefulness of intensive voice treatment for patients with Parkinson's disease (Scott and Caird, 1983; Robertson and Thompson, 1984). Application of these treatment concepts to selected individuals with multiple sclerosis, stroke, ataxic dysarthria has generated positive findings as well.

Summary

The past few years have seen a great increase in academic and clinical interest in neurological voice disorders. Knowledge of the neural bases and physiology underlying these disorders continues to grow. Surgical, pharmacological and behavioural treatments offer the potential to enhance speech production in individuals with these disorders. The combined efforts of the speech–language pathologist, neurologist and otolaryngologist can provide optimal speech intelligibility for individuals with neurological disorders of the voice.

Acknowledgements:

Some of the material in this chapter has been modified from a previous review (Ramig et al., 1996). Supported in part by NIH R01 DC01150 and P60DC00976

CHAPTER **10**

Vocal fold paralysis – paresis – immobility

JANINA K. CASPER

Introduction

Disorders of vocal fold mobility are complex problems with various aetiologies, diverse manifestations and significant implications for the functions of respiration, phonation and deglutition. Vocal fold paralysis is a well-known entity that, due to technological advances, has been the subject of recent increased attention. Advances in laryngeal imaging, new surgical and non-surgical treatment procedures, the use of laryngeal electromyography and improved methods of measuring phonatory function, have all served to change our understanding of, and approaches to, the diagnosis and treatment of disorders of vocal fold mobility.

Normally functioning vocal folds act as a valve opening appropriately and adequately to allow the inhalation and exhalation of air in sufficient quantity to sustain life. This valve also functions to sustain life by preventing airway penetration by any foreign object, and by acting to clear matter from the lower respiratory tract and lungs. For the purpose of phonation the vocal folds engage in a highly co-ordinated, exquisitely timed activity that allows them to approximate and oscillate producing the sound we refer to as voice. Their length, mass and tension can be adjusted and, in co-ordination with the responses of the vocal tract, the varied richness of normal phonation and the control and beauty of the singing voice are produced. Paresis, paralysis or immobility of one or both vocal folds may have a deleterious effect on any or all of these functions. In addition, it can have significantly negative effects on an individual's social, mental and vocational status (Smith et al., 1996).

Paresis is the term used to describe weakness of a vocal fold in the presence of partial movement capability. Videolaryngoscopically, that weakness can present as bowing of one or both vocal folds, as reduction in adduction and abduction, as a difference in speed of movement between the two vocal folds and as some glottal incompetence. The only observable movement in a completely paralysed vocal fold is the aerodynamically induced motion described by Hirano (1977) as similar to that of a flag flapping in the wind. Both of these terms, paresis and paralysis, imply a disruption of the transmission of neural impulses and disruption of neuromuscular innervation. Vocal fold immobility, however, may result from fixation or dislocation of the cricoarytenoid joint or from posterior scar bands that restrict joint movement. These aetiologies have nothing to do with the integrity of the neuromuscular system. In this chapter the term paralysis will be used routinely in discussing the neurologically based impairment, unless it is important to specify a paresis. Immobility will be used in describing other than neurologically based vocal fold movement problems. Furthermore, because bilateral vocal fold paralysis typically has different aetiologies, presents unique problems and specific treatment, and is significantly less prevalent, it will be discussed in a separate section at the end of the chapter. The main focus of the chapter will address unilateral vocal fold mobility problems.

Neurolaryngology

It is not within the purview of this chapter to delve at length into neurolaryngology or phonatory physiology. (Those interested in pursuing these areas are referred to Titze, 1994 and Benninger and Schwimmer, 1995.) However, it is necessary to have a basic understanding of the innervation of the intrinsic laryngeal muscles and the nature of the disruption that results from their impairment.

The Xth cranial nerve, the vagus, innervates the intrinsic laryngeal muscles. The vagus exits the skull through the jugular foramen and divides into three branches. The pharyngeal branch supplies nerve fibres to the pharynx and much of the palate. The superior laryngeal nerve branches off at the level of the inferior ganglion and contains both sensory and motor fibres. It descends along the pharynx and the motor fibres innervate the cricothyroid muscle, which is active in tensing and relaxing the vocal folds. The third branch, the recurrent laryngeal nerve, also carries both sensory and motor fibres. It does not follow a bilaterally symmetric path. Indeed, it is this difference in anatomic course of the nerve that makes the left recurrent, whose course is convoluted and longer, more vulnerable to trauma and explains the higher incidence of left unilateral vocal fold paralyses over right-sided paralyses. The right recurrent nerve passes into the upper chest looping around the subclavian artery before entering the larynx. The left recurrent laryngeal nerve follows a path that extends well down and deep into the upper thorax passing anteriorly, under and then behind the aorta then superiorly, within the tracheo-oesophageal crease to the larynx where it enters near the cricothyroid joint. The recurrent laryngeal nerve innervates all of the intrinsic laryngeal muscles with the exception of the cricothyroid.

Central (intracranial) or skull base lesions are most commonly implicated in bilateral vocal fold paralysis; however, unilateral problems may occur. Unilateral paresis may result from a brain stem stroke, for example, and present as reduction in speed and range of movement of the affected side. The nature of an upper motor neuron based paresis would be spastic as opposed to the flaccid paralysis of a lower motor event. Thus, in addition to the reduced movement noted above, a pulling of the posterior glottis towards the normal side occurs with onset of phonation.

A high vagal lesion, at or above the inferior ganglion, might result in combined superior and recurrent nerve involvement. Isolated superior laryngeal nerve paralysis would result in disruption of innervation to the cricothyroid muscle. Because this muscle controls the tensing/relaxing function of the vocal fold, the effect of such a lesion may present visually as a slight tilting of the posterior commissure to the affected side during phonation, with a normal appearance at rest (Benninger and Schwimmer, 1995). A combined paralysis would result in sensory and motor impairment of the hypopharynx and larynx with implications for both swallowing and phonation.

Low vagal peripheral lesions result in either unilateral or bilateral vocal fold paralysis with impairment in the ability of the vocal folds to either adduct or abduct. Although the position of the affected vocal fold (or folds) had been thought in the past to be indicative of the site of lesion, more recent information (Benninger and Schwimmer, 1995) has shown that these factors are not highly correlated. Nevertheless, varying degrees of glottal incompetence can be expected in these types of paralyses with implications for both phonation and swallowing (aspiration).

Paralysis of the posterior cricoarytenoid muscle (PCA), the primary abductor of the vocal folds, typically results in both vocal folds remaining in an adducted, median position and unable to open. This condition, with the vocal folds in a posture that obstructs the airway, has much more significant immediate implications for respiration than for phonation. However, treatment options will frequently result in some worsening of the voice in favour of improving airway. (See section on bilateral vocal fold paralysis at end of chapter.)

Incidence, prevalence and aetiology

There are no reliable figures of incidence of vocal fold paralysis. There are several reasons why such figures are difficult to obtain. In infants who are born with a vocal fold paralysis the condition may be undiagnosed and, in some cases, function may be recovered spontaneously. Thus the condition remains unknown. Similarly, this may occur in adults who have a paralysis of a transient nature for which services are never sought. Increased prevalence of vocal fold paralysis in the older population is related to the higher incidence of progressive neurological diseases and various non-laryngeal malignancies in this group, both of which are highly implicated in disruption of recurrent laryngeal nerve function. The effects of the primary conditions in these cases may often be more debilitating and of more urgent concern than the voice symptoms. Thus, actual diagnosis of the existence of the paralysis may be bypassed or overlooked unless aspiration is of concern. Because vocal fold paralysis is more prevalent in the older population, and because that sector of the population continues to be fast growing, it would seem reasonable to conjecture that the incidence of vocal fold paralysis may be rising.

In a review of 113 patients with vocal fold paralysis, Terris et al. (1992) reported that 74% had unilateral paralysis of which 68% involved the left vocal fold. Mean age of onset was 58 years. Percentages for specific causes of vocal fold paralysis vary to some extent. However, nonlaryngeal malignancy, primarily pulmonary, is now reported as the primary cause (Terris et al., 1992; Benninger et al., 1994a; Wippold, 1998), having overtaken thyroid surgery and iatrogenic causes. Surgical trauma occurs most frequently secondary to thyroidectomy, but thoracic, cervical spine, carotid artery and cardiac procedures may also result in damage to the recurrent laryngeal nerve. The second most common aetiology of vocal fold paralysis is trauma, surgical and nonsurgical. Included in the latter category are traumas resulting from motor vehicle accidents, intubation, penetrating injuries, or other neck injuries. Nonsurgical trauma is believed by some to be increasing as a cause of vocal fold paralysis (Tucker, 1993). Idiopathic aetiology, inflammatory causes, and central pathology occur with much less frequency. A number of progressive neurological diseases such as Parkinson's disease, Shy-Drager syndrome, multiple sclerosis and ALS, and neuropathies such as Guillain–Barré, diabetes, etc. may have a component of vocal fold movement disability as part of the course of the disease.

It is believed by some that vocal fold paralysis is an underreported problem (Benninger et al., 1994a). As previously noted, this may be particularly true in the case of idiopathic or virus induced paralysis that may recover spontaneously within a relatively short time period, obviating the need for the individual to seek medical attention. Indeed, our understanding of the degree of recovery possible in such cases is no doubt coloured by the fact that those seeking medical attention may be the group that fails to recover.

Some conditions may result in transient vocal fold paralysis that resolves in a month or less. Postma and Shockley (1998) describe cases of myasthenia gravis, meningitis and surgical trauma in which vocal fold mobility was clearly impaired for a very short time period. In each of the cases they described, normal return of function was restored following appropriate treatment of the underlying condition.

Another way to consider aetiology of vocal fold paralysis is to examine congenital versus acquired problems. The causes noted above appear to be primarily acquired. Congenital vocal fold paralysis, which has been estimated to comprise 27% of all vocal fold paralyses (Gereau et al., 1995), can be either uni- or bilateral. According to Gereau et al. (1995), bilateral paralysis occurs with greater frequency (38%) and is usually secondary to central nervous system problems or as part of other congenital abnormalities. In approximately 45% of these cases recovery occurs either spontaneously or secondary to treatment of the underlying condition. Although the paralysis may occur in utero, it is often difficult to determine whether the underlying aetiology is traumatic, secondary to the birth process itself, or developmental, secondary to an embryological disturbance. In a study of 113 cases of congenital vocal fold paralysis, deGaudemar et al. (1996) reported that 61 had unilateral paralysis (41 left and 20 right) while a smaller number, 52, had bilateral paralysis. The most common aetiology for this group was idiopathic, followed in decreasing numbers by paralysis associated with neurologic disorders, associated with heart malformations and difficult birth. More than 70% of unilateral paralyses of idiopathic, neurologic or difficult birth origin recovered spontaneously. The prognosis for spontaneous recovery in bilateral paralysis was poorer.

It has been reported that 10% of all congenital laryngeal lesions are paralytic (Gereau et al., 1995); however, the diagnosis may not be made immediately as the symptoms are often non-specific. Stridor is usually present in bilateral paralyses, but rarely in unilateral involvement. Vocal fold paralysis is the second most frequent cause of congenital stridor (Manaligod and Smith, 1998). Other symptoms might include weak, breathy cry, aspiration or choking during feeding.

Diagnosis

In a sizeable percentage of cases, the diagnosis of vocal fold paralysis can be made and the aetiology ascertained by history and appropriate physical examination. According to Terris et al. (1992) the primary objective in the evaluation of the patient with unilateral vocal fold paralysis is to determine the aetiology, with restoration of vocal function as the secondary objective.

This order of objectives may differ for the patient with bilateral vocal fold paralysis when the airway is compromised and its management becomes the primary focus. Aetiology of bilateral paralysis is also important to ascertain, but is perhaps more readily apparent based on history. Patients present themselves with a number of scenarios that should raise the examiner's index of suspicion that vocal fold immobility of some sort is present. Frequent complaints are: weak voice, inability to be heard, shortness of breath and running out of breath during speaking, instability of voice, hoarseness and choking on liquids or other foods. Many of these characteristics or signs may be noted perceptually during the interview.

Careful questioning of the patient may place the onset of the voice change in close temporal proximity to surgery involving the thyroid, the neck, the thorax, the cervical spine, the heart or a surgical procedure that required short or long-term intubation. This information strongly suggests the likelihood of recurrent laryngeal nerve injury or possible arytenoid dislocation. Indeed, in some instances it may be known that the recurrent laryngeal nerve was sacrificed during the course of the surgery. Another close tie-in may be the reporting of a viral infection preceding the voice problem. It is believed that viral infection may be implicated in causing unilateral vocal fold paralysis, particularly when no other cause can be verified.

Trauma, sufficient to cause vocal fold paralysis, is not uncommon. A thorough history should reveal the possibility of such an aetiology. Patients who present with a diagnosed neurological disorder or manifestations of such a disorder and complain of voice problems may present with vocal fold mobility problems associated with the underlying neurological disease. There are numerous other metabolic, inflammatory and auto-immune disease processes that may, on occasion, result in paralysis of the vocal folds.

It is important to rule out all other possible diagnoses through a process of differential diagnosis and to attempt to determine whether the mobility problem represents paralysis, paresis, arytenoid dislocation or ankylosis. It is also necessary to recall that the perceptual and physical findings in a patient with a psychogenically based voice disorder presenting with whispered speech may mimic a vocal fold mobility problem.

Diagnostic testing

The basic components of a competent and complete evaluation are always carried out for each patient (Colton and Casper, 1996). These components are: a complete history, a complete ear nose and throat examination (including laryngeal imaging), voice evaluations of both a subjective and an objective nature. These components of the examination help to establish and confirm the diagnosis, are essential for documentation of findings, are critical in determining the need for and nature of additional testing and in planning treatment.

Laryngeal endoscopy

Imaging of the larynx using endoscopic procedures is essential for determining movement characteristics of the vocal folds during phonation. The performance of non-phonatory acts such as whistle, cough, throat clear and swallow should also be observed. The rigid and the flexible endoscopes provide different and valuable information and the use of both is recommended. Videotaping the examination provides the opportunity for visualizing an enlarged image, for repeated study of the image, and for documentation and future comparison.

Stroboscopic examination adds the dimension of observing vibratory behaviour that sometimes can be helpful in making the differentiation between paralysis and immobility. The loss of tone of the body of the vocal fold resulting from damage to the motor fibres of the thyroarytenoid muscle is best appreciated with stroboscopy (Benninger et al., 1994a). 'The flaccid paretic fold opens laterally earlier in the glottal cycle and to a greater degree, but it does not have the normal undulating vibration that the normal fold exhibits' (Benninger et al., 1994a, p. 499). Stroboscopic signs of unilateral vocal fold paralysis pre- and post-treatment have been reported by Colton et al. (1998) for a group of 38 patients.

When the cause of the paralysis is known, such as severing of the recurrent laryngeal nerve during a surgical procedure, further tests, beyond videoendoscopy/stroboscopy, may not be necessary. When the history and physical examination fail to identify the aetiology of the paralysis or render it uncertain, further testing is mandatory.

Chest X-ray, CT scan, magnetic resonance imaging (MRI)

Because nonlaryngeal malignancy is the primary cause of vocal fold paralysis, it is imperative that exploration of that aetiologic possibility be pursued. A chest X-ray should be the first test to be performed. Lung tumours comprise the largest number of neoplasms that are implicated in laryngeal paralysis. A negative chest X-ray, however, is insufficient data on which to rule out the possibility of a malignancy. Thus, further imaging studies, such as CT scan or MRI (magnetic resonance imaging) from the base of the skull to the aortic triangle on the left and to the thoracic outlet on the right are necessary (Terris et al., 1992; Benninger et al., 1994a; Altman and Benninger, 1997).

Although vocal fold immobility in patients with rheumatoid arthritis had been thought to result from fixation of the cricoarytenoid joint, Link et al. (1998) report that cervicomedullary compression secondary to destructive arthritic changes and inflammatory processes may well be the cause. They provide data on three patients demonstrating the need for imaging studies that focus on skullbase, showing subluxation of the occipito-atlanto-axial joint and/or basilar invagination with brain stem compression. With appropriate treatment, the vocal fold immobility is reversible. Thus, the need for imaging studies that explore the route of the vagus nerve is further strengthened.

Laryngeal electromyography (LEMG)

Laryngeal electromyography (LEMG) is receiving increased attention and use in the examination of patients with vocal fold mobility and swallowing disorders (Woo, 1998). It is useful in making the distinction between vocal fold paralysis and vocal fold immobility due to mechanical fixation or dislocation of the cricoarytenoid joint. When action potentials are present despite the presence of an apparently immobile vocal fold, it can be inferred that the problem is one of mechanical immobility (Terris et al., 1992). Woo (1998) makes the claim that LEMG can be used to 'triage patients with immobile vocal folds' (p. 473) in a cost-effective and useful manner by directing the planning of further examination procedures or treatment approaches. The distinction between superior laryngeal nerve paralysis and recurrent laryngeal nerve involvement or the denervation of both nerve branches can be clarified when LEMG is used appropriately (Rontal et al., 1993; Woo, 1998). This constitutes site of lesion testing and also serves to direct the focus of further examinations. For purposes of prognosis and treatment planning, LEMG provides information about reinnervation. Comparison of tests performed at various times in the uncertain course of idiopathic paralysis or recovery from injury, helps to determine the timing and type of intervention required. Reinnervation can be detected via LEMG before it can be visually observed. This provides a refinement of treatment planning based on objective data that is not otherwise available.

However, it must be recognized that LEMG is a tool requiring precise technique and considerable experience and skill. There are numerous limitations and concerns about its reliability and the reproducibility of test/retest results (Benninger et al., 1994a; Ludlow et al., 1994; Ford, 1998; Woodson, 1998). Interpretation of the signal is subjective and thus reflects the skill and knowledge of the interpreter.

Airflow and air pressure studies

Although not diagnostic as such, measures of airflow and air pressure during phonation most objectively reflect the effects of paralysis on glottal closure. The results of airflow studies may add significant information that is not observable in other testing. For example, high leakage airflows (the flow during phonation) may suggest the presence of a significant posterior glottal gap that cannot be visualized due to the forward posture of the arytenoid cartilage on the paralysed side. Similarly, such a finding in the presence of fair vocal fold approximation may suggest that the vocal folds may be at different vertical levels. These measures are also useful in documenting the effects of treatment or the course of reinnervation.

Other tests

Other tests may be ordered when there is suspicion that systemic or other disease processes may be contributing to the vocal fold paralysis. These decisions must be made on an individual basis.

Diagnostic practices and cost effectiveness

There is not a standard protocol for evaluation of vocal fold paralysis that is agreed to and practised by all otolaryngologists. Indeed, Terris et al. (1992) reported a wide diversity of test procedures used, and found that those laryngologists most experienced and knowledgeable about the larynx ordered fewer tests than less experienced physicians. Cost-effectiveness questions include the relative information yield of the various diagnostic procedures and what that information adds to the diagnosis or the treatment. These authors suggest that the diagnostic tests described in the preceding section are the most productive, that they are readily obtainable, relatively inexpensive and relatively non-invasive. Tests that they report to be unnecessary in most cases include: erythrocyte sedimentation rate, VDRL, glucose level, complete blood count, urinalysis, chemistry profile, or thyroid function studies. Thyroid scans and barium swallows are also felt to be unnecessary if CT or MRI studies have been done. When aspiration is a concern and requires further definition, a modified barium swallow study (MBS) would be an appropriate consideration.

Treatment

There are a number of treatment options available for the patient with unilateral vocal fold paralysis. Figure 10.1 presents schematic flow charts describing general treatment courses. It should go without saying that decisions about patient care must be made on an individual basis. However, there are some general considerations that may help to direct the choice and timing of treatment.

Treatment Options: Unilateral Vocal Fold Paralysis

Known Permanent Aetiology
Unknown Aetiology > 9 Month Duration

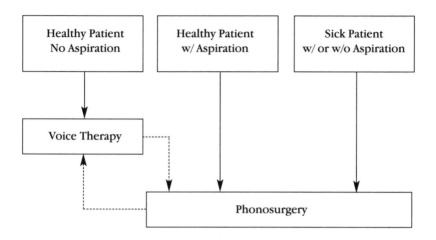

Temporary or Unknown Aetiology
< 9 Month Duration

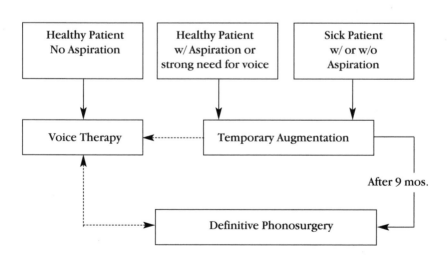

Figure 10.1 Flow chart of treatment options and course of treatment for patients with unilateral vocal fold paralysis. Dotted lines suggest possible options depending on individual patient needs while the unbroken lines suggest the typical course of treatment.

The first of these is an understanding of the patient's health status including the presence or absence of aspiration. Patients whose vocal fold paralysis results from the effects of a nonlaryngeal malignancy may be quite ill and debilitated, as may also be true of patients with other aetiologies. Aspiration is the primary concern for many. In such instances immediate intervention is required and should take the least aggressive, least invasive course possible. It is most likely that there will be improvement in the voice secondary to whatever procedure is done to control the aspiration. The presence of significant aspiration in any patient with vocal fold paralysis is of concern and demands prompt attention. However, if the patient is otherwise healthy, the choice of treatment to manage the aspiration may be different from that for the seriously ill patient. Assessment of the degree and severity of the aspiration relative to the time that the condition has been present is essential. Some patients may experience aspiration immediately following the onset of paralysis but may readily learn to control it through behavioural approaches. These approaches should be tried before other procedures are undertaken, particularly in an otherwise healthy person.

The second consideration is the certainty regarding the permanent vs. transient nature of the paralysis and the length of time since onset. As noted in previous sections of this chapter, knowledge of the aetiology of the paralysis will help to determine whether return of function or nerve regeneration is a possibility. If it is known that the nerve has been severed, it is usually a certainty that there will not be any spontaneous recovery of function. This knowledge will influence the choice and timing of treatment. There would be no need to postpone definitive procedures. However, if the paralysis is idiopathic in nature, some degree of functional recovery is possible for up to a year from onset. Thus, it is usually unwise to pursue a definitive treatment plan that might be incompatible with spontaneous recovery before at least nine months have elapsed.

The third consideration is the acceptability of the patient's voice. Although there are some 'typical' characteristics of voice in the presence of a paralysed vocal fold, the severity of the effects varies from individual to individual. In addition, there are varied personal vocal needs: the need to be heard easily, the need to be able to talk at length, the need to speak above noise, the need to have a pleasing voice, the need to communicate with the public, etc. The patient is the final arbiter of the adequacy of his or her voice to meet those needs. This assessment must be accepted by the professionals and must be taken into consideration in the planning of the timing and nature of treatment.

The available treatment options and indications for their use will be described in the following sections.

Voice therapy

Voice therapy is a non-invasive, behavioural treatment option that typically has no negative effects. Thus, a period of voice therapy has the potential of helping the patient even to the point of regaining functional voice, while doing no harm. When voice therapy fails to produce an acceptable degree of improvement, all other treatment options remain open and the only thing that may have been lost in some instances is a bit of time. Attempts have been made to devise a method of determining which patients would be most likely to benefit from a course of voice therapy and which would be better served by early surgical intervention (Woo et al., 1991; Heuer et al., 1997). Some authors simply state that patients who exhibit large glottal gaps are appropriate surgical candidates. However, such statements fail to specify at what point in the course of the paralysis the judgement relative to glottal gap size is made. We have seen patients whose initially large glottal gaps gradually reduced in size over the course of recovery of function. A functional staging approach was described by Woo et al., based on clinical symptoms and selected objective measures. The findings resulted from the study of 55 patients. Patients for whom surgery was felt to be the treatment of choice were those rated as having severe dysphonia, with significantly elevated airflow rates and decreased loudness and phonation times. The added presence of severe aspiration increased the need for surgical intervention. On the other hand, patients with mild dysphonia and no aspiration tended to respond well to voice therapy. It was determined that there is no clear-cut statement that can be made for the group in the middle, those with moderate symptoms and moderate dysphonia. Treatment decisions for those patients must be made on an individual basis. This study also found that objective measures of certain vocal functions are more sensitive to changes than are visible stroboscopic signs.

None of the proposed prognostic plans has assured a high enough level of accuracy to be universally accepted. However, numerous authors have reported very positive results for many patients following a course of voice therapy (Woo et al., 1991; Colton et al., 1992; Benninger et al., 1994a; Casper et al., 1996; Heuer et al., 1997). Casper et al. reported a significant decrease in mean severity of dysphonia rating from 6.06 at the initiation of voice therapy for 17 patients with unilateral vocal fold paralysis to a mean rating of 1.67 at the conclusion of therapy six to eight weeks later. The potential benefit of a period of voice therapy is given support in the following statement by the Committee on Speech, Voice and Swallowing Disorders of the American Academy of Otolaryngology Head and Neck Surgery (Benninger et al., 1994a)

Indeed, under good guidance, therapy sometimes produces astonishingly rapid improvements in voice quality despite persistence of the neurologic deficit. In any case, initial assessment is worthwhile to document vocal condition before surgery is considered and to get an estimate of how much the patient's voice can be improved without surgery.

We cannot ignore the contribution of spontaneous nerve regeneration in improvement of voice. There are no data available to prove that voice therapy speeds the rate of recovery or otherwise affects the recovery course in those patients with idiopathic paralysis. Certainly voice therapy cannot claim to restore nerve function. Nevertheless, we are strong advocates for initiating a course of voice therapy as soon as the paralysis is diagnosed. It is our belief that through voice therapy patients learn to use the mechanism to the best of its capability without adopting maladaptive compensatory behaviours. Thus, as spontaneous recovery occurs, they are able to gain greatest benefit from it through the manner of voice production they have been taught. A course of voice therapy in most settings today does not exceed weekly sessions for a 6–8 week period. The course of spontaneous recovery may last up to a year. Providing a course of therapy is helpful to patients in knowing that they have exercises they can do and continue to do throughout the 'waiting period'. Serial measures of vocal function taken over time are extremely important to track progress.

Another benefit of voice therapy for patients with vocal fold paralysis is an educational one. Patients learn about phonation and about the effects of a paralysis on the normal process. They gain an understanding of the nature of their specific problem and have more opportunity to explore and understand the various treatment options. It has been our experience that patients who understand their problem are better able to handle it, have higher motivation for improvement, and have more realistic goals.

The goal of voice therapy, and thus the techniques employed, must be decided on an individual basis. It is well known that when a body part becomes non-functional a variety of compensatory behaviours may arise. This is certainly the case when a vocal fold ceases to function. The classical description of the compensatory behaviour typical of patients with unilateral paralysis is that the remaining intact vocal fold overworks and crosses the midline in an attempt to contact the paralysed, nonmedialized fold. There has been some controversy as to whether this, in fact, takes place. Although we have observed occasional evidence of this behaviour, it does not happen in all cases, and indeed, even when it appears to happen it may not be sufficient to produce an adequate voice. Furthermore, there are numerous other attempted compensatory behaviours that are observed with some frequency and need to be recognized.

Excessive medialization of the ventricular folds – unilaterally on the affected side or bilaterally – is not uncommonly seen. It is not difficult to understand the mechanism for the development of this compensatory behaviour as the individual attempts to modulate the exiting airflow and produce the loudest sound possible. The presence of unilateral ventricular fold medialization does not usually present a problem. However, when seen bilaterally the entire laryngeal mechanism is being 'squeezed' in a hyperfunctional posture. This is a maladaptive compensatory behaviour (often referred to as ventricular phonation) producing a voice that is often unpleasant and fatiguing. Furthermore, this pattern can become so habitualized that it may persist even when the true vocal folds are increasingly capable of movement or when a surgical procedure has corrected the glottal incompetence. Thus, when bilateral ventricular fold medialization is observed, the goals of voice therapy should be to eradicate this hyperfunctional behaviour and teach a more gentle form of voice production.

Excessively high airflow and pressure measures are helpful in identifying those patients who are overworking the respiratory system and increasing air pressure in an attempt to better drive the phonatory system. In the absence of the bilateral vocal fold tensions and activity required to close the glottis and resist airflow, the increased pressure serves no useful purpose. Indeed, patients who engage in this behaviour complain of shortness of breath and an inability to speak more than a word or two per breath. This is very fatiguing. In such instances, the goal of voice therapy is to reduce the effort being expended to 'force' sound. Usually the resulting voice quality will be improved, the length of utterance capability will also improve and the element of fatigue will be significantly reduced. After this is accomplished the second goal of establishing the best voice of which the patient is capable becomes the focus of therapy.

Occasionally a patient may adopt the use of a high pitch as a compensatory behaviour. The use of a high pitch often results in a louder and clearer voice. Patients who do this have recurrent nerve involvement but the superior laryngeal nerve, which innervates the cricothyroid muscle and is most active in pitch regulation, is intact. When the intact motor units are brought into play, the tension of the vocal fold is increased allowing perhaps for slightly improved adduction and thus a stronger voice. If the 'new voice' is acceptable there is no need to suggest a change. However, an excessively high-pitched voice may be irritating and out of character for the individual. In such instances, the focus of voice therapy will be to lower the pitch while maintaining the best acceptable voice.

The most typical observation is incomplete glottal closure without effective compensatory behaviour. The goals of voice therapy are: (1) to help the patient identify the best voice he or she is capable of producing by exploring effects of pitch change, attending to respiratory dynamics, manipulating head position; (2) to begin to exercise the vocal folds using such activities as pitch extension exercises and trill (lip or tongue); (3) to increase the resonance characteristics of the voice which increases loudness without added laryngeal effort. The traditional 'pushing techniques' and effort closure of the glottis techniques should be under-taken with great care. Those techniques usually result in squeezing of all laryngeal structures, as they are incapable of isolating the true vocal folds alone. Thus, they may encourage the maladaptive ventricular phonation or other hyperfunctional behaviours (Casper et al., 1985). If these techniques are to be used, it is recommended that their physiological effect be assessed under endoscopic visualization to ensure that hyper-function of an unproductive type is not being introduced and reinforced.

A very short course of voice therapy may be indicated for patients who undergo a phonosurgical procedure to ensure that the patient is attaining the best voice possible with the least effort. Despite the changed anatomy, patients may retain learned maladaptive compensatory behaviours or may not adjust phonatory behaviour to the changed structure.

Many of the techniques mentioned in this section and rationales for their use are more fully described in Colton and Casper (1996).

Phonosurgery

The term phonosurgery is used to refer to all of the various surgical techniques that are primarily used to preserve or improve voice (see Chapter 17). This area has been the focus of much research and much growth over the past twenty years with constant improvement in techniques and results. The purpose of phonosurgery in the presence of unilateral vocal fold paralysis is to change the shape and/or position of the paralysed vocal fold, bringing it to the midline. There are two goals in doing this, i.e. to improve voice by allowing the intact vocal fold to come into contact with the impaired vocal fold, and to improve swallowing function by the same mechanism that provides greater protection of the airway. Injection procedures that augment the size of the affected fold or framework surgical procedures that either augment by surgical technique or surgically move the affected fold medially, or a combination of both, may attain these goals.

Intrafold injection procedures

These procedures began to be performed regularly in the 1970s with the reporting of intracordal injection of Teflon in 135 patients by Dedo et al. (1973). The use of Teflon has since gone out of favour because it has been shown to result in foreign body reactions with formation of Teflon granu-lomas. Teflon hardens, interfering with vocal fold vibratory behaviour and it tends to migrate, altering its position within the fold and moving to adjacent structures. However, there are several other materials that have been used to 'bulk up' the vocal fold: silicone, collagen, autologous fat and Gore-Tex (Wexler et al., 1989; Ford et al., 1992a). Gelfoam is another material that is used, but primarily for purposes of temporary augmenta-tion of the vocal fold, as it is a substance that dissolves spontaneously over a relatively short period of time. The materials most commonly used at present are autologous fat (Shaw et al., 1997) and autologous collagen. Both substances may be partially resorbed following injection, sometimes requiring repeated procedures. The method of managing these materials is constantly undergoing study and improvement in anticipation of a more predictable and stable outcome. The use of Gore-Tex is relatively recent, with no long-term reports available at this time relative to its efficacy.

Intrafold injection is used most commonly to correct the glottal incom-petence that results from unilateral paralysis. However, it is also used for vocal fold bowing, to correct sulcus vocalis defects or those caused by other surgery, trauma or scar tissue.

There are various methods of injection. Transoral injection using indirect laryngeal mirror visualization is possible with selected patients. The patient is seated in an examination chair and following topical anaes-thetization of the laryngeal and pharyngeal mucosa, a curved needle is used to administer the substance into the fold. Visual and auditory monitoring is possible as the injection proceeds. Transoral injection under direct laryngoscopic visualization using a microscope requires at least the use of local anaesthesia. If this is possible, auditory monitoring of vocal changes during the procedure is possible. However, general anaesthesia may be required, which eliminates the possibility of auditory monitoring of the voice. Transcutaneous injection through the cricothyroid space requires that the patient is supine and progress can be monitored visually via a flexible nasendoscope and auditorily as well. Flint and Cummings (1998) describe a 'lateral percutaneous approach through the thyroid ala at the level of the vocal fold' (p. 2075).

For correction of glottal incompetence due to paralysis, the material is injected lateral to the thyroarytenoid muscle and/or in the space between the thyroid lamina and the thyroarytenoid muscle. Fat is injected into the thyroarytenoid muscle. It is essential that the material not be injected into the mucosa overlying the vocal fold. The mucosa of the vocal fold must maintain its elasticity in order to ensure that vibratory behaviour will occur. The search is ongoing for a substance that will match the viscosity of the material in the normal vocal fold so that the resulting voice will be improved. Although these procedures correct the glottal defect, they do not necessarily restore 'normal' or pre-paralysis voice.

Laryngeal framework surgery

There are a number of framework surgeries that are done for various reasons. The particular ones that are appropriate for correction of vocal fold paralysis are those that medialize the affected fold.

The Isshiki Type 1 thyroplasty (Isshiki et al., 1975) is the most commonly performed procedure and one demonstrated to be effective in reducing glottal incompetence (Sasaki et al., 1990; Ford et al., 1992b; Gray et al., 1992; LaBlance and Maves, 1993; Netterville et al., 1993; Leder and Sasaki, 1994; Kieff and Zeitels, 1996). This procedure, performed externally through the neck, requires that the patient be able to respond and vocalize during the procedure. Thus, it is carried out under local anaesthesia with sedation. A window is prepared in the thyroid lamina lateral to the vocal fold through which a synthetic prosthesis (often a silicone wedge) is inserted, medializing and supporting the paralysed vocal fold. This procedure has several advantages including:

1. the ability to be performed under local anaesthesia;
2. preservation of the structural integrity of the vocal fold;
3. the individualization possible in customizing prosthesis size;
4. the reversibility of the procedure;
5. the minimal morbidity associated with it intra- and postoperatively;
6. the relative immediacy of the result;
7. the benefits that extend beyond voice to swallowing function, reduction of dyspnea and improvement of pulmonary toilet in sick patients allowing them to generate an improved cough.

Arytenoid adduction is another medialization procedure that can be done in conjunction with a Type 1 thyroplasty, or as a secondary procedure if the benefits of the initial thyroplasty were limited (Isshiki et al., 1978; Slavit and Maragos, 1994). It can also be done following intrafold injection, again to improve further on glottal closure and thus on voice production. The thyroplasty and injection medialization techniques are often incapable of providing adequate posterior glottic closure or in addressing differences in vertical level of the folds. In addition to improving posterior glottal closure, it is claimed that this procedure also makes it possible to adjust the vertical height of the paralysed fold and its length. However, Zeitels et al. (1998) have introduced a new procedure, adduction arytenopexy, in which the arytenoid is affixed on the cricoid facet. In animal studies and then in a series of patients this procedure resulted in a consistently significant increase in vocal fold length (2.1 mm) and a more normally contoured arytenoid in an optimal position for posterior glottal closure. Pre- and postsurgical comparisons of vocal function measures revealed improvement in all parameters following this procedure. These types of surgical refinements continue to improve the final vocal result for the patient.

Reinnervation techniques

The intent of these techniques is to correct the neuromuscular deficit by implanting adjacent functioning muscles. Tucker (1978), who is their primary proponent, provides the best description of these techniques. The techniques have not met with widespread acceptance or use.

Future direction

Neurolaryngology, an emerging field of increased research and interest, will probably provide improved understanding of vocal fold paralysis and improved methods for its treatment. We are just beginning to learn about the possibilities of electrical laryngeal pacing via implantable electrodes (Zealear et al., 1996). This holds much promise for future development.

Bilateral vocal fold paralysis

Bilateral impairment of vocal fold movement is much less prevalent than unilateral impairment. Improved surgical procedures for conditions affecting the thyroid and reduction in the need for that surgery due to improved medical treatment have reduced the frequency with which damage is iatrogenically done to the recurrent laryngeal nerve. Societal changes, on the other hand, have been responsible for increased incidence of laryngeal trauma as a result of mechanical injuries and perhaps injuries from violent confrontations. These types of trauma may result in bilateral vocal fold involvement. Increased survival of patients who suffer major head and neck traumas may also increase the numbers of patients seen with vocal fold paralysis, either unilateral or bilateral. Prolonged intubation often results in laryngeal trauma, with vocal fold immobility not an uncommon sequela. The cause of the immobility, whether dislocation of the arytenoids or posterior glottic scarring or paralysis, often presents a diagnostic challenge. Certain neurologic diseases may present with laryngeal findings. The presence of bilateral vocal fold paralysis in Shy-Drager syndrome and multiple system atrophy, for example, has been recognized as an early finding in some patients with these diseases, although still often overlooked (Williams et al., 1979; Wu et al., 1996; Hughes et al., 1998). Lack of recognition of the problem can be life threatening.

Bilateral impairment may involve both abductor and adductor function, with one or the other being predominant. When the impairment is primarily of the adductor type the patient's voice will be very weak and breathy, respiration will be unimpaired, but aspiration may be the most serious concern. Due to the potentially life-threatening concerns of intractable aspiration these patients require early intervention. Pou et al. (1998) report that of the patients they studied who presented with aspiration following high vagal injuries, 94% experienced improvement following medialization procedures, 79% who had required tracheotomy were decannulated and 90% were found to have subjective improvement in voice postoperatively. However, when the medialization procedures are not successful other surgical procedures may be required. In some instances patients have required total laryngectomy which is very effective in preventing aspiration but results in the loss of laryngeal function for voice production.

When abductor impairment is predominant, the vocal folds remain in a midline-adducted posture resulting in restriction of the airway, but good vocal function and no aspiration. Airway needs are of primary concern. The treatment for this condition is problematic. A tracheotomy may be required to provide an adequate airway while maintaining voicing capability by occluding the stoma. Phonosurgical procedures designed to improve the airway are somewhat successful in doing so, but often at the expense of the voice. Many of the procedures are surgically difficult and result in other problems. However, a laser cordotomy procedure described by Dennis and Kashima (1989) and Kashima (1991) holds promise. The procedure creates a wedge-shaped widening of the posterior glottis which adequately increases airway yet minimizes the dysphonia. Arytenoidectomy is another surgical option. There are reports on nerve anastamosis as a means of repairing the recurrent laryngeal nerve (Crumley, 1990) and also on proposed muscle transfer, specifically phrenic omohyoid transfer (Crumley, 1991), as a means of restoring abductory function. These procedures may hold promise for future development but have not been widely adopted.

Summary

Unilateral vocal fold paralysis is not, in and of itself, a life-threatening disability. However, we have come to understand that the impact of disease is not only physical, but also emotional, social and vocational. Smith et al. (1998b) studied three groups, patients with spasmodic dysphonia, patients with vocal fold paralysis and a control group, to determine what effect the voice disorder had on self–image and on work life demands. Of the group with vocal fold paralysis, 65% reported that their dysphonia had a moderately severe effect on their ability to advance in their careers and on future job options. Individuals reported a loss of self-esteem associated with their inability to perform up to expectations on the job. More than 50% of the vocal fold paralysis group reported moderate to extreme problems in communication particularly in noisy situations and on the phone.

Although we may have anticipated these results and understood them intuitively, the data validate the concerns and support the need for all forms of rehabilitation and treatment for these patients. An acceptable voice is a necessity in our society that is so heavily dependent on communication. As has been discussed in this chapter, the effects of the dysphonia that results from vocal fold paralysis can be treated effectively in a number of ways to restore acceptable vocal function. It is imperative therefore, that patients be examined early in the course of the problem, that they receive a complete and appropriate examination, that the diagnosis be correct and that an appropriate treatment course be initiated.

CHAPTER 11

Spasmodic dysphonia redefined: diagnosis, assessment and treatment

RENATA WHURR

Introduction

'Spasmodic Dysphonia'(SD), or as it was originally termed 'Spastic Dysphonia', has been one of the most poorly understood voice disorders. It has probably caused more controversy, confusion and contradictions than any other voice disorder. Since its original description in 1871, opinions about this unusual voice disorder have changed. First it was considered to have a psychogenic cause; the currently held view is that the cause is organic, with a neurological basis. There have been many methods of treatment ranging from psychotherapy, speech therapy and surgery, all of which proved to be ineffective. It is now recognized that there is no cure for spasmodic dysphonia, but there is symptomatic relief by means of intralaryngeal injections. For the speech and language therapist, spasmodic dysphonia (SD) requires a redirection of clinical skills.

What is Spasmodic Dysphonia(SD)?

Spasmodic dysphonia (SD) is a chronic phonatory disorder of unclear aetiology. It usually appears in adulthood and is characterized by frequent breaks in phonation, staccato-like catches, pitch breaks and variations in pitch, and is usually accompanied by effortful jerky, groaning or strained phonation. There are excessive spasms of the adductor muscles of the vocal folds and constriction of the glottic airway. This abnormal spasming or hyperadduction of the vocal folds is perceived by the listener as an unexpected change in voice quality – as a squeezed or strangled quality, or even a choking-off voice. This qualitative change may be very brief and widely spaced among otherwise normal phonation, or it may occur so frequently that the overall impression is of a strangled voice, interrupted only occasionally by more normal voicing. The listener is also aware of the effort that the patient is putting into forcing voice through a restricted glottis. These vocal symptoms are often accompanied by visible signs of struggle such as grimaces, eye blinking and contraction of thoracic and abdominal muscles. Patients, without exception, confirm the effort and fatigue that comes from extended speaking (Stoicheff, 1991).

Background

The condition was first described by Traube, in 1871, who suggested that spasmodic dysphonia was an hysterical illness. Others also regarded it as a hysterical conversion disorder (Heaver, 1959; Bloch,1965; Brodnitz, 1976). For over fifty years it was viewed by many as a psychiatric disorder (Beck, 1918; Berendes, 1938; Heaver, 1959; Bloch, 1965; Kiml, 1965; Brodnitz, 1976). A physical cause of SD was first proposed in 1874 and 1885 by Schnitzler (1885) who described two patients with 'cramping of the vocal cords and forced voice'. These patients were noted to have synkinesis of the facial muscles and abnormal movements of the arms and legs. Schnitzler called the entity 'spastic aphonia'. Gowers (1893) saw the condition as a functional laryngeal spasm, whereby the vocal cords were brought together too forcibly while speaking. In 1939 Critchley, a neurologist, described two patients with a vocal disorder who had neurological signs and concluded that the site of the pathology was likely to be the cerebellum or the basal ganglia. The vocal disorder was then described by Critchley as 'inspiratory speech'.

Current thoughts

Critchley's observation influenced the search for an organic cause for SD. Neurophysiological investigations have demonstrated some evidence for a neurological basis for the disorder. These have included abnormal electro-encephalograms(EEG)(Robe et al., 1960), abnormal responses to vagal stimuli (Feldman et al., 1984), altered evoked potentials (Shaefer et al., 1983; Finitzo and Freeman, 1989), hypersensitive blink reflex (Cohen et al., 1989) and deviant vocal reaction times (Reich and Till, 1983; Ludlow et al., 1987).

Redefinition of SD

More recent studies of spasmodic dysphonia have linked SD with dystonia. Oppenheim (1911) introduced the term dystonia to indicate that muscle tone was hypertonic on one occasion and in tonic spasm on another, usually, but not exclusively elicited upon volitional movements. It was the association of SD with Meige's syndrome which led to the disorder being redefined as a focal form of dystonia, one of a group of movement disorders which are characterized by prolonged muscle contractions with twisting spasms which may have additional myoclonic or tremulous components (Jacome and Yanez, 1980; Golper et al., 1983; Marsden and Sheehy, 1982).

It was not until recently that SD was generally accepted as a disease of neurological origin, (Aronson et al., 1968a; Dedo, 1976; Feldman et al., 1984; Hartman and von Cramon,1984; Brin et al., 1989). Now, the term laryngeal dystonia is used widely. Marsden and Quinn (1990) consider it an action-induced laryngeal form of focal dystonia. The term spastic dysphonia is considered erroneous and has been rejected. Blitzer et al. (1985) state SD is not a spastic disease, and should be differentiated from vocal tremor and myoclonus. No signs of spasticity have been delineated in the vocal folds of patients with SD (Aronson 1985a).

Incidence and prevalence

Spasmodic dysphonia usually presents during middle age, onset being insidious. Problems may first appear with a specific task, gesture or posturing of the larynx. At first, severity fluctuates with intervening periods of normal voice. Gradually, more laryngospasms intrude, taking a chronic course until a plateau is reached, beyond which there is no significant change (Ginsberg et al., 1988; Aronson, 1990). Onset often follows an upper respiratory tract infection, laryngeal injury, a period of excessive voice use, or either occupational or emotional stress (Ludlow, 1994).

Epidemiology

There is lack of agreement regarding onset of symptoms, as well as of sex ratio, age, ethnic group, genetic disposition or health histories (Izdebski, 1993).

Symptomatology

There is a plethora of terms to describe adductor spasmodic dysphonia, although there is universal agreement that the strain-strangled voice quality is present in adductor SD. Controversies prevail regarding physiological correlates, or the mechanisms responsible for symptom generation, and what constitute primary, as opposed to compensatory, symptoms.

Asymptomatic vocal behaviour

Many patients can use their voices normally in some situations, possibly a reflection of the task-specific nature of dystonia. There are many reports that patients with adductor SD have been observed to produce a normal laugh, to sing, to whisper or produce normal voice in the falsetto register. Moments of improved speech are noted in joy or anger states, ingressive speech, following yawning, in non-speech vocalization, and during paralinguistic utterances such as 'uh-uh'. Some authors find symptoms to be more severe in loud than in soft phonation and to be exacerbated when the patient is under stress (Bloch 1965; Blitzer et al., 1988; Izdebski, 1993). In some patients, spasmodic movements extend beyond the larynx into the hypopharynx and oropharynx (McCall et al., 1971; Parnes et al., 1978), into the oral cavity, (McCall et al., 1971) and may occur even during respiration as well as speaking (McCall et al., 1971; Parnes et al., 1978; Salassa et al., 1982).

The mechanism of dystonia

The patterns of abnormal muscle activity in spasmodic dysphonia reflect patterns seen in other types of dystonia. The amplitude, timing and co-ordination of contraction of groups of muscles are affected, and the pattern suggests faulty co-ordination of afferent and efferent signals, possibly in the basal ganglia. The basal ganglia are thought to be responsible for automatic execution of motor programmes, and influence the weighting and timing of movements. Excessive muscle activation can be generated if there is an imbalance in the timing, or reduced reaction to incoming sensory signals. This theory may explain why simple functions may be spared, while specific and more complex motor programmes are impaired. In adductor spasmodic dysphonia, the primary overactivity is of the vocalis adductor complex. It is thought that the brain may misread the adductor state of the glottis and respond with inappropriate, sudden efferent discharges. Many of the other features could be compensatory and involve cortical adjustment (Brookes, 1995).

Voice characteristics of spasmodic dysphonia

According to Freeman and Ushijama (1978), the main diagnostic distinction between the different forms of SD lies in the behaviour of the vocal cords such as hyperadduction, hyperabduction or the presence of a benign vocal tremor, together with the different possible aetiologies. Blitzer et al. (1988) distinguish between adductor and abductor SD using the following definitions:

Adductor spasmodic dysphonia

In adductor spasmodic dysphonia, patients have intermittent choked, strain-strangled voice quality with abrupt initiation and termination of voicing, resulting in uncontrolled short breaks in phonation, or changes in pitch. Ludlow et al. (1988) viewed the strain-strangled component as the primary component (as in action dystonia), where there are subjective signs of vocal 'spasms', with primary arrests which are glottal-like on adduction of the vocal cords, and aspirate on abduction. Other vocal features noted are hoarseness; breathlessness or air waste; irregular vibrations; amplitude variations; turbulence; noise; glottal fry and tremor. As a result of the over-adduction of the vocal cords, other parameters affect speech flow, demonstrated by changes in mean air flow rates, mean phonation time, maximum phonation time, pause time, percentage of voice and unvoiced time, subglottal air pressure, glottal resistance and laryngeal resistance.

Physiological behaviour of adductor SD

Ludlow et al. (1988) point out that in adductor SD, groups of muscles are impaired, rather than peripheral nerve organization. Adductor SD is found primarily to affect the action of the thyroarytenoid (TA) and the interarytenoids in the vocalis complex. Much controversy surrounds the explanation for the physiological correlates of the above symptoms. Some authors describe the vocal arrests and strain as being generated by the hyperadduction of the true and ventricular folds (Ginsberg et al., 1988; Aronson, 1990). Others believe that approximation of the ventricular folds occurs only in severe cases, and/or may indicate phonatory compensation (Izdebski, 1993). Fibreoptic observations have shown rapid twitch-like movements of the vocal folds, with forceful spasm-like jerking of the vocal folds and oscillations of the arytenoids. Forceful rapid jerking spasms have been noted in the velum as well as in the superior pharynx and tongue. Abnormal movements may be evident during quiet respiration, and these are exacerbated during phonation (McCall et al., 1971).

Electromyography (EMG) is used for muscle location in the diagnosis of SD. Blitzer et al. (1985) and Ludlow et al. (1986), using EMG, have shown that minimum and maximum peak activation levels in both the thyroarytenoid (TA) and cricothyroid (CT) muscles are significantly increased during normal respiration, as well as in phonation. They noted abnormal resting EMG levels in the thyroarytenoid and the cricothyroid muscles, with an imbalance between these muscles, possibly causing excessive adduction and shortening of the vocal folds during phonation, resulting in strain, overcome by increases in subglottic air pressure. In many patients, hyperfunction of the extrinsic muscles causing laryngeal tremor is also found (Rosenfield et al., 1990; Woodson et al., 1991; Zwirner et al., 1991, 1992). Finitzo and Freeman (1989), Freeman et al. (1984), and Ford et al. (1990) reported that transglottic airflow can also be reduced in many SD patients. Quantitative measures of EMG amplitude for thyroarytenoid activity have demonstrated that laryngospasms are specific to phonated speech (Freeman et al., 1984; Ford et al., 1990). Only complex rapid sequential movements are impaired. Simple laryngeal movement initiation is not delayed. Although it is not possible to judge SD on vocal output alone, Cannito (1989) compared SD speakers to matched normal controls on clinical ratings of oral-facial motor and extralaryngeal motor tasks and found that motor function was most affected in the tongue, labiofacial and velar structures of the SD speakers.

Abductor spasmodic dysphonia

Blitzer and Brin (1991) describe abductor spasmodic dysphonia as a whispering weak breathy effortful voice quality, particularly on voice onset with abrupt termination of voicing, resulting in aphonic, whispered segments of speech. Additionally, there are abnormal involuntary contractions of the posterior cricoarytenoid muscles resulting in sustained abduction of the vocal cords. Cannito (1989) found the diadochokinetic rates differed between adductor and abductor SD, with the latter having slower articulation time.

Compensatory modes

According to Schaefer (1983), many patients with SD developed compensatory modes of speaking, which tended to mask underlying phonatory symptoms. Inspiratory speech, whispered speech, high-pitched voice, breathy voice and glottal fry phonation were among the compensatory voices adopted by patients in his study. In many cases, it was difficult to differentiate between the compensatory strategies and the vocal symptoms of the disorder. The overall quality of each patient's voice was dependent on (a) the type of spasm, (b) the frequency, intensity and duration of spasm, and (c) the compensatory strategy adopted.

Strain-strangled quality, hoarseness, breathiness, inappropriate pitch, vocal tremor and glottal fry were the most frequently noted abnormalities. In addition to laryngeal spasms, abnormal respiratory inspirations during speech were noted. Abductor SD patients required frequent inspiration as so much air was wasted during spasms. The adductor SD patients appeared to use quick inspirations as a means of terminating the adductor spasms of long duration or pronounced intensity. Patients may use these manoeuvres to compensate or mask spasmodic dysphonia, and it can be difficult to distinguish between compensatory strategies and the primary vocal symptoms.

Degrees of severity

According to Aronson (1990), the common denominator underlying all types of adductor spasmodic dysphonia is adductor laryngospasms. The degree and frequency of adductor laryngospasms vary. The following have been observed during videofluoroscopy and videofibreoptic laryngoscopy, (McCall et al., 1971; Parnes et al., 1978) and provide a useful framework for delineating the degree of disorder:

1. *Mild:* In mild adductor SD there are adductor spasms of the true vocal cords only. Hyperadduction of the true vocal folds alone occurs in mild cases.
2. *Moderate to severe:* In moderate to severe cases, there are adductor spasms of both true and false vocal folds. There is closure of the false or ventricular folds which obscure the true vocal folds.
3. *Severe:* In severe adductor SD, there is strained voice or voice arrests, with supraglottic constriction, including the inferior pharyngeal constrictor just above the level of the false vocal folds. The more severe the adductor laryngospasms, the greater the vertical extent of intrinsic muscle participation. Constriction progresses superiorly from the true vocal folds to involve the ventricular folds and the pharyngeal constrictors. Severe laryngospasms are accompanied by synchronous movements of the entire larynx, involving the strap muscles responsible for moving the body of the larynx. Aronson (1990) points out the neuroanatomic implications, in that not only the Xth nerve, innervating the intrinsic laryngeal muscles, but also the IXth nerve to the pharynx and the cervical spine nerves to the extrinsic laryngeal muscles transmit nerve impulses, must be responsible for spasm.

Overview: one disorder or many?

In view of the disparities in symptomatology, aetiology, epidemiology and pathology, the question often posed is whether spasmodic dysphonia is one disorder or many. Izdebski (1993) argues that the symptoms in SD are not vague, random, disorganized, enigmatic or haphazard, but rather predictable and systematic. He claims that the symptoms can be explained by the physiological rules governing production of phonation. Izdebski states that SD symptoms are 'phonotopically organized' and provides a physiological model symptomatology to support this claim. The model is based on the notion that over-pressured phonation is generated because of faulty afferent-efferent motor control of the larynx in phonation (but not in vegetative tasks). This is thought to be due to faulty reaction of neuronal pools in the basal ganglia, to arriving sensory signals resulting in excessive adductor forces applied to the vocal folds. Other symptoms that occur are compensatory in nature, coexisting with the underlying over-pressure feature. In this model, it is evident that SD is a uniquely organized disorder.

The assessment of spasmodic dysphonia: differential diagnosis

Otolaryngological investigation

As Ludlow (1994) observes, the diagnosis of vocal fold movement disorders depends on observation of the vocal folds during a wide variety of movements. The larynx must be visualized by an otolaryngologist, to rule out other disorders that could account for the symptoms. Fibreoptic nasolaryngoscopy enables the voice team to rule out laryngeal lesions (vocal fold nodules, polyps, carcinoma, cysts, contact ulcers) or inflammation and vocal fold paralysis.

The otolaryngologist conducts a full laryngological examination, which will include indirect laryngoscopy and rigid laryngoscopy, to view the vocal folds at rest and during phonation. However symptoms are not always present during these activities in SD. Fibreoptic nasolaryngoscopy allows extensive observation and videotaping during a variety of tasks. The symmetry, range, speed and control of vocal fold adduction and abduction can be observed during non-speech tasks (at rest, quiet breathing, sniffing, throat clearing, coughing, breath holding, whistling, laughing), as well as in a wide variety of speech tasks, ranging from the production of vowels, voiceless consonants, voiced consonants in words and connected speech, where symptoms become evident particularly in connected speech and in all voiced sentences (Brookes, 1995).

Neurological examination

The neurologist conducts a full neurological examination, including a medical and social history, to establish the neurological status of the patient and exclude neurological diseases which can produce vocal cord abnormality.

The neurological examination is carried out to exclude motor neurone disease (amyotrophic lateral sclerosis), where a reduction in movement, range or speed involving one or both vocal folds should be consistent across tasks, regardless of whether or not the tasks are volitional, emotional or reflexive in content (Hartman and von Cramon, 1984).

Parkinson's disease, supranuclear palsies, multiple system atrophy or Shy-Drager syndrome can all present in reduced range of adduction and abduction of the vocal folds on all tasks (Aronson and Hartman, 1981; Hartman and Aronson, 1981; Hanson et al., 1983; Hartman 1984; Bassich and Ludlow, 1986; Ludlow 1994). Some degree of laryngeal tremor may co-exist with the hyperadduction and hyperabduction of the vocal folds. These are usually included as a subtype of laryngeal dystonia. Aronson et al. (1968b) found that in 31 patients with SD, 58% had a voice tremor in contextual speech, and 71% had tremor on vowel prolongation.

Many centres perform routine laboratory tests such as chest X-ray, blood count, sedimentation rate, biochemistry screen and copper screen, although these are unlikely to be abnormal unless the clinician suspects an underlying disorder.

Psychiatric assessment

A psychiatric assessment may be needed if the above battery fails to establish an organic cause for spasmodic dysphonia. Examination for psychogenic dysphonia must include an extensive history and psycho-social interview. Aronson (1990) stresses the importance of the psychosocial interview in the diagnosis and treatment of all 'functional' voice disorders. Often patients may have developed secondary emotional or psychological reactions to having a communication disorder by the time of professional diagnosis, which confounds the clinician's ability to differentiate idiopathic spasmodic dysphonia from psychogenic conversion disorders through history and interview (Whurr and Moore, 1994). Many patients with SD report social withdrawal, avoidance of the telephone, or loss of occupation due to aberrant voice (Barnes, 1992). The main differentiating features between spasmodic dysphonia and psychogenic dysphonia, according to Aronson et al. (1968a), is the consistency of symptoms which are constant in SD, while in psychogenic disorder the symptoms are episodic.

In spite of the evidence supporting a neurological basis, there are patients with this vocal symptomatology where the basis is psychogenic (Aronson and De Santo, 1983). The patient with a psychogenic cause usually reports a sudden onset to the voice disorder, as well as periods of remission lasting days or weeks or months. In patients with psychogenic aetiology, it is possible to trigger voice free of the strained quality in voice testing (Stoicheff, 1991).

SD Associated with hyperfunctional voice disorders

The main difference in patients with hyperfunctional voice disorder and SD lies in the intermittent character of the strained voice and the more continuous straining quality of ventricular or hyperfunctional dysphonia. The strained quality is a function of muscular tension, rather than unexpected laryngospasms. Patients in this category frequently complain of throat pain, which is due to excessive muscular tension of the extrinsic muscles of the larynx, creating the constriction which produces the strained voice quality. Unlike patients with SD, patients with hyperfunctional symptoms respond well to voice therapy (Stoicheff, 1991).

Idiopathic spasmodic dysphonia

Aronson (1980) has summarized the characteristic features of idiopathic SD:

1. Presence of intermittent strained and/or strangled phonations and breaks in the voice;
2. no laryngeal lesions;
3. no abnormal speech signs in the rest of the peripheral speech mechanism;
4. brief periods of normal voicing during singing, laughter, shouting or anger;
5. resistance to treatment.

Speech and language therapist's assessment

The speech-language therapist's assessment usually includes a voice interview where the patient is asked to describe the onset, history and pattern of the vocal problems. A sample of a case history format is in Appendix 11.1. This is followed by an audio and video recorded voice protocol, later submitted for perceptual and objective analysis (Chevrie-Muller et al., 1987; Zwirner et al., 1992; Izdebski, 1993; Whurr et al., 1993; Ludlow, 1994; Whurr and Moore, 1994; Stewart et al., 1997).

Voice protocol

In the Whurr et al. (1993) study, the voice protocol commenced with the reading aloud of a passage ('The North Wind and the Sun') which was used for later acoustic analysis. The voice protocol included the investigation of a variety of vocal gestures, including vegetative function as in coughing and non-phonatory tasks, as in deep inspiration, and whisper, plus a wide variety of phonatory tasks which include pitch and volume alterations. The authors found, as did Izdebski (1993), that these tasks could generate adductor symptoms in a predictable and systematic fashion and demonstrate that symptoms occur predominantly in loud modal phonation or within approximately one to two octaves above the basal voice fundamental frequency (F_o) level. Symptoms diminish or are absent at high F_o levels and in whisper, regardless of loudness levels. An example of the voice protocol can be found in Appendix 11.2.

Other acoustic parameters may be investigated such as shimmer, jitter, signal to noise ratio, and a voice break factor, all of which are abnormal in spasmodic dysphonia as compared to controls (Zwirner et al., 1992).

Objective voice measures

There are no international standardized methods for voice evaluation. Hirano (1989) found from his study into the main methods of the investigation of laryngeal function that tests and examinations could be classified into nine major categories:

1. tests related to the aerodynamics and glottic efficiency;
2. tests related to fundamental frequency (F_o), sound pressure level (SPL) and vocal register;
3. tests related to vocal fold vibration;
4. acoustic analyses and perceptual evaluation;
5. visual inspection of the larynx;
6. x-ray and magnetic resonance imaging;
7. electromyography (EMG);
8. tests related to respiratory function;
9. audiometric tests.

Methods of voice assessment of spasmodic dysphonia have varied. Evaluation has commonly included subjective speech/video recordings. Ludlow et al. (1986) and Zwirner et al. (1991, 1992) included objective acoustic analysis of speech, using protocols which included the production of a sustained vowel, and reading aloud a sentence. They assessed the number of pitch and phonatory breaks, sentence duration and phonatory aperiodicity by spectrographic analysis. Zwirner et al. (1991) identified a Voice Break Factor (VBF) which is defined as the number of voice breaks, divided by the maximum phonation time.

Chevrie-Muller et al. (1987) highlight the need for acoustical and electrophysiological description of the symptoms in SD. They proposed the use of an instrumental method with simultaneous recording of the speech signal and electroglottograph (EGG). This is achieved by a two track magnetic recorder and later analysis of the oscillographic trace of both signals. The recorded materials used were:

(a) reading aloud a list of words, two sentences and a text of 175 words;
(b) spontaneous self-formulated speech;
(c) sustained vowels (/a/, /o/, /e/, /i/)

A computer method of analysis was used to determine measures of pitch, amplitude and duration. From this, Chevrie-Muller and colleagues (1987) discovered four objective cues:

1. Voice stoppages during phonemes of words. Most of these stoppages were longer than 4 seconds.
2. Irregular lengthening of acoustic and EGG waves. This kind of glottal aperiodicity was described as 'laryngealization' by Freeman et al. (1984), and is an indication of hypertonic modification of the vocal folds. These irregular acoustic waves exhibit a damped aspect.
3. The simultaneous lengthening of the EGG waves corresponding to a longer closed time in the glottal cycle.
4. Breathy phonation or glottal friction. This is attested by a non-periodic and high frequency acoustic component (aperiodic turbulence) superimposed on the acoustic periodic waves in vowels or voiced stops or replacing them. Simultaneously the EGG waves are of small amplitude or disappear. They claim these are objective signs of widening of the vocal folds during phonation with a decrease of the contact area of the vocal folds. Periodic variations of amplitude in sustained phonation. Periodic variations of amplitude were considered a cue for tremor.

These quantitative methods of assessment allow for the measurement of the degree of severity as well as providing a base line for the measure of improvement.

Other authors have insisted on the value of acoustic criteria using spectrographic analysis (Freeman et al., 1984). In the Whurr et al. (1993) study, the Visispeech analysis package (RNID) was used. The Visispeech analysis programme measures the fundamental frequency of the voice over the duration of an entire speech sample. The data are scaled into 85 'bins' or compartments, and measures of central tendency, variance and standard deviation are calculated. This measure can be taken as an indicator of regularity of pitch of voice; thus, a voice with many pitch breaks and variations in pitch has a high standard deviation value.

Perceptual voice ratings

According to Laver (1980), voices are described as the product of perceptually distinguishable components, and the articulatory, acoustic and physiological correlates of these components need to be specified. Perceptually, voice quality is an accumulative abstraction, which involves laryngeal and supralaryngeal features contributing to voice quality. Laver

(1980) provides a system applicable to normal vocal anatomy, based on the principles of phonetic analysis, to the description of voice quality (see Wirz, in Chapter 12, for examples). However, when attempting to apply perceptual analysis to disordered voice, the number of distinguishable components become reduced and thus less amenable to organized descriptive analysis.

For the clinician, the perceptual characteristics of voice disorders provide a useful tool when attempting to assess and diagnose spasmodic dysphonia. Specific perceptual descriptions of SD have ranged from concepts such as strain-strangled, squeezed, hoarse, choked, effortful, jerky, staccato, low-pitched, hostile sounding and laborious. Zwirner et al. (1992) demonstrated that in their study of the interaction of perceptual-acoustic relationships in SD, perceptual results were related to the standard deviation of fundamental frequency and the voice break factor, which is defined as the number of voice breaks divided by the maximum phonation time.

Izdebski (1993) employs a minimal diagnostic vocal test battery which includes sustained phonation at varied frequency and intensity levels, voice and voiceless speech tasks, modal, falsetto and whisper modes, as well as vegetative tasks.

A Unified Spasmodic Dysphonia Rating Scale (USDRS) is currently being standardized. Stewart et al.'s (1997) tests include reading aloud, picture description and various automatic voice and speech tasks. Raters have a seven-point scale corresponding to seventeen parameters including overall severity, rough voice quality, breathy voice quality, strain-strangled quality, abrupt voice initiation, voice arrests, aphonia, voice loudness, bursts of loudness, deviated pitch, atypical intonation, voice tremor, expiratory effort, speech rate, speech intelligibility reduced, and related movements and grimaces.

De Langen (1996), speculates about the motor-programming systems in SD and distinguishes between propositional and non-propositional speech. He examines spontaneous speech, diadochokinesis, vowel prolongation, repetition, voicing start, voice quality, fundamental frequency-intensity profile, contrastive stress, sentence stress, speech respiration, posture of head and trunk, mobility of jaw, lips and tongue, motility in chewing and swallowing. Additional tasks are completion of word pairs, antonyms, proverbs and sentences. De Langen (1996) concluded in a single case study that SD is restricted to propositional speech. He further states that phonation in propositional expressions involves endo-evoked movements, which imply a considerable participation of the projectional system in the central nervous system, including the basal ganglia and supplementary motor area (SMA).

Video recording

Video recordings of patients provide an invaluable record of the before and after treatment status of the patient. A video recording provides an excellent overall impression of the patient's facial expression, as well as any concomitant movements associated with dystonia, such as grimacing, tics, tremor, external laryngeal movements and other intrusions which may distort speech production. Most centres use video recordings as part of their assessment protocol.

Psychosocial assessment

Whurr et al. (1998) assessed patients before and after treatment on three self-report inventories to evaluate attitude and mood. The assessments were the Beck Depression Inventory (BDI: Beck, 1970), which has been employed in epidemiological research and has significant correlations with anxiety. The Crown and Crisp Experiential Index (CCEI: Crown and Crisp, 1966) provides scores on six scales: anxiety, phobic, obsessional, pychosomatic, depression and hysteria. The Mood Adjective Check List (MACL: McNair and Lorr, 1964) is a self-report questionnaire with 24 mood-associated adjectives rated on a four-point ordinal scale.

Overview: the multidisciplinary team provide improved diagnosis

The evaluation and consequent differential diagnosis requires the co-operative efforts of the multidisciplinary team. Assessment involves the combination of subjective observation, perceptual and objective measures utilizing instrumentation and clinical judgement. The speech and language therapist's role is described in Appendix 11.3.

Although the aetiology of spasmodic dysphonia is still unclear, and the pathophysiology still needs objective quantification, the methods available for assessment and diagnosis are constantly improving. They are dependent on a multidisciplinary approach, with the use of both instrumentation and acoustic analysis, to provide objective information to complement skilled clinical judgement. It is essential to include perceptual voice ratings as well as objective measures to identify idiopathic adductor and abductor spasmodic dysphonia.

Dedo and Izdebski (1983) have indicated that a major problem with SD is misdiagnosis. It is often confused with disorders that present with similar symptoms. Salassa et al. (1982) urged clinicians to use spasmodic dysphonia as a 'voice sign' rather than a diagnosis and look at the total symptomatology for a differential diagnosis.

The treatment of spasmodic dysphonia

Previous methods of treatment

As yet there is no known cure for laryngeal dystonia. Approximately 5% of other forms of idiopathic dystonia may show spontaneous improvement or go into complete remission (Marsden and Quinn 1990).

Non-medical treatment

In the past, most patients with dystonia were referred to psychiatrists; clinical management was therefore directed along psychological lines. With few exceptions, treatment with psychotherapy, hypnotism, acupuncture, homeopathy and biofeedback relaxation techniques proved to be unsuccessful (Levine et al., 1979). Moreover, the majority of evaluations of these types of treatment were anecdotal in nature.

Voice therapy

Stoicheff (1991) reported techniques that were directed towards decreasing vocal cord contact. Therapy for two patients was directed towards slight elevation of pitch level, vocal loudness and easy voice onsets combined with 'light' voice. These techniques helped to alleviate the symptoms, but improvement was not sustained.

Surgical treatment

Early surgical approaches included transsection of laryngeal muscles, and excision of the posterior part of the false cord and lateral fixation of the arytenoid (Segre, 1951). The rationale was to induce scar tissue lateral to the vocal cord or fibrosis of the cricoarytenoid joint on one side. In 1976, Dedo introduced the operation of unilateral recurrent laryngeal nerve resection. It was thought that unilateral vocal fold paralysis would result in compensation, due to the strong adductive forces in the unparalysed contralateral side. Laryngeal nerve resection provided initial relief, but relapses were common. Long-term results were disappointing, with reports in some cases of symptoms being made worse (Aronson and De Santo, 1983). The cause for the relapse was thought to be due to the hyperadduction of the non-denervated cord, with exaggeration of the dystonic spasms or reinnervation on the surgical side (Brin et al., 1989; Fritzell et al., 1982). Other forms of surgery have included recurrent laryngeal nerve crush, arytenoid replacement, laser therapy, spinal cord stimulation, and even thalamotomy, all with no benefit or only transient effects (Brookes, 1995).

Pharmacological treatment

Pharmacological intervention has included the use of anticholinergics, benzodiazepines, baclofen and carbamazepine. Only mild benefit from clonazepam and anticholinergics has been reported (Brin et al., 1989). Although levodopa preparations or anticholinergic drugs such as benzhexol have a therapeutic role in some patients with more generalized dystonia, they are more likely to be efficacious with the young, but not older patients. Unfortunately, focal laryngeal dystonia that usually commences in middle age either does not respond to these drugs, or they cause intolerable side effects (Brookes, 1995).

Treatment with botulinum toxin

Botulinum toxin acts presynaptically to block calcium dependent release of acetylcholine. When injected in low doses, the toxin causes local weakness in the muscle into which it is injected. This eliminates the abnormal muscle contractions, while preserving functional ability. The effect of the toxin is temporary, due to re-sprouting of axons which form the new neuro-muscular junction. Botulinum toxin has been used in the treatment of certain focal dystonias for several years. (For further information about botulinum toxin see Appendix 11.4).

The initial use of local injections of Type A botulinum toxin was for the treatment of strabismus (Scott, 1981). The intention was to block certain neuromuscular junctions and thus rebalance neural input to the rectus muscle in an effort to enhance convergence. This therapy proved to be very effective, and since then local injections of botulinum toxin have been used for many focal dystonias with dramatic improvements (Elston 1988; Marsden and Quinn, 1990). The promising results of botulinum toxin injections in the treatment of dystonia, combined with the acceptance of the neurological aetiology of spasmodic dysphonia, led to a change of direction in the treatment of adductor spasmodic dysphonia.

Blitzer et al. (1985) were the first group to inject toxin into the vocalis muscle complex. Blitzer and his colleagues had acquired considerable clinical experience in performing percutaneous laryngeal EMG of the vocalis muscle, and it was therefore a relatively straightforward transition to inject toxin through a hollow monopolar needle electrode under EMG control. The rationale was not to paralyse the muscle, but to induce sufficient weakness to abolish the tonic spasm. Although the toxin is injected into the thyroarytenoid muscle, there is probably some migration to the lateral cricoarytenoid muscle which is in close proximity and is a strong adductor of the cord (Brookes, 1995). Since 1985, this group has published several accounts of their technique and results (Blitzer et al., 1988; Brin et al., 1989; Blitzer et al., 1992).

Troung et al. (1991) have since validated the efficacy of botulinum toxin in the treatment of adductor spasmodic dysphonia, by a double blind controlled study. A significant improvement was noted in the toxin treated patients compared to the placebo group receiving saline only. The use of botulinum toxin A in the treatment of spasmodic dysphonia has been tested in several centres internationally since 1986 and is now considered to be the treatment of choice.

A systematic review of the published research on the use of botulinum toxin treatment for spasmodic dysphonia was carried out to provide a summary and synthesis of this method of treatment (Whurr et al., 1997). A total of 26 studies that had been published since 1985 were identified. All the studies reported improvements in patients' voice quality after treatment with botulinum toxin. The treatment took an average of four days to take effect, with an average duration of vocal benefits of 10 weeks. Transient mild side effects, consisting of mild dysphagia on liquids and breathy voice or hypophonia (mean duration of 10 days) were reported. The evidence shows that botulinum toxin treatment improved vocal symptoms in all the studies (Whurr et al., 1997) and demonstrates that in both the USA and UK, botulinum toxin is the treatment of choice for SD. In a meta-analytic study providing a 'best synthesis' systematic summary of existing research, the average treated SD patient in the 22 studies subjected to meta-analysis obtained 97% improvement as a result of treatment with botulinum toxin (Whurr et al., 1998).

There is a difference between the potency of the American botulinum toxin 'A' produced by Allergan and the UK botulinum toxin 'A' produced by Ipsen Pharmaceuticals. The differences are outlined in Appendix 11.4.

Methods of evaluation

The methods of evaluation of the results on vocal quality after botulinum toxin treatment have varied. These have included the otolaryngologist's examination with fibreoptic laryngoscopy to view vocal fold vibration (Brookes, 1995), tests of aerodynamic and glottic efficiency measures of intrathoracic pressure; Valsalva manoeuvres (Miller et al., 1987); the neurophysiologist's EMG investigations, and the neurologist's x-ray and magnetic resonance imaging (MRI). The speech and language therapist's evaluation of results has commonly included subjective ratings of speech/audio recordings, as well as perceptual and acoustic analysis (Ludlow et al., 1988; Zwirner et al., 1991; Whurr et al., 1993). Acoustic analysis of speech may include the measures of the standard deviation of fundamental frequency (Fo); sound pressure levels (SPL); vocal register; jitter and shimmer. Other subjective methods have included the use of patients' diaries (Blitzer and Brin, 1991; Whurr et al., 1993).

Results of botulinum toxin treatment

Botulinum toxin was used to inject 31 patients who had adductor spasmodic dysphonia (Whurr et al., 1993). Injections of 3.00–3.75 units of botulinum toxin were performed bilaterally into the thyroarytenoid muscle. The treatment significantly decreased the standard deviation of the fundamental frequency of the speech sample, indicating a reduction in the variability of pitch among patients. A total of 96% of patients' subjective diary reports showed an improvement with a median of 7-day to peak effect and a 5-week duration of peak effect. Only 25% of patients reported any negative side effects; these were transitory in nature. Only one of the 31 patients failed to gain an improvement following initial injection. In this report, only data pertaining to the effects of the first injection have been analysed. All patients received follow-up injections. The majority of treated patients derived the most dramatic effect after the first injection of botulinum toxin. Most patients require subsequent multiple injections at varying intervals, to maintain spasm free voice.

Initially the volume of fluid injected into each thyroarytenoid muscle was 0.15 mls. To avoid complications of localized submucosal oedema, the volume of toxin/saline was reduced, changing the concentration of toxin; Brookes (1995) found that patients receiving lower volume injections had fewer side effects of shorter duration. The duration of benefit also increased with this modification.

The maintenance schedule varied between 2.5 UK mouse units into one cord and 3.75 UK mouse units injected bilaterally. The titration was adjusted to each patient's needs (Whurr et al., 1993; Brookes, 1995).

Injection technique

Although the treatment of adductor laryngeal dystonia is usually straightforward, on occasions injections do not achieve 'ideal' results. Brookes (1995) suggests that the reasons for 'not ideal' injections may be due to:

1. local anatomical difficulties (size or shape of larynx);
2. movements such as swallowing at time of injection;
3. obtaining a satisfactory EMG signal;
4. operator 'learning curve'.

Vocal change post injection

The pattern of vocal change post injection involves three stages (Whurr et al., 1998) which are as follows:

Stage 1: 1–10 days post injection

Reduced adduction of the vocal cords
Hypophonia
Breathy voice
Dysphonia
Lack of pitch control
Mild breathlessness
Mild dysphagia on liquids

Stage 2: 2–10 weeks post injection

Gentle adduction of the anterior two-thirds of the vocal cords
Fewer spasms and increased smoothness on phonation
Fewer concomitant movements of the neck and pharynx
More pitch control
Improved respiratory control
Aerodynamic stability
Improved respiratory and phonatory co-ordination

Stage 3: 10 weeks plus post injection

Increase in number of spasms
Less variability in pitch
Less adductive pressure-Bernouilli effect
Some voice onset mistiming and overadduction, but less forceful than
   pre-injection
Reduced volume
Mild ingressive phonation

Pitch related changes were typically on medium volume, high pitch, high pitch/light volume and monopitch. Problems were noted on loud volume and low pitch with increasing return of spasms. At this stage, patients should consider re-injections.

Psychosocial aspects

Therapy with botulinum toxin has enabled patients with spasmodic dysphonia to use their voice effortlessly and to communicate easily, in some instances for the first time for many years, with very few and temporary side effects. Although it has provided many patients with an irreplaceable communication lifeline, the fact remains that many still continue to suffer the psychological consequences of their condition. A study of the psychosocial factors in 60 laryngeal dystonia patients, pre-treatment and six months following treatment, using three psychosocial profiles, demonstrated that patients were more depressed and anxious than controls. Although patients were less anxious after treatment, their degree of depression was unchanged (Whurr et al., 1998). This may be due to the realization that their condition cannot be cured, although it is alleviated by treatment. However, reports of depression and mood of patients with other forms of dystonia, pre- and post-treatment with botulinum toxin, demonstrate an upswing in the depression rating scales after treatment.

Patients with laryngeal dystonia who suffer a disrupted communication system may require considerably more help and counselling after treatment to offset their fear of communication failure. Understanding the concept of stigma is important in understanding the social dynamics and social construction of illness. A study examining the presence, the dimensions and the degree of stigma in patients with spasmodic dysphonia identified that the majority of patients felt some or severe stigma. Stigma was found to affect the patient's social, private and working life. As stigma is part of the experience of patients with SD, clinicians have to address it in everyday clinical practice, as a relevant parameter in the overall management of patients with SD (Papathanasiou et al., 1997). This support is usually provided by the speech and language therapist, but patients themselves have set up self-help groups in the USA and Europe. An invaluable source of information and help is the Dystonia Society, in the UK, and the Spasmodic Dysphonia Society, in the USA. These societies run telephone helplines, as well as supplying up-to-date information on all aspects of the disorder. Most patients value the enormous amount of support provided by these societies and appreciate being told about them.

Overview of botulinum toxin treatment: the evidence?

There are widespread reports of the beneficial effects of botulinum toxin treatment of adductor and abductor spasmodic dysphonia. There are differences in the reported techniques such as those used in the UK and USA including: the methods of storage, volume, concentration and potency of the toxin; the dosage, dilution, concentration and volume of the fluid used; the side, site and method of injection, which could be percutaneous or perioral; the type of needle used and whether administration is accompanied by EMG support and local anaesthetic. The composition of the assessment team, such as laryngologist, neurologist, neurophysiologist, speech and language therapist, varies. The methods of assessment, evaluation of results and rating scales for side effects and beneficial effects also differ; see Whurr et al. (1998) for a meta-analysis.

Long-term effects?

There are still many unanswered questions about the use of botulinum toxin, particularly in relation to the long-term effects of multiple injections. The long-term effects on muscle physiology are not yet known, nor the potential long-term complications of injecting potent toxins into the body. Botulinum toxin appears to affect the autonomic system and there has been evidence of cardiac effect in animal experiments. Garfield Davies et al. (1989) drew attention to the risk of developing anaphylactic shock after multiple injections. Patients with already impaired neuromuscular transmission may be supersensitive to the effects of other drugs which interfere with neuromuscular transmission, such as certain antibiotics and anaesthetics (Argov and Mastaglia, 1979). The mechanism of spread of the toxin is unknown, but is presumed to be vascular (Lange et al., 1988). Also, the human thyroarytenoid muscle has a diffuse distribution of motor endplates (Rosen et al., 1983). Age is found to be an important factor in determining normality of motor units during ageing. How this affects the responses of the neuromuscular junction to botulinum toxin remains to be elucidated.

The temporary nature of the effect of the injection, due to axonal sprouting whereby new neuromuscular junctions are formed, makes long-term use of botulinum toxin treatment questionable. There is a need for further research into an anti-sprouting factor, which could be injected into the treated weakened muscle to maintain the status of the muscle.

It is too early to know whether patients will become refractory to this form of therapy. There is no evidence to date that the formation of toxin antibodies may occur, although it has been documented in some other forms of treated dystonias. There is an urgent need for the establishment of more treatment centres in the UK and Europe, so that deserving patients may benefit from this innovative advance in the treatment of a previously intractable condition.

Although botulinum toxin is one of the most poisonous substances known to man, it is now a therapeutic agent, an ally rather than an adversary. The use of botulinum toxin is said to be one of the major advances in the pharmacological treatment of neurological disorders and has provided symptom relief for a considerable number of patients with spasmodic dysphonia.

Appendix 11.1 Sample case history

Onset:

When did the problem with your voice start?
How did it start?
Did you notice your voice change or did someone else?
Have you had any problems with your voice before?
At school or as an adolescent?
When is your voice at its worst?
Does anything make your voice better?
Does it make any difference who you speak to?
When you speak?
Any situations worse or better?
Do you avoid doing anything since you have had problems with your voice?
Do you use the telephone?

Social history:

What is your job?
Has your voice problem made any difference to you at work or at home?

Duration:

How long have you had this voice problem?

Family history:

Is there anyone in the family with a voice problem?
Is there anyone in the family with a neurological problem?

Description of symptoms:

How would you describe your voice?
Is it an effort to speak?
Can you point to where you feel the effort?
Have you noticed any shaking or tremor of your hands or any other part of your body?

Past history:

Have you had any illnesses in the past?
Have you had any shocks, upsets or traumas in the past?

Action:

What did you do when you first noticed problems with your voice?
What did you do after you saw your GP?
Then what did you do?
What treatment have you had for your voice?
Has anything helped you ?

Background information:

Has the word dystonia been mentioned to you?
Have you heard of the term spasmodic dysphonia?
Who mentioned it to you?
Have you had a diagnosis for your condition?
Has anyone mentioned treatment by some form of injection?
Has the phrase botulinum toxin treatment been mentioned to you?

Appendix 11.2 Spasmodic dysphonia voice assessment protocol

Using video recording and audio recording:

Task	SLT's assessment
1. Reading aloud: 'The North Wind and the Sun'	Check for impressions of pitch breaks, phonatory breaks, tremor, breathy voice, creak, harshness, prolongation of vowels, respiratory function, diaphragmatic movements and facial expression
2. Cough	Check whether throat feels cleared. If not ask about any swallowing problems
3. Breathe in and out	Note shoulder position and diaphragm movements
4. Sigh inwards and outwards.	Note sound quality in both conditions
5. Whisper counting from 1–5.	Note sound quality
6. Hum aloud on 'MMM' and hold the hum	Note breaks, consistency and tremor
7. Say /a/ on a low-pitched voice	Note pitch breaks, phonatory breaks, tremor
8. Say /a/ on a high-pitched voice	Note pitch breaks, phonatory breaks, tremor
9. Glide up the scale on /a/	Note pitch breaks, phonatory breaks, tremor
10. Glide down the scale on /a/	Note pitch breaks, phonatory breaks, tremor

11. Alternate your pitch, making your voice high and then low on /a/	Note pitch breaks, phonatory breaks, tremor
12. Alternate your pitch, making your voice low and then high on /a/	Note pitch breaks, phonatory breaks, tremor
13. Count aloud from 1 to 10 alternating your pitch. Start with a low-pitched number '1' and high-pitched number '2' and continue.	Note pitch breaks, phonatory breaks, tremor
14. Imagine you are out in the street and you want to hail a taxi. Shout 'Taxi'	Note volume, pitch breaks, phonatory breaks, tremor

Appendix 11.3 The speech and language therapist's new role in the assessment, diagnosis and treatment of spasmodic dysphonia

The speech and language therapist plays an increasingly important role as a member and co-ordinator of a multidisciplinary team. The role has expanded from one of unilateral diagnosis, assessment and treatment to that of specialist clinical team co-ordinator of all aspects of assessment, diagnosis, treatment and management of patients with laryngeal dystonia.

A. Assessment and diagnosis

1 The speech and language therapist undertakes the initial case history interview (see Appendix 11.1).
2. The speech and language therapist is also responsible for baseline audio and video tape recordings, using the specific voice protocol covering many different laryngeal gestures. A sample voice protocol is provided in Appendix 11.2.
3. The tape recording can be used for subsequent acoustic analysis.
4. The speech and language therapist is involved in the examinations by the laryngologist, neurologist and neurophysiologist, and can co-ordinate the opinions and facilitate an agreed diagnosis.
5. The speech and language therapist explains to the patient the reasons for each part of the examinations and procedures and acts as a link between the specialist departments and the patient.
6. The speech and language therapist also may explain the background to the condition, introduce the patient to the Dystonia Society leaflets and provide a Question and Answer leaflet about SD, which is given to the patient prior to treatment.

B. Treatment and management

7. The speech and language therapist can explain to the patient the nature of the treatment, including the fact that the injections are not a cure but will help to alleviate the condition for up to three months at a time. It is important that the patient feels informed and that he or she has a choice to accept, reject or postpone the treatment until feeling completely sure about it.

8. The speech and language therapist explains the post-treatment side effects. The patient should expect to have a breathy voice for ten days. The patient should avoid drinking liquids quickly for the first 24 hours after treatment.

9. The speech and language therapist should introduce the patient to another SD patient undergoing treatment. This can be done at the clinic and the patients should be given a quiet room for this purpose.

10. The speech and language therapist shows the patient where and how the injections take place.

11. The patient is given details of the speech and language therapist's hospital/clinic telephone number, which should be on an answerphone. The patient should telephone three days after injection and leave a voice message. However, if there is a problem, the patient should be given a contact number to request the therapist to telephone the patient before this; most problems can be handled by explanation on the telephone. The speech and language therapist has a trained ear and is the best person to interpret SD voices.

12. The speech and language therapist should ask the patient to keep a voice diary, particularly after the first injection, as reactions are idiosyncratic in spite of patients receiving the same baseline dose and site of injection.

13. Follow-up liaison is conducted on the telephone. The patient decides when he or she requires re-injection.

14. When patients attend the clinic for re-treatment, they should complete a questionnaire that asks questions about the results of the last injection. This helps the otolaryngologist decide on the best dose for the next injection. This is always discussed with the patient.

C. Post-injection voice therapy

15. The speech and language therapist is in a good position to advise on specific exercises for certain patients, particularly professional voice users. The course of exercises requires about six sessions of instruction, with regular follow-ups. Patients should be informed about the

mechanics of normal voice production and the changes in the vocal folds as a result of the treatment. Exercises should incorporate techniques for efficient respiratory support, accurate voicing and some pressure exercises to aid gentle vocal cord adduction during the hypophonic period ten days post-injection. This should be followed by general voice production and efficiency techniques, focused voice projection and accurate articulation. For many patients, it may not be convenient to attend the specialist centre for voice exercises and they may prefer to receive voice therapy locally. In such cases the specialist SALT can liaise with the local speech and language therapy services.

Appendix 11.4 Botulinum toxin

Botulinum toxin is a term used to describe at least eight different biological substances which have a common origin, structure and pharmacological activity. Although these substances are antigenically distinct, they have three features in common:

1. they are synthesized by the same species of bacterium;
2. they possess similar structure and molecular weights;
3. they block acetylcholine release from cholinergic nerve endings.

The seven antigenically distinct toxins have been identified (types A, B, C, D, E, F and G) (Simpson, 1981).

Botulinum toxin acts pre-synaptically to block calcium dependent release of acetylcholine. When injected in low doses the toxin causes weakness in the muscle into which it is injected. This eliminates the abnormal muscle contractions while preserving functional ability. The effect of the toxin is temporary due to the re-sprouting of axons which form the new neuro-muscular junctions.

British botulinum toxin is a purified form of type A. It is a freeze-dried preparation manufactured in the UK by Porton Products under the name of Dysport (TM), Ipsen Pharmaceuticals. The American equivalent is manufactured in the USA by Allergan International and marketed as Botox (TM), originally marketed as Oculinum. Although both products are standardized using a similar LD50 biological assay, the potency of the two products differs. The molecular weight of Dysport is 150 K. The crystalline form in the USA product is combined with haemagglutinin to give a molecular weight of about 900 K. The latter may be needed in large amounts to produce the same effect, as haemagglutinin may bind to non-neural sugar residue. Due to a larger molecule, the crystalline toxin may be more potentially antigenic.

Potency

Potency differences between the two commercially available toxins have been noted by various researchers (Jankovic and Brin, 1991). These differences have been estimated to be the ratio of 3 units of Botox = 1 unit of Dysport for laryngeal muscle (Whurr et al., 1998) and 3–1 for blepharospasm (Marion et al., 1995). A 5–1 ratio has been recorded for use in larger muscles (Sampaio et al., 1997). Jankovic and Brin (1991) state that a higher incidence of side effects has been reported when using the British toxin, Dysport, compared with the American toxin, Botox. They suggest this may be accounted for by the higher potency of Dysport compared with Botox (1 nanogram of Dysport contains 40 units whereas 1 nanogram of Botox contains 2.5 units, where a 'unit' is a standard measure of potency of commercially available toxin).

Both Allergan and Porton products use the LD50 Biological assay in the preparation of the toxin.

Preparation and dosage

The toxin Clostridium Botulinum Type A (Dysport) is obtained from Ipsen Pharmaceuticals as a freeze-dried toxin haemagglutinin preparation. Each vial contains 50 nanograms which is equivalent to 2000 UK mouse units. The toxin vial is first diluted in 10 mls of sterile normal saline. Then 1 ml of this solution is taken and diluted further into a concentration of 50 mouse units per ml.

CHAPTER 12

Managing voice with deaf and hearing impaired speakers

SHEILA WIRZ

Introduction

To be invited to rework a chapter written originally 12 years ago forces the author to reread the work in detail and to suffer a déja vu experience which is not altogether pleasant. For example, the title 'Deaf Voice', as used in the first and second editions of this book sounds very dated and in many ways, pejorative. Changes in thinking about whether 'normal' features exist and whether normalcy is the goal of deaf people, have raised therapists' awareness as to the sensitivity of labels such as 'deaf voice'. In reworking this chapter I am persuaded that there is some value in describing a technique for the perceptual analysis of deaf voice, but that the use of such a technique by therapists has changed considerably over the past 12 years. In this chapter I describe some of those changes as a prelude to the description of the technique, but the later part of the chapter describes the use of Vocal Profile Analysis (VPA) as a technique in much the same way as earlier editions.

Thinking in rehabilitation circles has changed considerably in the last decade. Ten to fifteen years ago speech and language therapists, in common with other rehabilitation professionals, were engaged in a process of reductionism. Excited by new technologies, they sought to describe features such as voice in ever greater detail; encouraged by advances in understanding from cognitive and neuropsychology, they sought to explain the nature of breakdown or difference and were in danger of focusing upon the impairment rather than the person with the disability. Wirz (1995) expands upon this deconstructive approach to assessment and therapy planning. More recently, forces outside the profession have forced therapists to re-evaluate whether there is a danger that overspecialism can detract from the basic skills of a therapist.

Voices, primarily from disabled people's organizations (DPOs), have been raised over 20 years to challenge an impairment-led deconstructive approach to therapy (Morris, 1991; Swain et al., 1994). These warnings from DPOs, together with the publication of the WHO classification of Impairments, Disability and Handicap (World Health Organization, 1980) – plus the inevitable timelag between publication and readership by practising professionals – began a shift away from reductionism. It was not until the mid to late 1980s that large numbers of speech and language therapists began to question whether their activity was directed towards clients' impairments or disabilities (Wirz, 1996). The answer to this question has to be that a good therapist has responsibilities to address the needs of each client appropriately, and this will sometimes mean disability focused therapy and at other times the need will be to address the impairment. Hallberg and Carlsson (1993) discuss the relationship between hearing impairment, the disabling consequences and the potential handicap, and stress the need for preventative action to inhibit the move from disability to handicap.

A chapter which demonstrates how accurately to describe the vocal characteristics of deaf speakers must do so in the context of why the disabled person's voice is different and whether he wishes to change it. The use of VPA as a technique for analysing the vocal characteristics of those deaf speakers who want to change their voice patterns remains, however, unchanged.

There are a plethora of reasons why a deaf person's voice may be different from those of his hearing peers. These include the degree and type of deafness; age at which the person became deaf; type and appropriateness of amplification; the educational regime and the communication system that the person used in his or her education, and the amount of speech therapy. There is, of course, an enormous difference between the speech characteristics of a hearing impaired person who has had a period of normal hearing (and normal auditory feedback) and another who has never heard. Deaf people themselves refer to the former as hearing impaired and the latter as deaf.

This chapter is primarily concerned with vocal characteristics of congenitally deaf speakers. Parker and Irlam (1995) outline the difficulties of speech production occurring after the onset of a hearing impairment and divide those changes in speech production affecting the 'naturalness' of speech production from those affecting intelligibility. They refer to problems that may arise in the breathing patterns for speech of deafened adults, related or unrelated to increased tension, and the effects that this can have upon phonation. Parker and Irlam point out that deafened speakers have disruption at a phonetic level – illustrated by difficulties of controlling volume, rhythm or the smooth and appropriate pitch changes necessary in intonation – but that phonological disruption is unlikely among speakers who have learned the rules of speech before the onset of their hearing impairment.

The data reported in the later part of this chapter are from a group of congenitally deaf speakers who were aged between 18 and 23 years when the data were collected in 1979. That is, they had been born between 1956 and 1961, when hearing aid technology and early detection of deafness were much less advanced. Since the 1960s, hearing aid technology and early detection have improved considerably, leading to a situation where the auditory signal received by young deaf children is greatly improved.

It can be assumed that congenitally deaf people who use auditory signals may have less marked vocal differences than those given in Table 12.2 (below), but there is no reason to suppose that the relative distribution of vocal differences (as measured by the VPA) between deaf and hearing speakers will be any different.

There is, of course, a new client group who seek help with their vocal quality. Clients who have had cochlear implants seek normalcy in their spoken output, and this includes phonological, articulatory (including vocal) features. It is perhaps a further change in thinking since the first version of this chapter 12 years ago that it is more likely that a therapist will consider therapy directed to the vocal characteristics of a deaf speaker as part of that deaf speaker's articulatory performance, rather than as a separate entity.

The second major change that has occurred since these data were collected is the importance of choice in the education of young (and older) deaf children. This choice between total communication medium or spoken medium, between monolingual or bilingual education, has had considerable impact on the development of language skills among deaf children. With improved language skills, it may be that there is a different client group choosing to seek help with their spoken output, including those profoundly deaf sign language users who wish (often in young adulthood) to improve their spoken intelligibility.

The vocal characteristics of deaf speakers may impact upon intelligibility but, more importantly, they impact upon the listener who, on hearing a different voice quality, anticipates difficulties with listening. Wirz (1986) contrasts acceptability features of voice – those features which change the listener expectation – with intelligibility features. It is the contention of this author that to change vocal characteristics of some deaf speakers can improve the acceptability and thus, the naive listener's response to the deaf speaker's spoken output.

The third, and perhaps greatest, change since the first version of this chapter is society's greater acceptance of diversity and the greater acceptance that speakers who are deaf will sound different. In the earlier version of this chapter in 1986, I wrote: 'deaf speakers have abnormal voices'. Such a statement now sounds crass and insulting as well as being inaccurate. A more accurate way of expressing this would be that deaf speakers frequently have different vocal characteristics from hearing people. Received wisdom and casual observation support this view, yet the literature is confused and confusing in its description of deaf voice. It is difficult to establish whether an author refers to laryngeal function as voice or uses the term 'voice' or 'voice quality' to refer to the overall product of a deaf speaker's vocal apparatus.

In this chapter, the definition of voice that will be followed is one that includes those parameters at laryngeal, supralaryngeal, and subglottal levels, which interact to affect a speaker's voice.

A brief review of the literature

In this review, the relevant literature has been divided for convenience into three sections:

1. a review of that literature referring to the laryngeal performance of hearing-impaired speakers;
2. a review of those studies referring to the velopharyngeal incompetence disturbing the resonance characteristics of deaf speakers; and finally
3. a consideration of those studies that have looked at other prosodic aspects of the speech of deaf people.

There is, of course, considerable overlap between the various parameters of deaf speech which can be disturbed, and any division of the literature in an arbitrary way like this leads to problems of classification. For example, does one classify loudness as a comment on the laryngeal performance of a deaf speaker or as a reflection of his disturbed prosody? 'Over fortis' is frequently cited (but seldom defined!) in the literature as a feature of deaf speech. Is 'over fortis' synonymous with loudness, or is it an articulatory feature?

Laryngeal features: the speech of deaf and hearing impaired speakers

The inability of hearing-impaired speakers to control their laryngeal performance results in different voice quality and poorly controlled pitch and intonation. Jones (1967) lists the attributes of voice quality which are most commonly cited as: 'tense', 'flat', 'breathy', 'harsh', 'throaty', 'monotone', 'lack of rhythm', 'poor resonance', and 'poor carrying power'. Calvert (1962) also noted that none of the adjectives used by teachers of the deaf to describe the voice of deaf speakers suggested pleasing quality; all were unpleasant. Poor laryngeal control was often attributed in the early literature to abnormal breathing patterns (Rawlings, 1935; Hudgins, 1937), with observations that deaf speakers had less breath control in speech than did hearing speakers. This was picked up by research in the 1960s, when Calvert (1962) studied harsh and breathy voices of deaf speakers, compared with simulated voices of hearing speakers. He concluded that deaf voice quality was identified not only by fundamental frequency and subsequent harmonies, but by information from the articulatory timing of the speech. Stark (1972) studied the vocalizations of young (preverbal) deaf children and one of her observations was that young deaf children did not acquire control over voicing, pitch and intensity variation as did hearing children.

A variety of terms, then, such as hoarse, breathy, weak, harsh, huskier, strident have been used to describe the voice quality of deaf people (Fairbanks, 1960; Zemlin, 1968; Nickerson, 1975). While there appears to be general agreement about the meaning of these terms, there have been very few efforts to study how these perceptual features can be related to acoustic aspects or to the actual respiratory and phonatory dynamics responsible for the quality.

In attempts to describe voice quality in deaf speakers, many studies have used perceptual ratings but few have gone on to demonstrate that the use of such ratings is replicable and can be used with good interjudge reliability. Markides (1983) asked 30 teachers of the deaf and 36 lay people to rate the voice quality of 85 hearing-impaired children. It is not clear from this study, however, whether the teachers were using terms such as 'deep', 'throaty', 'hoarse' or 'soft', 'fairly normal' in a similar way, or whether they were using different terms to describe the same phenomenon.

One of the qualities commonly cited as characteristic of deaf speakers is a tense/harsh voice quality. At the National Technical Institute for the Deaf (NTID) between 10% and 12% of students entering college education have tense/harsh voice quality. This term is used in the voice classification scheme employed by the speech pathologists at NTID, where there is high reliability of perceptual judgements by experienced judges (Subtelny 1975). Wirz et al. (1980) examined the acoustic features which allowed this high interjudge reliability. Spectrographic examination of deaf speakers' production showed that tense phonations of the vowels of hearing-impaired speakers were characterized by increased distribution of higher amplitudes of sound energy in the higher frequencies of the spectrum.

There continues to be lack of agreement in the published literature about voice quality in hearing-impaired speakers, even when care is taken in the research design to ensure objectivity with perceptual ratings. Commonly, the literature refers impressionistically to 'high pitch' among deaf speakers (Martony, 1966; Miller 1968; Levitt, 1971) without attempting to define the pitch level more closely. Rather than apply impressionistic labels, other writers have described the laryngeal performance of deaf speakers with reference to the pitch and intonation. Voelker (1935) was the 'father' of such research.

Gilbert and Campbell (1980) studied the fundamental frequency characteristics of deaf and hearing children and found, in a subject intra-group analysis of variance, there was no significant difference between the deaf and the hearing individuals. Their work suggests that there is a trend for some hearing-impaired speakers to have a higher pitch than their hearing peers when compared with the norms provided by work of Michel et al. (1966) and Hollien and Shipp (1972).

Not only is the fundamental frequency of hearing-impaired speakers reported to be different, and usually thought to be higher, but the frequency range is also reported to be narrower. Monsen (1978) noted that there is no correlation between the speech intelligibility of hearing-impaired adolescents and either mean fundamental frequency or mean change of fundamental frequency. He notes that while it is 'commonplace that poor control of fundamental frequency detracts from the speech intelligibility of the hearing impaired, it is not entirely clear how the pitch control of hearing impaired differs from normal in ways that affect voice quality' (Monsen, 1978).

Velopharyngeal features

Nasal voice quality is frequently cited as one of the characteristics of deaf speakers. Hudgins (1934), in his classic study, was the first to describe 'excessive nasal resonance' as a feature of deaf speech. However, it is always difficult to establish the features that influence the perception of 'nasality'. This search for a relationship between degree of hearing loss and degree of perceived nasality is followed by Seaver et al. (1980). They investigated the velopharyngeal characteristics of 19 hearing-impaired subjects who exhibited nasality. One of their results was a non-significant relationship between degree of perceived nasality and degree of hearing loss. This led them to conclude that: 'in terms of anatomical physiological attributes, the hypernasality observed in the speech of many hearing-impaired speakers is not analogous to the hypernasality observed in the craniofacial cleft population' (p. 246). Thus, although the nasal resonance features of the deaf may be perceived to be similar to those of the velopharyngeal insufficient population, they are of a different origin. Boone (1966) raises the question of how deaf speakers achieve their characteristic quality and suggests that the deaf use 'cul-de-sac' resonance, by using pharyngeal tension and lowering the body of the tongue.

Other prosodic aspects

Other suprasegmental parameters affecting the vocal characteristics of deaf speakers include intensity, intonation, and frequency. Frequency disturbances affecting pitch have been reviewed above in the discussion of laryngeal parameters. Stoker and Lape (1980) posed the question 'is it possible to determine a [hearing-impaired] child's competence in speech with measures other than articulation?' Among the parameters they examined in their sample of 42 hearing-impaired children were breath duration and suprasegmental competence. 'Pitch', 'loudness modulation', and 'duration modulation' were rated by four speech pathologists. Only items with an interjudge reliability coefficient of 0.05 level of confidence or better were included in their study. In this respect the methodology of this study was much more rigorous than many others using ratings. They found that 'pitch modulation', and 'loudness modulation' correlated with hearing loss and intelligibility at a 0.001 level of significance, and breath control and duration modulation correlated at a 0.05 level of significance. Interestingly none of these four suprasegmental features had a significant correlation with hearing aid use, age or sex.

Levitt (1971) comments on the excessive effort that deaf children use in speech. This excessive effort he refers to as an 'over fortis' of breathing and phonation, which is manifest as poor pitch control and rhythm.

It can be seen from the above review that many aspects of voice among deaf people have been studied, using different methodologies to examine different parameters. What all these studies have in common is that they study one, or in some cases a few, parameters of voice in deaf speakers, frequently drawing comparisons with hearing speakers. These studies do not attempt to be assessment procedures, but rather descriptive activities.

One of the problems of reviewing existing assessment procedures, or descriptions used, is that there is a lack of common agreement as to what constitutes voice. As Monsen (1978) says, voice quality is a rather ill-defined term.

> For the phonetician 'voice quality' is a technical term and refers to perceptual attributes pertaining to the way the vocal folds vibrate for example, to laryngeal gestures. In this technical sense it is separate from qualities of speech which derive from articulation. However, while it may be true that the phonetician can listen to a word and separate the poorly executed gestures of the larynx from those of the other speech articulators, most listeners probably cannot!

Here, Monsen is probably expressing a concern felt by many listeners and going some way to explaining the inefficiency of some of the perceptual assessment procedures reviewed above.

The Vocal Profile Analysis (VPA) scheme

One of the problems leading to the confusions identified above is that phonetic theory has provided us with few tools with which to attempt the task of describing parameters (or groups of parameters) such as voice

quality. Laver (1968, 1980; Laver et al., 1981) is one of the few phoneticians who has addressed this question. He says:

> if it is the legitimate business of general phonetic theory to take on the task of
> describing phonetic realisations not only of phonological elements but also of
> paraphonological attitudinal signals and of the learnable features of voice
> quality that signal membership of a given community, then a more comprehen-
> sive scheme for accounting for phonatory quality has to be available than that at
> present utilised in linguistic description (Laver, 1980).

Laver (1980) provided this phonetic description of voice quality by specifying laryngeal and supralaryngeal parameters of voice quality. Laver et al.
(1981) devised an assessment procedure, the Vocal Profile Analysis (VPA)
scheme, which can be applied to both normal and non-normal speakers.
The VPA scheme is a system that allows description of those parameters at
laryngeal and supralaryngeal levels affecting voice, and which cannot be
readily described using traditional phonetics.

The VPA scheme is based on the fact that a speaker's voice quality is
derived from those laryngeal and supralaryngeal features which are
idiosyncratic to him. Such idiosyncrasy is the product of both the anatomical make-up of the individual and his learned phonetic settings. The
anatomy of a speaker's vocal tract will affect his vocal characteristics.
These differences in anatomy may be at a supralaryngeal level – for
example, a speaker with a class 3 orthodontic bite will have different oral
resonance characteristics from a speaker with a class 1 bite. Or, more
obviously, a speaker with an inadequate velopharyngeal sphincter will
have a different oral/nasal resonance balance from a speaker who is able to
achieve adequate velopharyngeal closure.

At a laryngeal level, too, anatomical differences will affect phonation.
An extreme difference will be the way the increased length and bulk of the
vocal folds of an adult male speaker produce a very different phonation
from the shorter, less massive folds of a woman or child. Similarly, the
change in mass of slightly inflamed oedematous folds will change the
phonation characteristics of a speaker.

As well as the physical differences that lead to marked differences in
voice, the way in which a speaker habitually uses his vocal tract will also
affect his voice quality. A speaker who has learned, and habitually uses, a
forward tongue body posture will have a different oral resonance from a
similar speaker who has a habitual back posture of tongue body. Thus, a
speaker's voice quality can be said to be affected by learned muscular bias
and by his anatomical make-up.

The VPA identifies those supralaryngeal and laryngeal features which
are affected by either long-term muscular bias or by skeletal idiosyncrasy.
These features are muscular bias or skeletal differences at the lips, the jaw,

the tongue tip, the tongue body, the velopharynx, and the larynx. As well as identifying the posture of those articulators, the VPA also notes the range of movements of lips, jaw and tongue, the efficacy of phonation and the degree of muscular tension.

The degree of habitual tension will affect the long-term muscular tension at laryngeal and supralaryngeal levels, and thus voice quality. The phonetic theory developed by Laver (1980) suggests that by specifying a neutral point for each of these supralaryngeal, laryngeal features and tension characteristics it is possible to measure displacement from these specified neutral points. Measurements from neutral can be made acoustically or physiologically and they can, of course, also be perceived.

The VPA scheme, then, provides a perceptual rating scheme based on neutral settings of supralaryngeal and laryngeal parameters and allows measurement and perceptual rating of a speaker's deviations from the neutral points. The resulting profile of these deviations from neutral is a specification of the characteristics of a speaker's voice. Table 12.1 shows the parameters included in a VPA.

A trained user listening to a speaker makes a first judgement as to whether the speaker deviates from neutral for each of the supralaryngeal, laryngeal or prosodic parameters. If there is a deviation from neutral, the listener judges whether this is a deviation within or outside the normal range. Having made that judgement the listener then identifies the precise nature of the deviation on a six-point rating scale.

The application of the VPA can be illustrated by describing its application to the vocal characteristics of hearing-impaired speakers. Forty profoundly hearing-impaired young adults, aged between 18 and 23 years, in tertiary education and with an average hearing loss (over the speech frequencies in their better ear of 85 dB) were recorded reading the Rainbow Passage from Fairbanks (1960). Three trained listeners then rated these recordings using the VPA, and had an interjudge reliability of 80% over the 287 scalar degrees of the VPA. They also listened to recordings of 40 hearing speakers. The results of these analyses are presented in Table 12.2.

Differences between vocal profiles of deaf and hearing groups

It can be seen from these data that the differences between the vocal profiles of the deaf and hearing groups can be divided broadly into four groups:

1. ratings relating to the range of movements;
2. ratings relating to pitch and loudness;
3. ratings relating to tension;
4. ratings relating to laryngeal factors.

Table 12.1 Parameters included in a Vocal Profile

Supralaryngeal features	Labial features	Rounded or spread
		Labiodentalized
		Extensive or minimized range
	Jaw features	Closed or open
		Protruded
		Extensive or minimized range
	Tongue tip	Advanced or retracted
	Tongue body	Fronted or backed
		Raised or lowered
		Extensive or minimized range
	Velopharyngeal	Nasal or denasal
		Audible nasal escape
Tension features	Pharyngeal tension	
	Supralaryngeal features	Tense or lax
	Laryngeal tension	Tense or lax
	Larynx position	Raised or lowered
Phonation type		Harsh
		Whisper
		Creak
		Falsetto or modal
Prosodic features	Pitch mean	High or low
	Pitch range	Wide or narrow
	Pitch variability	High or low
	Tremor	
	Loudness mean	High or low
	Loudness range	Wide or narrow
	Loudness variability	High or low

Range of movements

The deaf speakers were markedly different from the hearing speakers in terms of the range of articulatory movements.

- 97.5% of deaf speakers had minimized tongue movement compared with 5% of hearing speakers;
- 60% of deaf speakers had minimized jaw movement compared with 12.5% of hearing speakers;
- 55% of deaf speakers had minimized lip movement compared with 7.5% of hearing speakers.

In direct contrast to this are the significant differences between the occurrence of extensive ranges of lip and jaw movements among the deaf speakers:

- 25% of the deaf speakers had an extensive range of lip movements compared with 5% of hearing speakers;

Table 12.2 Percentages of hearing and hearing-impaired speakers exhibiting non-neutral supralaryngeal, laryngeal or prosodic features, using the Vocal Profile Analysis scheme

	Control group speakers exhibiting the parameter (%)	Deaf group speakers exhibiting the parameter (%)
Lip rounding	45	55
Lip spreading	5	15
Labiodentalized	0	2.5
Extensive lip range	5	25*
Minimum lip range	7.5	55**
Close jaw	37.5	15
Open jaw	10	40
Protruded jaw	5	17.5
Extensive jaw movement	2.5	20*
Minimum jaw movement	12.5	60***
Advanced tongue tip	45	25
Retracted tongue tip	12.5	48
Fronted tongue body	37.5	20
Backed tongue body	52.5	65
Raised tongue body	42.5	40
Lowered tongue body	15	27.5
Extensive tongue body	0	0
Minimum tongue body	5	97.5***
Nasal	100	95
Audible nasal escape	0	12.5
Denasal	0	5
Pharyngeal tension	47.5	87.5***
Supralaryngeal tension	57.5	85.0
Supralaryngeal laxness	2.5	7.5
Laryngeal tension	72.5	95.0*
Laryngeal laxness	0	5.0*
Raised laryngeal position	17.5	55.0**
Lowered laryngeal position	30.0	27.5
Harsh	25.0	72.5***
Whisper	97.5	92.5
Creak	77.5	67.5
Falsetto	0	20.0***
Modal	100.0	97.5
High pitch mean	30.0	40.0
Low pitch mean	42.5	40.0
Wide pitch range	0	7.5
Narrow pitch range	27.5	90.0***
High pitch variation	0	5.0
Low pitch variation	7.5	87.5***
Tremor	25.0	25.0
High loudness mean	17.5	10.0
Low loudness mean	2.5	47.5
Wide loudness range	2.5	2.5
Narrow loudness range	5.0	90.0***
High loudness variation	0	0
Low loudness variation	5.0	90.0***

*** $p = 0.001$ ** $p = 0.01$ * $p = 0.05$.

- 20% of the deaf speakers had an extensive range of jaw movements compared with 2.5% of hearing speakers.

Pitch and loudness

In these parameters, too, there is a highly significant difference between the pitch and loudness characteristics of deaf and hearing subjects.

- 90% of deaf speakers showed narrow pitch range compared with 27.5% of hearing speakers;
- 87.5% of deaf speakers showed low pitch variability compared with 7.5% of hearing speakers;
- 47.5%. of deaf speakers showed low loudness mean compared with 2.5% of hearing speakers:
- 90% of deaf speakers showed narrow loudness range compared with 5% of hearing speakers:
- 90% of deaf speakers showed low loudness variability compared with 5% of hearing speakers.

Surprisingly the pitch means of the deaf and hearing groups were not significantly different even at $P = 0.05$ level.

Tension

Here the following results were noted:

- 87.5% of the deaf speakers were characterized by pharyngeal constriction compared with 47.5% of hearing subjects;
- 95% of the deaf speakers showed laryngeal tension compared with 72% of hearing speakers;
- 5% of the deaf speakers showed laryngeal laxness but no hearing speakers showed this characteristic.

These figures are difficult to interpret. We can see that nearly all deaf speakers show laryngeal tension, but so do a large number of the hearing speakers. However, the difference between the deaf and hearing groups is significant. No hearing person shows laryngeal laxness, but all the deaf speakers who did not show laryngeal tenseness show laxness. The difference in the incidence of the laxness too is significant.

Finally, a highly significant group of deaf speakers showed a non-neutral degree of pharyngeal constriction.

Laryngeal factors

Of the deaf speakers, 72.5% show harshness, compared with 25% of hearing speakers; this is probably interrelated with the high incidence of laryngeal tension. Among the deaf speakers, 20% used falsetto, while none of the hearing speakers did. Both harshness and falsetto are highly kinaesthetic laryngeal performances, and it is possible that the high incidence among deaf speakers is related to this fact. Of the deaf speakers 55% had raised larynx position compared with 17.5% of normals.

The reported results showing the percentage of deaf and hearing speakers who exhibited a non-neutral setting of a parameter goes some way towards indicating whether a feature is common among deaf speakers, when compared with hearing speakers. Where the occurrence is greater for the deaf group than for the hearing there is some justification for calling such parameters 'typifying features' of deaf voice. In the results reported above, it can be seen that there are several features in the vocal balance of these 40 deaf speakers that were significantly different from those of the 40 hearing speakers.

Other factors affecting the voice of deaf speakers

The discussion above describes the voice characteristics of congenitally deaf speakers. It does not account for the other factors that may affect the vocal characteristics of deaf people. These 'other factors' may be organic voice disorder, secondary voice disorder, or functional voice disorder. Organic voice disorder, where there is an organic problem of the laryngeal assembly, laryngeal tract, or of the velopharynx, may occur in deaf speakers as readily as in hearing speakers. Non-organic voice disorders arising from emotional stress or from vocal abuse may also occur among deaf speakers. Following Aronson (1980) and Boone (1983), it is useful to consider non-organic vocal pathology as a continuum, with the disorders related to vocal abuse resulting in secondary changes to the larynx at one end of the continuum, and disorders where there is no observable laryngeal pathology at the other (Wilson, 1987).

Secondary voice disorder arises from misuse of the vocal apparatus. Changes in healthy patterns, posture and voicing, as well as extraneous irritants combine to cause laryngeal distress and subsequent laryngeal changes. Chronic laryngitis, vocal nodules, Reinke's oedema and polyps are the four commonest changes in laryngeal structure associated with misuse (Bennett et al., 1987; Damste, 1987; Van Den Broek, 1987; Lancer et al., 1988).

Deaf speakers as a group have increased tension of pharynx and larynx, increased harshness and raised larynx position (Wirz, 1987). It is tempting to suppose that deaf speakers may therefore, as a group, be more vulnerable to secondary voice disorder than hearing speakers. A literature search suggests that such a study has not been published. Clinical experience does, however, suggest that some deaf speakers have frequent periods of chronic laryngitis, which raises questions about whether is this a manifestation of secondary voice disorder.

There is increasing evidence that secondary voice disorder is related to certain personality characteristics (Greene, 1980; Yano et al., 1982; Wilson, 1987). Aronson comments that speakers with secondary voice disorders frequently exhibit emotional stress. It was common to find attempts to describe the personality traits of the deaf population in the literature of the 1950s and 1960s, suggesting a homogeneous view of personality in deaf people. Since the 1970s, the diverse nature of personality traits among deaf young people has been recognized and it is this diversity that the clinician must remember when dealing with deaf speakers with secondary voice disorders. He or she must be aware that the stress-related features of secondary voice disorder are as likely to appear in deaf as in hearing speakers.

Organic voice disorders and secondary voice disorders will occur among deaf speakers. So too will functional voice disorder, where there is no observable laryngeal pathology, but discernible voice change.

In addition to the characterizing vocal features of deaf speakers, to their vulnerability to secondary voice disorder or functional voice disorder, therapists must also consider the effects that ageing has upon deaf voice. Hollien (1987) reviews the vocal changes that occur with ageing, which he attributes to biochemical, aerodynamic and laryngeal changes. Ringel (1987) introduces the concept of biological ageing as the important concept in any considerations of ageing voice. He stresses that although there are inevitable changes in larynx and phonation as well as the general anatomical and physiological changes of senescence, this decline varies considerably in rate and extent.

It is important, then, for a clinician to consider the totality of voice among deaf speakers. As well as commonly occurring characteristics related to the hearing impairment, other voice problems may occur as a result of organic voice disorder, secondary voice disorder, or as a consequence of ageing.

This review has attempted to show that there are features which distinguish the voice quality of hearing-impaired speakers. However, because voice is seldom clearly defined, it is difficult to make cross comparisons from the literature as to precisely which are these distinguishing features. The Vocal Profile Analysis scheme (Laver et al., 1981), which provides a comprehensive labelling procedure for the supralaryngeal and laryngeal components of voice, is a very useful tool for identifying vocal difficulties among deaf speakers.

Summary

The communication of hearing-impaired speakers is different. The difference in language skills is the primary difficulty for most hearing impaired children, and not unreasonably becomes the primary teaching objective for teachers and therapists. However, the effects that poor voice quality can have upon the listening 'set' of a naive listener to a hearing-impaired person should not be underestimated. If the teacher or therapist can encourage easy relaxed phonation among young hearing-impaired children, voice problems should not develop in later years. However, there will be many hearing-impaired speakers who do develop aberrant voice patterns where specific voice therapy will be applicable.

CHAPTER 13

Mutational disorders of voice

ROBERT FAWCUS

Introduction

The process of phonation is the first complex motor act that heralds the infant's entry to the world and is not uncommonly the last an individual achieves at the end of human life. The nature of the phonation produced changes significantly throughout life. The rapid transient changes conforming to the linguistic and communicative needs of the individual occur against a backcloth of phonatory function that alters slowly throughout our speaking lives. Most of these latter changes occur so gradually that they are hardly noticed by either speaker or listener. A few, however, have a dramatic impact, such as the shift from a boy's voice to the mature male pattern of phonation.

As the mass of the vocal cords increases during childhood there is a steady, often imperceptible, decrease in the fundamental frequency of phonation. In the female this process usually continues by infinitesimal decrements until the menopause when, in a number of individuals, a marked shift can occur, bringing the fundamental frequency well within the male range. The sudden nature of the change in the pubertal male leads to the occasional occurrence of a maintenance of the former fundamental frequency of phonation. This is commonly achieved by a shift, of which the individual is usually unaware, from modal voice to loft register (falsetto).

Physical and physiological causes of puberphonia

Greene (1980; Greene and Mathieson, 1989) outlines the range of physical and physiological causes of puberphonia suggested in the literature.

1. Unusually early breaking of the voice, leading to self-consciousness and habitual continuation of a high-pitched voice (West et al., 1957).
2. A desire to retain a successful treble voice that has brought distinction (Seth and Guthrie, 1935).
3. Fear of assuming a full share of adult responsibility. (Greene rejects the oft-quoted alleged link with the Oedipus complex, but comments on her frequent observation of a strong bond with the mother and the relative prevalence of puberphonia in boys without siblings.)
4. Hero worship of an elder boy.
5. A natural tenor voice or small larynx with short vocal folds.
6. Delayed pubertal development (Luchsinger and Arnold, 1965).
7. Severe deafness (Greene, 1961).
8. Congenital abnormalities and asymmetries, paralysis of one vocal fold (Arnold, 1961) or congenital web (Baker and Savetsky, 1966).

Aronson (1980) would add to the list the effect of 'general debilitating illness during puberty, which not only may delay overall growth during puberty but, because of the physical restrictions of being bedfast, may reduce the range of respiratory excursions and consequently, tidal air volumes, preventing the development of adequate infraglottal air'.

He goes on to enumerate laryngeal-respiratory postures and movements that have been noted as bases for high-pitched mutational falsetto voice.

1. The larynx is elevated high in the neck.
2. The body of the larynx is tilted downward, apparently having the effect of maintaining the vocal folds in a lax state.
3. With the vocal folds in a flabby state, they are stretched thin by contraction of the cricothyroid muscles.
4. The vocal folds are thus in a state of reduced mass and offer little resistance to infraglottal air pressure.
5. Respiration for speech production is shallow, and on exhalation infraglottal air pressure is held to a minimum, so that only the medial edges of the vocal folds vibrate and do so at an elevated fundamental frequency.

The first of these characteristics was noted by Makuen in 1899 (cited in Luchsinger and Arnold, 1965) and is quoted in almost every work on the subject of puberphonia.

Evidence derived from simple observation of laryngeal excursions during normal phonation and falsetto suggests, however, that the reported high elevation is associated with the typical upward shift in pitch that occurs when a male speaker demonstrates the switch from true cord phonation to falsetto. This usually involves a pitch change of at least an octave. If the transfer is made at the same pitch level the elevation is much reduced.

Despite the wide range of alleged causes of puberphonia there is an alternative explanation that matches our own experience and many of the accounts occurring in the literature. The former typically ignore the possibility that a pubescent male may blunder into an alternative mode of phonation during the initial period of vocal mutation and then be unable to escape voluntarily.

The fact that an individual is apparently unable to shift from one mode of phonation to another should not be at all surprising. After the successful transfer from falsetto to true cord phonation, it is often just as difficult for the former puberphonic to achieve falsetto voice. The flexibility that some individuals appear to have in control of their phonatory and articulatory behaviour is not universal. The range of skilled behaviour evident in such activities as mimicry and singing suggests that a significant proportion of those with a normal speech mechanism are unable to achieve even average performance (Fawcus, 1980).

Luchsinger and Arnold (1965) comment that 'while their peripheral auditory perception is usually normal many of these [puberphonic] patients are not musical'. They also note the influence of auditory factors, reflected in the occasional occurrence of falsetto voice in profoundly deaf males.

It is often not appreciated that falsetto phonation is employed by the normal speaker. It is a feature of war cries in many cultures, and can also be heard on Army parade grounds, in the issuing of orders during drill. More peaceful phenomena include giggling, laughing, yawning, sighing, yodelling, and the singing of the counter-tenor.

At the London Conference of the International Association of Logopaedics and Phoniatrics in 1959, Moses traced the swings in fashion which were associated with the castrato singing voice over the previous 200 years and made the confident prediction that male singing styles were about to enter a new phase in western culture. Many in the audience, including the present writer, found this prediction difficult to accept. With the possible exception of a single popular male alto, Alfred Deller, the overwhelming majority of male singers rarely strayed into falsetto phonation. On the popular stage as well as the concert hall, male singers exuded as strong a masculine image as possible.

For the past quarter of a century, successions of highly successful popular singers have laboured consistently to lend credence to Moses' prediction. The Beatles, the Beach Boys, Tiny Tim, the Jacksons, and hosts of others have spent a major portion of their time producing falsetto phonation to the evident delight and full acceptance of their followers.

Gutzmann (1897) described the role of the cricothyroid in the production of falsetto voice in the normal larynx by means of a 'functional over-contraction'. Arnold (1961) investigated the operation of the laryngeal musculature by means of electromyography and confirmed that the external vocal cord tensor (cricothyroid) is the muscle chiefly involved in falsetto phonation. Hirano et al. (1970) studied the regulation of register, pitch, and intensity in the larynges of a small group of singers using hooked wire electrodes.

Traditionally, falsetto voice has been considered as the main component of head register and part of the constituent pattern of the mid-register or mixed register. It is not held to be involved in the highest range, known as the whistle register, or the lowest described as chest register. The Hirano recordings show most differences occurring in the trace derived from the vocalis muscle of one of the authors (Vennard), an accomplished bass as well as a speech scientist.

Fawcus (1986) reported on a group of young men seen at both the Middlesex Hospital and Guy's Hospital, over a period of two decades. All were reported to have laryngeal structures within normal limits and there was no evidence of endocrine disorders. None of the young men gave cause to either the referring ENT surgeon or the speech therapist to consider the necessity for psychiatric referral. Their complaints centred on the basic acceptability of the high-pitched voice and in no case did this seriously affect social adjustment. The group bears strong resemblance to subjects in studies by Hammarberg (1987) in Stockholm, and Green (1988, personal communication) in Sydney, Australia.

Treating puberphonia

Diverse techniques, as well as accounts of their success, abound in the texts devoted to voice disorders. Greene (1980) suggests a number of activities, principally concerned with postural adjustments and relaxation. Gutzmann's pressure test, for example (cited in Luchsinger and Arnold, 1965), is recommended by Aronson (1980) as a successful therapeutic technique. It requires digital pressure on the thyroid cartilage during attempts at phonation.

After one has taken the necessary case history, it is obviously important to investigate the patient's pitch range. The first problem encountered is that he is very likely to be able to produce falsetto voice at, or near, the normal adult male fundamental frequency. This is, however, clearly different from the normal male voice. It usually has a slightly breathy tone, tends to be weak and somewhat flat. However, depending on how long the individual has been using falsetto, the stage of growth of his vocal cords and idiosyncratic factors related to phonation patterns, it is possible that he may have achieved a reduction in breathy quality and more power than is usual for a puberphonic voice. This can be seen most clearly in the male alto who can typically achieve considerable intensity with a minimum of breathiness.

The principal test is to listen to conversation or reading aloud to determine whether or not the low pitch is maintained and whether the transition to a higher pitch is a smooth one without voice breaks. Many individuals find singing scales difficult or embarrassing, and it is just as satisfactory to proceed in simple steps to pairs of notes up to the top of his comfortable range and then down to the lowest point. The therapist who is not a musician may find it simpler to employ a small electronic keyboard which is usually nowadays portable and inexpensive. This has many applications with other types of dysphonic patient as well as offering a broad range of opportunities in work on listening skills with young children.

A laryngograph (Fourcin and Abberton, 1971) can provide the therapist with a visual display of the pattern of phonation. The puberphonic does not produce the typical saw-tooth output of the normal speaker, but a wave-form that closely approximates to a sine wave. The absence of the characteristic bursts of laryngeal output is responsible for the weaker almost ethereal tone of the falsetto. The tissues of the vocal folds are vibrating with reduced mass and a lower level of tension in the closed phase. They are behaving like a tuning fork or the air in a flute and the resulting voice is reminiscent of these sounds.

It is preferable not to attempt to alter the mode of phonation too quickly in the session. The abrupt change in voice which is relatively easy to achieve is usually very difficult for the patient to adjust to. It is important to determine if he has been aware of any occasional shifts into true phonation. These can occur accidentally, but it is not usually possible for the puberphonic male to reproduce them at will.

The exploration of range of falsetto may have resulted in production of 'creaky voice' particularly in the lower frequencies. It is very useful to assess how easily the patient can achieve creak, or glottal fry as it is known in the American texts on dysphonia. Of all techniques suggested the most effective with the above group of persistent puberphonic cases at the Middlesex Hospital and Guy's was the transfer from falsetto phonation first to glottal fry (creak) and then into true cord phonation.

The voice therapist should ask the patient to imitate 'creaky voice', and when he is comfortably producing this mode of phonation, ask him to raise the pitch gradually. There is a reasonable chance that he may shift dramatically into normal phonation immediately. If this does not occur, then it is necessary to attempt the task two or three times and then divert to a relaxation task. If there is repeated failure (see Greene 1961, 1980) after an interval, the technique may be repeated. Many authorities, however, report success within a few minutes of commencing the process.

Such success leads almost without exception to one of the major paradoxes in the field of speech therapy. A young man has come to the clinic, complaining that his voice is too high-pitched and that he is often upset by people mistaking him for a woman when speaking on the telephone. Within a matter of minutes it is possible for him to achieve true cord phonation. The pitch drops accordingly and he has achieved exactly what he requested. The most common, initial reaction is to reject the new voice. The reasons given differ from individual to individual, but with very few exceptions this is a typical response.

In the past, this behaviour only served to confirm the views held by psychoanalysts, and those therapists who were inclined to their philosophy, that the young man actually preferred his original state and that it was the result of a process of 'symptom-choice'.

Establishing the new voice

Although disconcerting to the therapist, even if the response is anticipated, it would be a serious mistake to interpret the rejection of the new voice as anything but a normal and temporary reaction. It is very similar to the panic described by some stammerers when they realize for the first time that they can approach speaking situations with a low risk of stuttering (Dalton and Hardcastle, 1977). This is usually the result of a rapid response to a specific therapy procedure, which can leave him feeling 'naked and vulnerable', as a stammerer once described it. Another example is the response of the adult patient who requests therapy because he or she habitually uses a lateral /s/ or uvular /r/ and wishes to learn to speak 'normally'. In both such cases it is possible to achieve, sometimes with singular difficulty, the performance which they claimed to desire, only to find that they dislike the result.

Appropriate advice and counselling can usually overcome this very human, quite normal reaction to change. The most effective approach can be to accept the negative response as a normal reaction. It has to be remembered that if the therapist is disconcerted, the individual himself is not unaware of the paradox and is likely to feel even more uncomfortable about his protestations than he does about the quality and 'feel' of his new voice or new articulatory pattern.

In the case of the puberphonic male it is helpful to work on developing and establishing the new voice in spite of the initial protests. This entails exploring the vocal range, and encouraging the young man to experiment with the new mode of phonation. He should be encouraged to use his new voice as often as possible with strangers before he encounters his family, friends or colleagues at work. Some gain great benefit from talking on the telephone or having a face-to-face conversation with a sympathetic friend prior to approaching a situation which may be potentially threatening.

It can be emphasized that, contrary to his expectations, people in the patient's environment are not likely to notice the change. Furthermore it should be pointed out that he himself will be much more aware of any difference, as most people will tend to listen to *what* he says rather than *how* he speaks. It helps to keep the volume of the voice down at first, as this aids the maintenance of stability and tends to limit the attention paid by others.

Strong reassurance can be given but this will be greatly reinforced if some assignments are attempted. These can include telephone calls to strangers, and being interviewed by a colleague of the therapist unfamiliar with the original puberphonic voice. Often the young man is more anxious about the reaction of parents and siblings than strangers.

Case history 1

KS, a young man whose family were immigrants from Pakistan, had been criticized and ridiculed for up to a year by relatives, particularly his uncles. He was very concerned about their reaction to his new voice but found that they did not notice the change until he brought it to their attention some weeks later.

Case history 2

TJ, a young man in his early twenties, showed a particularly distressed reaction to achieving a very serviceable male voice in the first session of therapy. 'Well as you know, I work for a construction plant hire firm, and have to deliver and demonstrate vehicles on site. I often get a bit of leg pulling about my voice but this will be terrible. Tomorrow I'm getting married and when I get back from my honeymoon, they will all fall about laughing.'

He resigned from work that day and sought a similar post in another district after his honeymoon.

Case history 3

PM was referred in his mid-forties after an ENT examination, following a period of laryngeal discomfort. His father had undergone laryngectomy a few months previously, and he was, understandably, very conscious of his own larynx.

His response to therapy employing a glottal fry initiation was rapid and effective, and he showed less concern about the change than the younger cases mentioned previously. It was agreed that he should return after a few days to make a laryngographic recording, so that we could examine the transition from falsetto to true cord phonation and obtain a visual record. When he returned to the clinic, he was quite unable to achieve falsetto voice, he was now as locked into the normal mode of phonation as he had been trapped into the former phonatory pattern since puberty.

Case history 4

CT was very self-conscious about his high-pitched voice. He was lightly built and of small stature and his voice only added to his general dissatisfaction with his persona. Surprisingly, the ENT surgeon found that his larynx had grown satisfactorily at puberty and was within the normal range for a male in his late twenties. His voice sounded distinctly feminine and he was continually upset by the response of strangers on the telephone.

Although highly motivated he was unable to achieve the transfer to creak or to low-pitched modal voice. He was able to achieve a fundamental frequency of 140 Hz for brief periods but could not maintain it. His laryngograph traces showed modal patterns and although his fundamental pitch was typically 250 Hz, his voice had few of the characteristics of loft register.

After many months of frustrating attempts to help him achieve the voice to which he aspired he was finally discharged. Opinions differed about the reasons for his inability to achieve a lower fundamental frequency. These ranged from the inevitable explanation that he had a deep seated desire to maintain a high-pitched voice, to the suggestion that the small size of his resonating cavities tended to enhance the high frequencies.

Other mutational and related problems

Few, if any, mutational disorders of phonation share the dramatic nature of persistent puberphonia. Most of the disorders are so rare and so subtle that they have even avoided acquiring a specific label. A very small number of children may be referred to a speech therapist with problems relating to their fundamental frequency, well before the anticipated effects of puberty. The few cases in my own experience were associated with growth problems, and observation of the children over a number of years showed little significant change in the tendency to use a fundamental frequency markedly higher than their peers. On the single occasion when a six-year-old was referred because his voice was virtually an octave below normal it was found that he had a major chronic infection pervading his vocal cords. The ENT surgeon had not been able to view the larynx by indirect laryngoscopy and the diagnosis was later confirmed by direct laryngeal examination.

Boliek et al. (1996, 1997) are engaged in both cross-sectional and longitudinal studies of the relationship between breathing and vocalization in young children. This work will provide important bench marks for the study of both normal and disordered phonatory patterns in the developing child.

Female adolescents

The problems of the female adolescent whose fundamental frequency remains at a pre-pubertal level have received little attention, either as a clinical problem or in the literature. Within the range of females in the population, at any age, there is inevitably a proportion whose voices lie even more than two standard deviations below or above the mean. It is the lack of severe social stigma attached to the possession of a high-pitched voice by a female which reduces the conspicuousness of such individuals and their referral is very rare. This is not to say, however, that the problem is unimportant, because for some women a fundamental frequency which deviates from the norm may be a source of considerable embarrassment and concern.

Biever and Bless (1989) investigated the acoustic and aerodynamic characteristics of the phonation of 20 geriatric and 20 young female adults and contrasted these findings with videostroboscopy. They found that the elderly women showed a greater degree of shimmer and more intersubject variability in fundamental frequency and mean airflow rate. Videostroboscopy revealed a profile including greater aperiodicity, incomplete glottal closure, mucosal wave alterations and a relative reduction in the amplitude of vocal fold vibration. It was perhaps misleading to describe the elderly women as geriatric. Their mean age was 69 (range 60–77 years), their hearing was better than average for their age group, they had no known neurological disease and were non-smokers.

Sulter et al. (1996) studied over 200 subjects with different degrees of vocal training and an age range from 17 to 44 years. The most marked differences in vocal fold function and appearance were gender related. Female subjects tended to have thinner, wider, shorter and slacker vocal folds. They confirmed a tendency for fundamental frequency to decrease with increasing age.

Linville (1996) found that listeners were able to make reasonably good estimates of the age of speakers from recorded samples. She examined a wide range of factors including speech rate and the stability of the fundamental frequency. She comments that in a number of studies, elderly men have been observed to have a significantly higher incidence of glottal gaps than young men, whereas elderly women have a lower incidence than younger women. Slower reading rates in elderly speakers were found to correlate with reductions in maximum intensity level. Linville claims that this provides support for the notion that changes in the respiratory system associated with ageing and/or inadequate laryngeal valving are responsible for this phenomenon.

Max and Mueller (1996) have investigated speaking fundamental frequency and periodicity of voicing in the conversation of a single subject aged 105 years. They caution that previously reported group trends regarding ageing effects on the mean speaking fundamental frequency of the female voice cannot be attributed to all women. Their subject had a higher mean speaking fundamental frequency than the literature would have suggested and less periodicity than a 35-year-old female subject.

Therapy for individuals who exhibit phonatory dysfunction due primarily to mutational factors is inevitably very similar to the basic principles outlined by Oates (Chapter 7 of this volume), with particular emphasis on the pitch component of the problem.

Male–female differences

As men and women pass through their middle years there is a tendency for them to show evidence of a gradual reduction in fundamental frequency of phonation. This is undoubtedly more evident in the amateur or professional singer who is constantly aware of the parameters of the singing voice, but it is nevertheless a feature of the vast majority of speakers. Hollien (1987) and other authors have noted a tendency for a rise in fundamental frequency in male speakers during the 6th and 7th decades of their life, and Hirano et al. (1983) suggest that elderly females tend to show oedema of the vocal folds which has the effect of maintaining a lower fundamental frequency. Histological changes associated with ageing are reported widely but there is little clear evidence as yet to show whether or not such changes are associated with factors such as smoking, exposure to irritants or patterns of vocal use.

As our understanding of hormonal influences develops we shall be in a better position to monitor and possibly control the changes which occur during development (Abitbol et al., 1989). MacCurtain's (1990) initial

investigations into the possibilities of Magnetic Resonance Imaging also
offer prospects of the co-ordination of anatomical studies in vivo with
other pertinent acoustic and physiological information. Crary et al. (1996)
report on the use of a dynamic version of this technique for studying vocal
tract configuration.

CHAPTER 14

The voice of the transsexual

JUDITH CHALONER

Introduction

It may seem a departure from the traditional view of the speech therapist's role in the treatment of voice disorders to include a chapter on voice work with transsexuals (people who feel they have been born into a body of the wrong gender). After all, the only 'disorder' of the voice is that the speaker feels it does not fit the sound of the persona and image he or she is presenting to the world. But it is now recognized by the medical team working with these clients that successful adjustment and transition into a new sex role needs a total approach, and that voice work is generally a very important element in this treatment.

Therefore speech and language therapists working in the area of adult voice work may very well find themselves being asked to help people in this client group. Consequently they should be aware of the medical programme involved when sexual reassignment is considered, be conversant with the transsexual condition and the ramifications that work of this type entails. This is in addition, of course, to any appropriate therapy procedures needing to be undertaken.

The object of this chapter is to give speech and language therapists a background knowledge about transsexualism, guidelines for approaching voice work with these clients, and suggestions about general management.

Transsexuals can, of course, be of either sex, but it is the male to female transition that is being discussed here. This is by far the most common situation, in any case, and it will be widely acknowledged that female to male clients will have the advantage, for them, of the effects of hormone therapy, a lower voice, and face and body hair. Hormone therapy for male to female transsexuals does not have any effect on the voice.

The speech and language therapist does not have to have a deep knowledge of psychiatry, counselling, psychology, fashion, or beauty therapy to work with these clients. The client is usually far better served to seek the advice of those trained in those areas, if they want long in-depth help with a particular problem. What is needed is knowledge of voice, knowledge of communication skills, a balanced psychological personality with an ability to detach oneself from the situation and a sense of humour that can be shared with the client. Above all one must like and enjoy working with this client group.

Most transsexuals want to have a sex-change operation and, with a view to possibly qualifying for this very serious undertaking, they must undergo rigorous screening. Part of this preoperative period may include help to make their voices sound as convincingly feminine as possible.

Much of the discussion in this chapter is based on personal experience gained over a period of 20 years. During this time, much of the initial work was with groups of male to female clients who had been referred through the Gender Identity Clinic at Charing Cross Hospital in London. Although the groups eventually had to be abandoned due to lack of funding, they formed the basis for valuable insight into ways to tackle both voice work and presentation skills. Now, the majority of clients are seen individually, both privately and as NHS patients. Over the years I have been referred approximately 250 transsexual clients.

The group work was held in the evenings on the hospital premises, and was particularly useful because it offered the mutual support represented by membership of the group, in addition to the speech therapy itself. It was conducted in a leisurely fashion, which was an ideal way to consolidate ideas; it worked then, but would never be tolerated in the modern streamlined NHS. It should be pointed out that although all the referees were NHS patients, the classes themselves were paid for as 'evening classes' by what was then ILEA (Inner London Education Authority).

Each group consisted of ten people, with a weekly two-hour session in ten week blocks. Many clients came back several times. At all times a total approach was aimed at, with a beauty therapist working closely with the speech therapist, and voice work was always coupled with communication skills. Clients learned from one another – what to copy and what to avoid – and unconsciously seemed to develop strategies to cope with any public criticism they might encounter, because they found they were not alone in their situation. There was also the back-up of a psychiatric social worker, who often worked with troubled family members and helped with practical matters like talking to employers and advising about legal rights.

Final results regarding how well the voice work had succeeded were in general very satisfactory, at a subjective level. Approximately a quarter of these clients went on to have an NHS sex-change operation. Some are still waiting for a referral for the operation, some decided to go privately rather than wait for what might be years, and approximately a quarter dropped out of the programme, or were encouraged to leave for various reasons. It is always accepted that many individuals in a situation of this kind are simply not able to satisfy the rigid requirements imposed during this trial period. It is also worth pointing out that now relatively few gender-reassignment operations in the UK are paid for by public money, and the majority are privately funded by individuals who have, of course, had a psychiatric referral to a surgeon. It is not possible to give an exact cost to the gender reassignment operation, as procedures vary, but one would probably be considering something between £7,500 and £9,500.

Long-term contact has been kept with many group members who it was felt achieved satisfactory voice results, and, in general, their own attitude to their voices is now one of ease when speaking, with little attention to the mechanics involved. They feel, for the most part, that their voices are acceptable, and no longer cause them personal concern. This is the goal that the therapist hopes to achieve for the client – a convincing sounding voice and a confident, unselfconscious speaker.

The first referral of a transsexual client to a speech and language therapist may well present as a daunting prospect. This is not surprising, as it is unlikely that there will have been much reference to work of this type during training; consequently it will probably be a situation far removed from both clinical and personal experience.

In England, one of the leading centres of work with transsexuals as NHS patients is at Charing Cross Hospital, so this will be used as a model in discussion. People from all over the country travel to the Gender Identity Clinic to take advantage of the psychiatric and psychological expertise and usually, if suitable, they will embark on a programme of hormone therapy. This will usually produce modest breast development, increase body fat and lessen beard growth.

To even be considered as a possible candidate for gender reassignment the client has to have lived successfully for at least a year in the female role, and be able to earn a living as a woman. He must also satisfy the psychiatric panel that he is stable and well-adjusted before the operation, and does not feel that the answer to all emotional and psychological difficulties will be instantly solved post-operatively. There is usually a long wait for National Health surgery. It is at this time that a speech and language therapist living within the client's local catchment area may be asked to help in the voice training.

Therapists exploring this area of voice work may be interested in various research projects involved in measuring fundamental frequency and intensity differences between the male and female voice. This will be discussed later in the chapter. It is hoped that any therapist who feels that he or she has a client who is a suitable subject for self-monitoring work with instrumentation techniques or if the precise progress needs to be recorded, will exploit the possibilities in this area.

This chapter's discussion is largely a very basic and practical guide based on empirical observation. It is to be expanded by individual therapists as their own experience and expertise in this area increases with confidence, and adjusted to suit each particular situation.

The transsexual condition

The term transsexual was coined by an American psychiatrist, Harry Benjamin (1966), who reported on a number of cases and became one of the first workers to initiate serious study of the subject. In her study on bisexuality, Charlotte Wolff (1977) defines transsexuals as people who believe that their mind is trapped in the wrong-sex body. She explains that some people are satisfied with hormone therapy alone, but when there is a violent clash between their sexual and gender identity, some will only be satisfied with surgical gender reassignment. It is the sense of belonging to the 'wrong' or opposite sex that disturbs them, rather than the qualities of 'masculinity' or 'femininity'.

For years, those involved with the subject have been struggling to elucidate the cause of transsexualism, but to date, all that is clear is that we do not know for sure what the causality is, while biological and psychological theories seem to trip over one another. As little is probably known about ultimate causality, as in the analogous area of homosexuality. In both conditions, there is certainly no simple anatomical cause, nor is any chromosomal abnormality securely implicated. The problem is fundamentally psychological. We understand little enough about the programming of 'normal' psychosexual differentiation, and less still about that of its deviations. Money and Erhardt (1972) aptly comment that 'the programming of psychosexual differentiation is [...] a function of biographical history'. More significantly, they go on to suggest that 'there is a close parallel here with the programming of language development'. It is hardly surprising that coping with the linguistic aspects of the transsexual's presentation proves, in its way, to be quite as important as the surgical, in creating a survival strategy for the individual.

The onset of sexuality in the developing foetus is controlled by the inherited sex chromosomes. This blueprint determines the physical development of the sex organs, and the ensuing secretion of foetal hormones from the developing gonads takes over the wider expression of sexual differences. As Money and Erhardt (1972) explain 'the testicular secretions account not only for the shape of the external genitals but also for certain patterns of organisation of the brain ... that will subsequently influence certain aspects of sexual behaviour'. But at present, there is no evidence of chromosomal or hormonal abnormality to explain the transsexual condition; yet interestingly, hormonal treatment is very widely used in supplementing the surgical treatment involved in sexual realignment!

It appears that the differentiation of the sex organs in both males and females operates on a hormone controlled pattern, superimposed on a basically female template. If no male hormone secretion makes its imprint, the foetal development follows a female path. It is less clear how far the development of the brain operates along the same lines. It is not relevant to the present chapter to pursue any further the matter of the underlying clinical cause of transsexuality, but an understanding, even in the broad terms presented here, forms a useful background for therapists working in this field.

An interesting aspect of this whole subject was discussed by Chaloner (1991) when pointing out Money and Erhardt's comparison of gender identity and language. It was mentioned how they compare 'Being bilingual from early exposure to two languages and the "learning" of sexual identity'. This leads on to the theory that 'early exposure to conflicting language signals may occasionally result in a poor version of both languages'; problems with gender identity may have a similar causality.

Whatever the aetiology, these people feel overwhelmingly that they are in the wrong-gender body, an obsession that may have dominated their life since early childhood. Mentally and emotionally they completely identify with the opposite sex and feel that their body is a tragic mistake. In their study on gender identity, Money and Erhardt (1972) explain that the transsexual is driven by a compulsion to have the appearance, body and social status of the opposite sex.

A footnote to this is that although the majority of transsexuals do wish to have complete surgical gender reassignments, some feel that although they want to live and be perceived by society as members of the opposite sex, they do not want the actual surgery possibly for reasons of health, fear of operations, or even moral reservations. It is also the case that some transsexuals choose castration only.

The sex-change operation involves castration, and the penis is then modified to form an artificial vagina, which requires a considerable period of dilation after the patient leaves hospital, usually in about a week, although recuperation often takes a month or six weeks. Breast implantation is sometimes carried out under the same general anaesthetic, but it is more commonly a secondary procedure. Although hormone therapy is generally part of both the pre- and post-operative treatment, the resulting breast development is only moderate, and not enough to satisfy some individuals' quest for their own feminine ideal image.

There is often some confusion about transvestism and transsexualism. Transvestism is the act of male to female cross-dressing, often in connection with sexual arousal, but sometimes just as a chance to indulge exhibitionist fantasies and act out another side of their personality, although the transvestite does not actually wish to assume the identity of the opposite sex. However bizarre some members of society may view the practice of transvestism, it is in fact usually totally harmless play-acting and is remarkably common. Transsexuals and transvestites often attend the same social groups and mix at clubs and parties where they feel accepted and comfortable, but the boundaries are well understood between the groups.

There is also the question as to whether there is a homosexual quality in the transsexual's desire to change sex. Most male transsexuals deny this although some wish for a permanent relationship with a man at some future time after the operation. One should be aware that in many cases, the question of gender identity has led the individuals to experience a variety of sexual experimentation. However the 'true' transsexual wants above all to appear, and be accepted, as the opposite sex; all other sexual considerations are very much secondary to this.

It is impossible to generalize, but the progress of most transsexual clients follows a certain pattern. Most say they have always felt different and uncomfortable in their developing bodies, particularly at puberty, but of course did not have the experience or knowledge to understand why these feelings existed. Rarely was the child or adolescent able to discuss his or her worries openly and in doing so, it would be the very unusual adult who would encourage the young person to follow a path alien to expectations.

So in early adulthood most try to conform to accepted social customs and fit into their gender role. Many have deliberately taken on a very masculine job in the hope it might resolve their conflicting feelings. Quite a number of transsexuals say they joined a branch of the armed forces for this reason.

A continuation of this pattern is that many transsexuals marry and have children, but in most cases they say sexual acts were performed out of duty rather than pleasure. The emotional rapport with their wives is often warm and loving; there is frequently a feeling of guilt in later years that their obsessional feelings have destroyed the marriage and caused the partner pain and distress. Many wives remain ignorant of the situation for years, while others are aware of the problem, but try to live with it.

It is very surprising that in this sexually enlightened age it is not uncommon for a transsexual to reach adulthood and be unaware that his sexual dilemma is not unique. These people are generally those who read little and have been unwilling or unable to discuss their personal feelings and experiences with others. Some of the experiences and problems that may be encountered by transsexuals are illustrated in the following cases.

Case history 1

Richard is a 57-year-old former civil servant in a government office in London. From childhood, he felt confused that he seemed different in attitude to his contemporaries, felt that his male body was a terrible mistake and that he should have been a girl, like his sisters. He dressed in their clothes whenever he could and identified in every way with the opposite sex, although he felt very guilty and was unable to stop doing what he sensed were deviant, and even possibly evil, actions. He was a good student and was good at games, but had few close friends. He was essentially a solitary person, who never discussed his feelings or sexual identity with anyone.

His entire early life was coloured by the anxiety that he must be going insane, because of these persistent feelings about being a woman. The fact that he is an extremely masculine looking person, tall, with heavy dark facial and body hair and a deep voice, made his predicament seem, to him, compounded, and all the more ridiculous.

As a young man he had a successful army career, and in spite of his lack of interest in sex, a companionable married life with three children. He began to cross-dress increasingly when he was alone and became convinced that he must be a transvestite even though he did not seem to fit the definition of that state.

It was at that time that he happened to read the book *Conundrum* by the journalist Jan Morris (1974). This was the account of Jan's life as James Morris – writer, mountain climber, father of four sons and happily married man – who also felt that he should have been born female. The book details her unhappiness as a male and her fierce struggle with problems of sexual identity. It then goes on to describe her sex-change operation and her adjustment to a new way of life as a woman. It also tells of the effect this change had on her wife and family.

Richard realized that his feelings were not unique and once told the Charing Cross transsexual group of the feeling of joy and relief that this realization gave him, even though nothing was resolved and he never told his wife of his dilemma. It was at this time that he was unexpectedly widowed, and he made the decision that he would seek medical help through his GP, who referred him to the Gender Identity Clinic.

From there he received counselling, and decided to begin to live full-time as a woman with a view to the operation. As his employers were not happy with this situation, he was retired on medical grounds. At this point, one of his three children refused further contact with his father. However, Richard was still determined to pursue this path, started electrolysis twice a week and joined the group at Charing Cross. Surprisingly, he managed to achieve a satisfactory voice against all expectations, for he was a very inhibited man who found it hard to communicate easily.

After 18 months he was referred to an NHS surgeon, and was bitterly disappointed because the surgeon refused to operate on the grounds that he could never pass visually as a woman. In the end, the surgeon has the right to refuse to perform what is, after all, not an essential operation.

One must remember the great responsibility that falls to the psychiatrist and surgeon when taking the decision to irrevocably alter another human being's life in this way. The long and often difficult 'trial period' required before any surgical referral is made is necessary for this reason, as well as being in the patient's long-term interest. Ability to pay should not be a factor in this moral dilemma, although there are enough issues involved here to qualify as a subject in a university debate.

It is interesting to note that not all psychiatrists view surgery as the answer. Benjamin (1966), for example, viewed it as a last resort – to be considered only if the patient was felt to be suicidal. He felt that more conservative therapy was often the more appropriate course.

Richard continues to live in the female role and to be active in various voluntary local organizations, where his background is well known. He has more friends and a more active social life as Edith than he had living as a man, and professes to be happier and more contented than ever before, although he claims to feel great disappointment not to have had final surgery, and thinks he was very unfairly treated by the system.

The majority of transsexuals seek help much earlier than Richard, but many wait until middle age or later, and it is often a trigger like a death or divorce that forces the decision. One group member who went forward for surgery was nearly seventy, but the average age would probably be in the early 40s.

During the assessment and trial period, hormone therapy will begin unless there is some medical reason against it. The refusal of hormone therapy often produces panic and depression in the client, but the fact remains that many transsexuals, particularly older ones, manage perfectly adequately with no drug therapy at all.

As discussed earlier, the client must live at least a year as a woman before even being considered for the operation. This involves in many cases a complete change of lifestyle and, if one considers the upheaval that would be caused if this situation occurred in one's own workplace or social circle, it is easy to appreciate the stress involved. In theory, a change in sex role should not pose a problem in a tolerant environment, but in reality, the difficulties can be immense and some employers will simply not accept the new situation. Also, in some very male dominated workplaces like a building site or an engineering works, it is difficult to accommodate a lone female. These are all real issues, and are often not thought through adequately.

It may seem very obvious to say so, but the successful organized perceptive man does not lose these qualities with a change of gender. One high-powered business manager in his male role decided to retrain as a secretary and take what he considered a gentler more feminine job. Within months she had been promoted to management level and rapidly went up that ladder.

Case history 2

Iris is now in her middle 50s; a short, slim, bright, attractive and articulate woman with a warm outgoing personality and a keen sense of humour. Iris attended one of the first groups at Charing Cross and long-term contact has been maintained with this client. She has an excellent, rather gentle voice with a slight regional accent and dresses suitably for her age. There is really no sign that this woman lived for more than forty years as a man. As well as gender reassignment Iris has had plastic surgery to her nose, and has had extensive dental work and a painful jaw realignment operation in addition to breast implantation.

The early history reflects the usual unhappy feelings of being in the wrong gender, but in spite of this Bill (as he then was) became a productive dynamic salesman, married and had six children. All his life he cross-dressed and, as he was often away from home staying in hotels, he experimented with going out in the female role and he found that not only did he seem to 'pass', but he found it more and more difficult to go back to the male role. At this point he confided in his wife, who had no idea of his feelings and began to seek psychiatric help for depression. It was at this point that he began the group classes and also began to live apart from his wife. He approached his employers, who said they would not consider keeping him on in the female role.

Bill had a remarkable wife, and after the initial shock, she decided to help him through the transition. He began to retrain and eventually moved to a country area, started a business, and he and his wife lived as sisters, bringing up the family together. This domestic situation continues, and an outwardly congenial home life has been maintained. There can be no doubt that the family suffered as a result of Bill persisting in his gender-reassignment, and it would be easy to be judgmental. However, the majority of clients in this situation say they had no choice psychologically, and their sanity depended on making the change.

It is worth mentioning that, strange as it may seem to most outsiders, many transsexuals do continue with their former wives or partners for a variety of reasons, and sexual needs and customs are adapted to meet the new situation. Not surprisingly, some relationships fail in spite of initial promises to tolerate the new situation. But it must be accepted that the majority of marriages do break up when the man begins to live openly as a woman. What might have been tolerated in the privacy of the home proves too difficult to share openly with society.

Case history 3

Simon, 42, was luckier than Bill, so far as his job was concerned, at the time of his sex-change. He was a highly paid scientific officer with a large company where his expertise was very much valued. He had lived a double life for years, until with the support of his wife he approached the firm's company director with his problem. It is interesting to note that prior to this step Simon had weighed up all sorts of alternatives about his future, from retraining to trying to 'disappear' and take on a new identity in a new location.

As it developed he had a sympathetic boss, and the decision was made to allow him a period of leave during which time his colleagues were fully briefed about his situation, and he returned to work as Wendy. He was fully aware that not everyone felt comfortable with his new persona, but he had enough support to feel accepted and occasionally even openly admired for his courage.

He has now had the operation and has moved up the job ladder. His wife did not feel that she was able to tolerate her husband in the female role, and they have parted.

At one time it was a condition before referral for surgery that the client must be divorced, but this is no longer the case. As long as the psychiatric panel is satisfied that the client is mentally stable and able to have a reasonable chance of living successfully as a woman, they can be put forward for surgery. Not all transsexuals, even those considered suitable for surgery, elect to have it. One extremely convincing-looking and sounding client who satisfied all the criteria, and had, in fact, lived as a woman for many years never wanted referral for the operation. He explained that counselling had enabled him to come to terms with the situation, and help with voice and grooming had boosted confidence. However, he felt that the operation would be an act of mutilation that would not in his case change his lifestyle. He continues to live with apparent success as a woman.

Physical appearance has not any real bearing on the transsexualism of an individual. Of course the work of the beauty therapist would be much simpler if all transsexuals were of short or medium stature, had small hands and feet, fine delicate features and minimum beard growth. Sadly this is not the case, and many extremely masculine looking men feel inwardly feminine. Appearance seems to act neither as a deterrent nor an impetus in those people wanting a sex-change.

Acoustic and linguistic considerations in transsexual treatment by speech therapists

It is appropriate at this time to discuss research work done in this area. Oates and Dacarkis (1983) give a very full review of the rather scattered and inconclusive literature on communication problems of transsexuals. As those authors emphasize, 'the validity and efficacy of management proced-ures remain limited, until a more comprehensive data base on sex markers in speech is delineated.' In this connection they discuss the important distinction between male and female 'speech markers' (on which there is little valid published data) and 'speech stereotypes'. The former are those features of speech, both segmental and non-segmental, that constitute the clues by which we consciously or unconsciously assign gender to a speaker when other (for example, visual) clues are lacking or ambiguous.

The 'speech stereotypes' are the subjective expectations of the average person as to what they expect the speech of one or other sex to be. The speech gender indicators are at present still ill-defined. What makes us identify an unknown voice on the radio as male or female? Even those who have carefully studied the subject of such 'markers' produce inconclusive results. For the purist the speech markers are the important attributes about which we need to know more, and on which further research is clearly needed. Of course fundamental frequency is the most obvious of these markers. Oates and Dacakis (1983) summarize the findings of the funda-mental frequency of adult speech as follows: adult males from 20 to 29 years have an approximate mean of 138 Hz with a range of 60–260 Hz. Females of the same age span have a mean of 227 Hz, with a range of 128–520 Hz. They conclude 'thus although female voices averaged 1.7 times higher in funda-mental frequency than those of males, the ranges for males and females overlap considerably'. It is also mentioned that in older people there is a considerable reduction in the difference between the fundamental frequen-cies of male and female speakers, although no figures are given.

Perhaps 'stereotypes' are more important to the fulfilment of the trans-sexual's expectations than the fundamental speech markers. As Oates and Dacarkis (1983) record, 'the client's goals often arise largely from stereo-typical beliefs'. In other words, it is more important that the client thinks he is creating the expected image than that he is actually reproducing the precise idiosyncrasy of the intended voice.

In summary, the help that a speech and language therapist can give to the transsexual is still based on empirical observations. Until more funda-mental research on absolute speech markers has been carried out, the therapist will be guided by subjective criteria.

Responsibility of the speech and language therapist

Voice work

The therapist gives help and practical advice on voice modification to help the client sound and project as acceptable and plausible a result as possible to the receiver.

Encouraging general communication skills

There cannot be too much emphasis on the need to develop a confident manner. This must be coupled, of course, with as convincing an appearance as possible. Expectation in the listener of hearing a female-sounding voice, because the speaker appears at ease and looks feminine, is often enough to defy the critical ear.

Referral to other agencies

This entails referral to the appropriate source for additional help if it is indicated. Advice is often sought regarding grooming, clothes or makeup. Obvious basic suggestions can be made, but referral to a beauty therapist is more satisfactory. In London there is a very comprehensive service available at La-zarus Training P.O. Box 4701 London SE1 4XL Tel. 020 7207 8473. This is run by a post-operative transsexual who is fully trained as both a make-up artist and as a model, and has appeared often both in the press and on television. This is a reputable agency aimed at helping the transsexual through the initial stages of change. It offers lessons in make-up, supplying the products if requested. This is often very useful as special needs such as beard growth, cover etc. are often needed. The prices are competitive, as are the consultation fees. The agency also offers classes in fashion and deportment.

It is sometimes difficult to make the distinction between giving help with voice and communication skills and assisting with other aspects of the client's presentation. Each therapist will feel differently about the ability to advise in these other areas, and should be guided by common sense rather than a rigid code of rules. The transsexual is often a very troubled individual who will value suggestions if made tactfully.

Information about the formalities of changing names by deed poll and queries about documents and other matters of a legal nature can be obtained from any solicitor or from the Citizens' Advice Bureau. Transsexuals should be advised to carry some sort of proof from their psychiatrist that they are undergoing medical treatment, in case they are questioned by the police, as for example they are in a traffic accident, and appear in female dress with a male driver's licence. It is also a fact that, seeking a sympathetic social setting, some transsexuals frequent gay bars and clubs. Unfortunately, these venues are apt to attract a disruptive crowd as well, and if trouble starts it is again important to have correct identification to prove a bona fide reason for being cross-dressed.

Nearly all male transsexuals need years of painful and expensive electrolysis. Information about this can be obtained from the beauty therapist mentioned earlier or from like-minded people on the Internet. Communicating with people on the Internet has proved a lifeline for many other socially isolated transsexuals.

The Albany Trust (24 Chester Square London SW1W 9HS) was set up about 30 years ago to provide information and a counselling service for members of sexual minorities and information about self-help groups and support services. The people answering the telephone are experienced in this area and nobody need feel embarrassed to make this contact.

The Trust can also put people in touch with the Beaumont Society which, although originally started to help transvestites, will also welcome transsexuals and, as wives are also welcome, it is often a valuable source of support at a possibly vulnerable time in family relationships. The Society also provides information about where to get wigs, shoes, clothes and protheses if wanted.

Refraining from personal involvement

This should be mentioned because it may be a temptation to try to undertake more in the way of counselling than one is qualified to give. Many speech and language therapists now have good basic counselling training enabling them to work very adequately with many of the clients on their caseload. But transsexuals are unique in speech therapy work and many may be under a great deal more stress and have many more deep psychological problems than may be immediately apparent, and require very specialized guidance. As Dalton (1994) points out, when discussing counselling clients with long-term psychological problems such as transsexualism, there has generally been a history since childhood of psychological stress, if not acute distress. She says, 'Here clearly, the clients' psychological needs go far beyond the issue of a change in voice' and she goes on to talk of their need for 'stringent psychological assessment to ensure that the choice they make to change their sex has been fully explored'.

Voice modification

It is assumed that anyone attempting voice work with these clients will be completely familiar with the mechanics of the normal voice and have had experience working with adult voice patients. The anatomical differences of the voice-producing apparatus of the male and female, such as size of larynx and length and mass of vocal tract, will be well understood.

The rationale, therefore, behind any techniques suggested will be self-evident, so it is expedient to outline the therapy programme in terms one would use in explanation to a client. All the following procedures have been practised without creating problems of vocal strain.

The only case of hoarseness (not including problems following vocal cord surgery) among the group members started when a client was about to have the gender-reassignment operation. The condition persisted to such a degree that she was seen post-operatively by an ENT surgeon. It was found to be an entirely functional problem, and gradually resolved itself in a few months. This client had had a period of several years caring for a terminally ill wife. Although her death had allowed the husband freedom to have the longed-for sex-change, it was still an emotionally traumatic period, and the voice suffered.

As was mentioned earlier, this is a guide to the straightforward techniques employed in the ordinary clinical situation. In other words, the answer to, 'But what do I *do* with the client?'. That there are more sophisticated methods employing instrumentation is well-known, and one such American case study of a post-operative client will be referred to at the end of the chapter.

It might be argued that as this is essentially an exercise in acting, it might be more expedient to send transsexuals to a drama coach. After all, the only 'disorder' of the voice is that the client views it as a hindrance to his ability to function successfully as a woman. However, these are not professional actors but troubled individuals who need the help of someone who is used to dealing with people under stress, and where there is medical back-up available.

The reference to acting may seem obvious, but it is not always easy for these clients to accept this idea. It has been my experience that, much as a transsexual may wish to produce a convincing female voice naturally, he often dislikes the idea of having to deliberately work to achieve it. To concentrate on how the voice sounds, and thinking about altering its production is sometimes, understandably, felt to inhibit thought and conversation.

It is the dislike of feeling they must 'put on an act' that worries the transsexual. This feeling does not extend to wearing female dress or make-up, because this is the natural taste and inclination. Clothes are simply part of the female image he wishes to impart on the world and to himself. Many preoperative transsexuals refuse to look at themselves undressed as they find it so distressing, especially when they are going through the process of change.

To openly defuse this worry about acting by talking it over is often a helpful step to move the voice therapy on. Tell the client that it is a difficult but achievable task, but unless he is remarkably lucky, considerable effort is necessary. My work has been almost entirely with pre-operative clients, who need a passable, if not a perfect, voice to qualify for surgical referral. In my experience the new female voice usually improves with use and in most cases is usually quite acceptable, so long as the rest of the presentation is reasonable. There are, of course, some natural actors who enjoy the process of vocal gymnastics. People with some singing ability, or at least an ear for music, usually do better than those with no ability to tell one note from another. Getting a client to develop even the rudiments of musical skills is often an opening to self-monitoring.

It is convenient to divide the plan for voice work into the following categories, and for these to be interwoven as appropriate:

1. assessment
2. relaxation
3. voice experimentation
4. breathing for speech
5. pitch establishment
6. elimination of chest resonance
7. intonation, peaking and lilt
8. role-playing and self-expression practice
9. non-verbal communication
10. personality projection and communication skills

Assessment

As assessment is our tool for drawing up a plan for treatment, the following outline is suggested as a useful guide. This is a subjective assessment based on the first meeting with this client. We assume that the client will present at the initial interview dressed as a woman and using his 'female voice' if he has one.

1. Is the voice already convincing enough to pass as feminine?
2. Does it need only minor adjustments?
3. Is it a light-sounding male voice?
4. Is it unmistakably masculine?

This impression will be influenced, of course, by how well the client presents and how at ease he is with his voice and his ability to communicate as a woman. Many clients have been playing this role successfully for years. There can be every permutation of looks and voice with no absolute categories.

I recently had the experience of having a musician referred, and when he made the appointment on the telephone the voice was so female that I said he really didn't need my services, but he wanted to come anyway. He was very masculine-looking and in person when relaxed the voice sounded noticeably affected with the almost 'camp' quality of the gay male, although of course this was not the case for this person. Removing the drawling quality of the voice and the affected facial expression that went with it, was all that my role required. His accent was a soft west country one, and he said he had made no alteration to it. This was borne out by his telling me at a later date that after he had had considerable help to soften his image and was living the female role full-time, an old friend who knew nothing about his new life heard his voice in a crowd, and recognized him solely by that.

The following things should be noted:

1. quality of voice
2. impression of the degree of chest resonance
3. pitch
4. method of delivery, e.g. hard or soft attack
5. manner of articulation
6. manner of speech
   Is it flat and unemotional? Is there a regional accent that can possibly be capitalized on? Has an attempt been made to feminize the voice by the affected quality just mentioned?
7. physical impression
   One needs to record how the client presents as a person, how intelligent he appears to be, and how realistically perceptive he is about the overall problems that may be encountered, no matter how good the appearance and voice may become. One also needs to note size, age, and appropriateness of dress and make-up. One should also record habits that detract from his appearing as a relaxed speaker, or communicator in general, as, for example, poor eye contact, rigidity of face, over-anxious manner, covering the face or Adam's apple and similar traits. Some of this may sound very trivial, but they add up to the overall impression. We must also be realistic ourselves, and realize that some things can never be improved as well as might be wished, so that it would be short-sighted to ignore those that can.

In general, of course, one expects the voice to be lower in pitch than that of the average female speaker, and although many females have reasonably low voices, they probably aren't usually mistaken on the phone for a man. This is because the male speaker is generally chiefly using chest resonance. This is, in fact, the most important single difference in the two voices, and the area where most work is needed.

It may sound very simplistic to state the following, but what one is attempting to do is to instruct the speaker in ways to modify only slightly his own speech production. In realistic terms this means that one should try to bring about as little vocal change as possible, and still carry off the illusion of a female voice. It is a rare client who has the discipline to work endlessly on trying to create a voice of mechanical perfection. The effort involved tends to create such a self-conscious speaker that pleasure in human communication is lost.

It may be of interest here to mention one of the more unusual clients that attended the Charing Cross groups. He was a totally convincing looking – and sounding – female, a South American journalist, with a charming manner and perfect dress sense, a small delicate man with premature grey hair and, at 43, both elegant and sophisticated. He had a soft contralto voice with a strong Portuguese accent. I repeatedly asked him if he would speak in Portuguese to compare the effect of his speaking a second language carefully and slowly and how he sounded in his native tongue. He totally refused to do this, and would give no reason, but I suspect that as he had come to England for the operation and it was only from his arrival here that he had totally assumed his new role, he simply did not want to interrupt the masquerade.

One glaring problem that Carlo did have was a total lack of animation. He had a rigidity of face and manner that called attention to itself, despite his perfection of visual presentation in all other aspects. As one might imagine, members of a group like this often establish warm friendships because of their common experiences, but Carlo was never able to establish rapport with anyone.

In this particular case we did spend time trying to break down barriers by role play and talking about the problem. There was some improvement, but even in the end he was very wax-dummy-like which unfortunately caught one's attention. Too much perfection is perhaps not totally feminine. In any case, he went on to have the operation and one might feel this was a success story, especially as he went on with his journalistic career when he returned home. As he worked from home and was at the time unmarried, his life was fairly solitary, as it always had been, although there was a mother, brothers and sisters.

I did, however, feel less satisfied with his ability to cope with the new lifestyle emotionally and with his family than I have with many others, who seemed more human in spite of their imperfection. This is, of course, not the speech and language therapist's problem, but it is almost impossible to separate the voice from the personality, and one is always aware of the total person. Some things are too deep-seated to try to correct in voice therapy sessions, and it would be inappropriate to try. Carlo's personal isolation was a personality problem, but although he was having counselling arranged by the psychiatrist, there was no evident change at all in this area.

Relaxation

Whatever the feeling about the use of relaxation as part of voice therapy one cannot deny that it is a useful aid in getting an individual to feel in control of his own body. It is also essential to be physically relaxed in order to breathe correctly. Progressive relaxation is effective, and it is important to suggest that the client concentrate on feeling the state of relaxation in order to try to return to it at times of alarm or great tension. Greene (1975) summarizes many of the various relaxation techniques; other excellent descriptions can be found in Boone and McFarlane (1988) and Butcher et al. (1993).

This ability to be 'in control' means that the client is not going to forget all about using the feminine voice whenever there is a stressful situation. One can readily understand the reasons for this, and giving them a tool like relaxation to use in time of panic is an investment in ensuring that the overall therapy programme succeeds as well as possible.

Vocal experimentation

Most individuals have no idea of the variety and range of sounds that the voice is capable of producing. It is often reassuring for someone to realize that it is possible to free the voice from rigid vocal habits, even if initially it feels embarrassing to try attempting it. To accomplish this, suggest that imitation is made of sounds that have no connection with speech, and so require no intellectual effort. For example, the copying of musical instruments, birds, sounds of nature or even animal noises. This type of exercise is very disinhibiting and encourages further voice experimentation. It can also be incorporated when trying to eliminate chest resonance, which will be discussed later.

Breathing for speech

Instruction in diaphragmatic breathing, with exercises to increase the efficiency of breath control, is extremely important. The ultimate aim is to gain control of this breath, much as a singer would, both to support and project the sound. The difference in the technique that the transsexual should try to employ is that, instead of using the full tank of air to speak with full-balanced power, he controls the flow so that no articulation begins until the air is centred in the mouth. He then manipulates the sound in the oral cavity so that the voice is 'smaller', and a shade more breathy.

What he is in fact doing is taking little 'tucks' of air from the full chest reservoir created by efficient diaphragmatic breathing, and then articulating. The articulation itself should be light so that there are precise lip and tongue movements and deliberate lip rounding.

The breathy sound mentioned needs careful monitoring to be sure it is barely noticeable. If done properly the softening result can be very effective.

Another very useful technique is to ask the client to sing an easy and familiar song and explain the quality of the singing is not important, but rather the fact that he should become aware of taking a breath before the phrase he is singing. Then suggest he take the breaths but speak the song so that the breath finishes on the phrase end and the whole effect is a breath supported musical voice. This breath support will enable the client to be able to slightly vary the pitch if necessary by sliding the pitch up or down without having to start again.

Pitch establishment

Something has to be said about pitch, but in fact it is not an area that one should interfere with too much unless some slight pitch elevation comes about very easily, is not too difficult to sustain and the ear is good enough to monitor its continuance. It was once thought that for a man to make his voice sound feminine he should raise the pitch to the falsetto. In reality, of course, all this accomplishes is to make the voice sound like a man speaking in a falsetto voice! In addition, even if it were effective it would be very difficult to sustain.

As was mentioned, there is considerable overlap between the pitch ranges of male and female voices. Often in the middle-aged speaker the pitch needs to be raised only slightly – often by mentally fixing an agreed note on the scale, such as /la/, and starting speech on that note.

One will remember that the fixation of a singer's pitch begins in the brain. From there, the signal is sent to the vocal cords, which tense to the appropriate size and shape. It is hoped that the transsexual can learn the rudiments of this technique.

I agree with Bryan-Smith's (1986) experience with her clients, that ear training and practice gradually bring about a gentle rise of pitch. It is also interesting to note that she had two clients xeroradiographed by MacCurtain at the Middlesex Hospital, and in both cases found that there was a change of laryngeal position when they used a female voice instead of a male one. It was found that both clients achieved an enlarged super-glottic space during female speech due to tilting back of the larynx but this was not done when they were speaking in the male voice. Apparently both these clients passed very well when speaking as females.

Elimination of chest resonance

This is one of the most vital areas of this work. It is useful to have the client think of his body as a series of empty spaces or echo chambers one on top of the other. He must then learn to move sound up and down through this series of chambers from chest to neck to head and down again until the feeling and sound of each is established in his mind and ear. This exercise may take some time and concentration. The ultimate aim with this is to establish the ability to produce sound from the head region. It is possible to suggest to the client that when he actually feels the vibration coming from the head region he concentrates on prolonging the sounds until he finds it easy to hum or intone various nasal or vowel sounds from this area. From there he should progress to the intoning of words starting with these sounds, as for example, 'my music', 'much money', 'many moons', etc. From there he can be asked to flatten the intoning into speaking the phrases and thus establish the pattern of using head resonance.

As this is an important part of the voice training programme it is necessary to take plenty of time working through this stage of therapy. Let the client hear the difference on the tape recorder and actually feel with his hands the vibrations moving from chamber to chamber.

Articulation techniques

As mentioned, emphasis should be on 'light' articulation with suggestions that the client should think of making delicate contact with the articulators as he reads a passage. He should focus speech forward in the face, thinking of pushing the sound forward to the lips, which should if possible be very slightly rounded. Suitable choice of material should be considered to let the client feel feminine during practice. One is not trying to produce a stereotypical female, but it is easier in practice to concentrate on gentle poetry or prose than militant or violent material.

Peaking, intonation and lilt

Peaking is a term used to explain the method of raising the pitch of the voice at intervals up high enough to break into the falsetto for an instant and thereby adding variety to the voice and giving the illusion of a higher pitch and lighter voice. This can be practised by marking a passage so that the client knows when to raise the pitch up, perhaps on every fifth syllable or as seems appropriate.

It should be noted that in general the female voice tends to end phrases with a rising intonation pattern while the male voice uses a falling pattern.

The female voice also has much more rise and fall and variety of pitch levels as opposed to the much flatter male monotone.

Role playing, non-verbal communication and personality projection

These last three items are areas that are combined together and there is considerable overlap. It is worth mentioning that one does not want to feel this is a charm school, which is certainly not our object, but to work solely on the voice and ignore obviously masculine personality traits and mannerisms is short-sighted. In the end the client can decide what he feels is worth noting and possibly making an effort to alter.

Dr Lillian Glass (1992) has written a fascinating study about the communication differences between the sexes; it is a useful reference tool in role play situations or just as a check list to discuss with the client.

To touch briefly on a few of the sex differences in this area;

1. *Body language:* in general men take up more space than women, use more forceful gestures, gesture away from the body and keep their gesturing fingers closed. Women do the opposite when gesturing. Women lean forward when listening while men lean backward and men provide less listener feedback in conversation than women.

2. *Facial language:* men use less eye contact, provide few facial reactions and use less animation than women.

3. *Speech habits:* men interrupt more, use more fillers like 'um'; do not open their mouth as widely and speak more slowly than women. Men ask fewer questions, rarely discuss their personal life, use fewer emotional verbs (like feel, love, hope, etc.) and use more slang and jargon than women.

4. *Differences in behaviour:* men give fewer compliments, are more critical, use more sarcasm, gossip less and tell more jokes than women.

For every statement one can find an argument, but these are some general well-researched sex differences. In my experience the clients who make the greatest success of living in the female role from the personality point of view are those who are warm and outgoing and interested in other people. Transsexuals are often made quite insular due to the circumstances of their lives and are often very self-absorbed, which makes it difficult to communicate in either sex role. This is a subject worth discussing with the client as awareness of these barriers is often a help to breaking some of them down.

Vocal cord surgery

This has become a far more common operation over the past few years and there are a number of transsexuals who feel it is an option they are determined to try. The surgery involved reduces the vibrating length of the vocal cords and thereby hopefully raises the pitch to a believable level with no long-term attendant hoarseness. The ENT surgeons doing these operations are very skilled and the number of satisfied clients is better than it used to be, but success in the new role depends on more than just the pitch of the voice being in normal parameters. An operation to reduce the laryngeal prominence can also be done with or without the vocal cord surgery.

Using instrumentation

Some speech therapists have used Visispeech to help their clients monitor their speech and help them to match their pitch contours with those of a female voice as displayed on the screen. Mount and Salmon (1988) give an account of changing the vocal characteristics of a 63-year-old post-operative patient, over an 11-month period, using this type of instrumentation with a high degree of success. This is an important study of an in-depth analysis of the measurable differences between the male and female voice. Any speech therapist who feels that he or she has a suitable individual client, and the facilities and time to work with him very intensively, should study this literature.

Summary

Most transsexuals can achieve an adequately unisex voice to enable them to be absorbed into the world as females provided they are intelligent enough to understand what is expected of them. Far more important, however, than the vocal mechanics is the building of a confident manner and a feeling of self-worth in the individual.

As was said earlier the reasons these clients want to change their sex are varied and deep-seated, and the therapist is not expected to try to unravel them, and should not attempt to do so. Sufficient to say that in some cases failure to achieve an adequate voice is not the failure of the therapist, but lies within the client's psyche. In a few cases, much as the clients insist they want to change sex, there seems a reluctance to let go the male voice, even when they have the ability to do so.

Not all transsexuals are going to blend completely into society as believable women, although many do and these are the ones we do not notice. Life for some will eventually have to be a great compromise. But even this compromise can often bring a greater degree of happiness and peace of mind than has ever been experienced before by these people.

As an individual opinion, I think the greatest fulfilment and happiness is experienced by those who continue in a life where they were known in the male role and accepted as someone with a problem who hopes for support and acceptance, but does not expect full understanding from everyone. The client who manages to get a reasonable voice and presents as a believable likeable woman usually finds that after the initial shock of friends and colleagues life can be fairly normal. It is a fact that many marriages fail and relatives cannot accept the new role, but it may be too much to expect in many situations.

Research is going to enable us to measure more accurately the differences between the voices of the sexes. It may be that even when there is fuller theoretical understanding of male/female discriminators this will not materially affect the present empirical pattern of therapy adopted in these cases.

Lastly, one can endlessly debate the moral issue of whether one should, in fact, help these people at all. They are, in the eyes of many people, acting immorally by going against nature, and should not be assisted in achieving this goal. This is a decision for the individual therapist and if it is wrong for him or her personally, that decision should be respected. I feel one should not be judgmental in these cases, and that the moral issue is not one for the therapist to decide. I also feel that no matter what our personal feelings, one must realize that these clients are going to go ahead and try to pass visually and vocally as women with or without our help. We are simply giving them the benefit of our expertise. The final decision about what they decide to do with their lives is out of our hands and lies with the individual.

CHAPTER 15

Post radiotherapy voice quality

EVA CARLSON

Introduction

An early symptom of cancer of the larynx is persistent hoarseness unresponsive to conservative treatment by antibiotics. If the patient is known to be a heavy smoker and possibly also drinker, the astute GP should promptly refer the patient to a local ENT department, for examination of the vocal folds for any mass lesion or mucosal changes to account for the hoarseness. Any irregularity or change in texture, mobility or colour of the laryngeal tissues observed may lead to further investigations, in the case of suspected malignancy, to direct laryngoscopy and biopsy of suspicious looking areas.

The fact that laryngeal cancer produces symptoms early, and metastasizes late, makes it a highly curable form of cancer by means of radiotherapy. It is only when patients wait to see their doctor, often for fear of what may be the matter, or are not being referred to the otolaryngologist in time that the cancer may spread superficially into the sub- or supraglottis and/or into deeper layers of the vocal folds. In such cases, the first line of treatment may be surgery and the patient may need a total laryngectomy with or without post operative radiotherapy. These tumours are more advanced and tend to be those classified as T3 and T4 tumours, often with palpable lymph nodes on the same or opposite side of the laryngeal tumour, which further decreases the likely long-term survival rate of the patients (see Table 15.1).

However, this chapter will review reports on the effect of radiotherapy on voice quality in patients with early glottic carcinomas, that is tumour stages T1N0M0 and T2N0M0. In Britain these are the tumours most likely to be treated with radiotherapy. In recent years successful outcomes have also been reported after laser resection of superficial early tumours.

The main aim of treatment in laryngeal cancer is survival, but as cure rates of early glottic carcinomas are excellent, another aim of treatment is to ensure a good quality of life for these patients. The early and late effects of radiotherapy on the laryngeal mucosa will be described, as will the effect on voice quality in the short and long term. Some evidence will also be offered of the beneficial effect of voice therapy and vocal hygiene advice.

Staging of tumours

The TNM system for classification of cancer has been regularly revised and updated to provide a system for clinical classification of the severity and extent of tumours (Sobin and Wittekind, 1997). The extent of each lesion is defined in terms of three parameters (Table 15.1). Such a system facilitates exchange of information and comparison of treatments and end stage results.

Table 15.1 TNM staging for glottic carcinomas

T1	–	Tumour is limited to vocal cords with normal mobility
T2	–	Tumour extends to subglottic and/or supraglottic region with impairment of vocal fold mobility
T3	–	Tumour as in T1 or T2 but with fixation of one or both cords
T4	–	Tumour invades through thyroid cartilage and/or extends to other tissues beyond the larynx
		—
N0	–	No lymph node involvement
N1	–	Ipsilateral single lymph nodes < 3 cm
N2	–	Ipsilateral single lymph nodes 3–6 cm
		Ipsilateral multiple lymph nodes < 6 cm
		Bilateral, contralateral lymph nodes < 6 cm
N3	–	Lymph nodes > 6 cm
		—
MX	–	Distant metastases cannot be assessed
M0	–	No distant metastases
M1	–	Distant metastases

Source: Adapted from Sobin and Wittekind, 1997.

Incidence of laryngeal carcinoma

Tumours of the larynx constitute 2% of all cancers diagnosed, and are among the most common tumours of the head and neck. In 1980, 1725 laryngeal carcinomas were diagnosed in England and Wales, which gives an incidence of 4 per 100 000. (Sikora and Halnan, 1990). An article by Cann and Fried (1984) cites a statistic from the United States that 2.3% of all cancers diagnosed in males and 0.4% in females are cancers of the larynx (Young et al., 1981; Flanders and Rothman, 1982).

In a large retrospective study of laryngeal pathologies by age, sex and occupation in a treatment-seeking sample Herrington-Hall et al. (1988) reported laryngeal carcinoma as the fourth most common diagnosis, in 9.7 % of a total sample of 1262 cases. It was distributed equally across the age range 45–64 and over age 64, and developed approximately at the same age in men and women. It was most common in retired people. The male to female ratio in their sample was 3/1. The West Midlands Cancer Registry reports an incidence of laryngeal carcinoma in the period 1988–92 of 4.2 per 100000, and a male/female ratio of approximately 7/1.

Certain factors combine or enhance the risk of people developing cancer of the larynx. The most important are sex, age, smoking, alcohol drinking, exposure to employment related risk factors such as inhalation of asbestos dust, and genetic susceptibility (Rothman et al., 1980).

The combined effect of smoking and alcohol drinking is not simply additive but the risk is about 50% greater than the risk of cancer developing as a result of one of the agents alone (Flanders and Rothman, 1982; Guenel et al., 1988).

There is obviously a strong tendency for laryngeal cancer to be more common in men. However, the incidence among women aged 50 and over has shown a marked increase over time, which is assumed to reflect the increased smoking habits among women (Cann and Fried, 1984).

Treatment for early laryngeal tumours

The most common laryngeal tumour is a generally well-differentiated squamous cell carcinoma. Vocal fold tumours tend to be of this type. Gerritsen and Snow (1991) report a tendency for glottic carcinomas to affect the anterior parts of the vocal cords and the anterior commissure.

For laryngeal tumours, stages T1 and T2, radiotherapy tends to be the primary form of treatment in Britain and surgical procedures are used for salvage in case of recurrence.

For T1 tumours with no involvement of the anterior or posterior commissures, laser excision may be used with good results (Strong, 1975; McGuirt et al., 1992). Cragle and Brandenburg (1993), in a literature review comparing cure rates of early glottic tumours by laser cordectomy or radiotherapy, found that both methods were just as effective in achieving cure, the voice quality was comparable and, important in these days of health care rationing, laser excision was considerably cheaper. They therefore advocate laser excision rather than radiotherapy for most early tumours. This may increasingly become the treatment of choice, and presumably avoid some of the inevitable normal tissue damage caused by the irradiation and the resulting acute and late radiation reactions that are reported.

However, radiotherapy is likely to continue to be extensively employed for many early tumours that are not well localized, and much research has been, and continues to be, devoted to finding the most effective treatment for control of such tumours.

Treatment is delivered in fractions of radiation doses per day until a maximum total tumour dose of 5000–7000 cGy has been given. The total dose depends on the tumour volume and radiosensitivity, and normal tissue tolerance. A number of different fractionation schedules have been employed over the years with the aim of achieving maximum control rate and survival of the patients with the least number of side effects. Cost in time and money to the health service providers and the patients is also an issue.

After diagnosis and staging of the glottic tumour the patient will be involved in careful treatment planning using a simulator, a diagnostic X-ray machine which allows the radiologist accurately to localize the volume of tissue to be treated in order to treat the tumour with as homogenous a dose of radiation as possible and minimize the dose to normal tissues. A transparent plastic shell, or mask, is produced, with markings indicating the areas to be irradiated. During each treatment session the patient is immobilized using this shell. Common radiation field sizes in early glottic tumours are between 5 x 5 cm and 7 x 7 cm. The smaller tend to be used for T1 tumours, the larger ones for more extensive T2 tumours.

Mendenhall et al. (1988) describe the extension of the radiation field for T1 lesions as usually extending from the thyroid notch superiorly to the inferior border of the cricoid anteriorly. The posterior border depends on the posterior extension of the tumour. The fields for T2 tumours are larger because of the larger extent of the tumour.

Once the tumour volume has been decided, careful computer calculations are made to arrange the distribution of the radiation fields to give a homogenous dose to the entire treatment volume.

Control rates

'Control rate' refers to the disease free long-term survival rates of patients after treatment for cancer. A number of studies are reported every year regarding control rates with radiotherapy treatment for early cancer of the glottis. To mention but a few, Mantravadi et al. (1983) report 87 % recurrence free survival, Shapsey and Hybels (1985) give a cure rate of 80–90% three year survival without recurrence. More recently a report by Chatani et al. (1993), studying a group of patients treated for T1N0M0 tumours, found a ten-year relapse free rate of 83% and ultimate loco-regional control using surgery for salvage in 97% of patients, with voice preservation in 86%.

A study by Medini et al. (1996) reported 97% disease free survival after three years in patients treated for T1 glottic tumours. Treatment was delivered in small fractions of 1.75 Gy in 40 fractions over 56 days and the total tumour dose was 7000 cGy. They recommended this treatment schedule for patients who show a low tolerance to irradiation with laryngitis, oedema and swallowing difficulties induced by larger fractions.

There is some evidence that prolonging the radiotherapy treatment, in cases where there is low tolerance, may allow tumour repopulation, or cell division during rest periods; the shorter the time over which the treatment is delivered, the better the chances of tumour control. Robertson et al. (1993) tested six different fractionation schedules and found that a total tumour dose of 6000 cGy, delivered in 25 fractions over a 35-day period was the most effective. This tends to be the most common schedule used in Britain.

Rugg et al. (1990) describe radiotherapy treatment over a shorter space of time than in the common 4–6 weeks of treatment five days per week. CHART (continuous, hyperfractionated, accelerated radiotherapy) gives 36 fractions of 140 cGy, over a 12-day period with three treatments per day at six-hourly intervals, up to a total dose of 5040 cGy (Rugg et al., 1990).

The effect of radiotherapy on laryngeal tissues and factors influencing recovery

Radiotherapy causes destruction of malignant disease both at the tumour site and at nearby microscopic extensions. It also sterilizes tumour cells within the local lymphatic system (Lo et al., 1985). Laryngeal oedema is the main side effect, as the radiotherapy causes an inflammatory response in normal tissues. This accounts for the hoarse or aphonic voice during the late stages of radiotherapy in some patients.

The duration of oedema after the end of radiotherapy treatment has been shown to be affected by:

- dose of radiation;
- volume of tissue irradiated;
- continued use of alcohol and tobacco;
- size and extent of the original lesion.

Mendenhall et al. (1988) found a serious complication rate of 0.5 % in 184 patients with T1 lesions. This rate increased to 3.4 % in their group of 119 T2 lesions.

A study by Fu et al. (1982) found that in a group of 247 patients irradiated for cancer of the larynx, oedema was common after radiotherapy but usually subsided in 4–6 weeks. Thirty-seven patients had oedema beyond this time and 17 of these were found to have recurrent disease. Mantravadi et al. (1983) report an overall incidence of laryngeal oedema of 18 %. Of these 54 % were free of cancer recurrence. This indicates that persistent oedema is an important warning sign of possible recurrence.

Acute and late complications of radiation e.g. dysphagia and persistent laryngeal or soft tissue oedema are associated with large radiation field sizes (Stell and Morrison, 1973; Fu et al., 1982). Optimum size seems to be an area of 6 by 8 cm for supraglottic tumours and as little as 5 by 5 cm for glottic tumours on account of their sparse lymphatic drainage (Wang, 1974; Botnick et al., 1984).

Inoue et al. (1992) studied the effect of field size on the control rates of T1 vocal fold cancers and found that a larger treatment field size resulted in a higher proportion of minor complication rates, such as persistent laryngeal oedema, without improving the local control rate. A field size 5 by 5 cm resulted in a 93 % control rate with 4 % persistent oedema. A field size 6 by 6 cm resulted in 95 % control but 21 % persistent oedema.

Rugg et al. (1990) using CHART, demonstrated the detrimental effect of continued smoking on mucosal recovery after radiotherapy. Mucosal reactions appeared on days 13–15 in the majority of cases and persisted for 8–24 weeks. They found that the duration of oedema was 13 weeks in those patients who stopped smoking and did not restart, as opposed to 21 weeks in those who smoked during and after treatment or started again 4 weeks after treatment. In patients whose mucosal reactions healed quickly, recovery of the mucosa to normal appearance often occurred. Prolonged reactions were associated with permanently thinned and atrophic mucosal appearances. Under conventional fractionation regimes the effect is likely to be present but less marked than when CHART is used.

Whittet et al. (1991) confirmed Rugg et al.'s (1990) finding of the detrimental effect on the mucosa of continued smoking during and after radiotherapy. They also found that a small group of non-smokers, who were heavy drinkers, developed significant mucositis (inflammatory reaction of the mucous membrane) during radiotherapy. Considering the findings reported earlier on the powerful contribution of alcohol drinking to increasing the risk of developing laryngeal cancer, this finding may not be surprising.

Karim et al. (1983) found significantly higher smoking habit scores among those patients who reported unsatisfactory voice quality post radiotherapy. In Benninger et al.'s study (1994b) smokers were significantly more likely to have poor voice quality than those who did not smoke. They also had a highly significant, sixfold increased risk of recurrence.

In some early studies (Mendonca, 1975; Stoicheff, 1975; Karim et al., 1983) patients were asked to rate the time the voice took to recover after radiotherapy. This varied between 2 and 6 months.

The effect of radiotherapy on vocal fold vibration

Stroboscopic observations

The effect of radiotherapy on voice quality has been the subject for study since the early days of radiotherapy treatment for cancer of the larynx.

Riska and Lauerma (1966) used stroboscopy to evaluate the effect on vocal fold function in a group of 24 patients who had radiotherapy as a primary treatment for early vocal fold tumours. Only three of these patients were deemed not to have any observable abnormality in vocal fold function. In all the others, irregular or asymmetrical vocal fold vibration was observed. The cord particularly affected by the tumour appeared red, thickened or atrophic resulting in deviant vibratory patterns. Despite this the majority (15) of the patients were deemed to have voice qualities that fell within the top two of five perceptual categories. However, of these, five were dissatisfied with their voices. These patients had gone back to work.

Werner-Kukuk et al. (1968) used ultra-high-speed photography for observation of the larynx at different times during and after radiotherapy in one subject. The mass lesion and inflammatory reaction of the laryngeal mucous membranes resulted in the restriction of the amplitude of vibration of the vocal folds and prevented their close approximation.

A comprehensive study by Lehman et al. (1988) compared a group of 20 male subjects, aged 55–80, 1–7 years after radiotherapy for T1 tumours of the vocal folds, to a group of normal age and sex matched subjects. Videostroboscopy showed that 12 of 20 irradiated subjects showed irregular closure of the glottis. The vibratory edge of the vocal fold margins was irregular in 17 subjects, often on the side contralateral to the tumour. The amplitudes of vibration were reduced and abnormal mucosal wave and phase abnormalities were observed. Some degree of extraneous supra-glottic activity was also observed in 13 subjects.

All the subjects had had at least one direct laryngoscopy and biopsy prior to irradiation and Lehman et al. (1988) suggest the explanation for the observed abnormalities may be radiation fibrosis and breakdown of elasticity. Depth of biopsy, or stiffness resulting from it, is also a possibility, but they found that patients who had stripping of the affected vocal fold did not show significantly worse acoustic perturbation measures than patients who had more localized biopsies.

Carlson (1995b) found the most common laryngeal observation after radiotherapy under stroboscopy was of vocal fold atrophy (thinning), a reduced mucosal wave over the irradiated vocal fold and asymmetrical vocal fold vibration. Hypertrophied false vocal folds were also often observed.

Verdonck-de Leeuw (1998), using stroboscopy to examine 60 irradi-ated early glottic cancer patients, found that the irradiated patients often showed glottic oedema and injection of the vocal fold. The vocal fold edge was often found to be irregular with a diminished mucosal wave. Occasionally a non-vibrating portion was observed. The effect of this was often incomplete vocal fold closure.

The effect of radiotherapy on perceptual and self-rated voice quality parameters

An early version of the GRBAS scale for perceptual evaluation of voice quality was used by Isshiki et al. (1969) to attempt differential diagnosis of hoarseness resulting from vocal cord polyps and nodules, as opposed to cancerous lesions.

The voice quality resulting from a cancerous lesion, of the same size and on the same site on the vocal cord as a benign lesion, was rated significantly more 'breathy' than the voice quality produced by the benign lesions. The voice of a patient with laryngeal cancer would have degrees of both 'rough' and 'breathy' quality as opposed to the benign laryngeal lesions that produced 'rough' quality. The acoustic correlate of 'breathy' quality, the 'B' factor, was characterized by a marked noise component in the spectrum, with reduced or negligible harmonic components. The acoustic correlate of factor 'R' (rough) was found to be fundamental frequency perturbation. The latter was assumed to be due to asymmetry of the vibrating cords.

Many early studies of voice quality after radiotherapy report a return to perceived normal or near normal voice quality in a majority of patients (Mendonca, 1975; Stoicheff, 1975; Karim et al., 1983).

Stoicheff (1975) carried out a comprehensive study of the effects of radiation treatment on patients' 'quality of life'. The patients made self-ratings of voice using the following categories:

1. Normal
2. Improved but not quite normal
3. Improved but still a problem
4. A definite problem

She found that patients tended to rate their voices more favourably with increasing time after radiotherapy. Despite a high proportion of patients in her study reporting 'normal' or 'near normal' voice after radiotherapy (83%), a majority (80%) also reported persisting problems with fatiguing of voice, difficulty in singing/speaking loudly or shouting, and hoarseness of the voice. This may be explained by Lehman et al.'s findings (1988) on the basis of their comprehensive objective measurements, among them measures of airflow and subglottic pressure, that voice production requires considerably more effort after radiotherapy. This was confirmed by observation of extraneous supraglottic activity on videostroboscopy, and patients' subjective reports of an increased effort required to speak (Lehman et al., 1988).

Numerous studies report perceptual ratings of voice quality by trained voice professionals. A number of different terms and scales are used to describe voice quality and the results are therefore often difficult to compare. They seem, however, to point in the same general direction of the post radiotherapy voice being better than the voice before radiotherapy, but not completely normal compared to controls (Lehman et al., 1988; Carlson, 1995b; Verdonck-de Leeuw, 1998)

Verdonck-de Leeuw (1998) used both trained and untrained judges, as well as the patients themselves, to rate the voice quality of her irradiated patients. Trained judges rated the voices as more 'breathy', 'rough' and 'tense' before radiotherapy than after. Voices 6 months after radiotherapy sounded more 'tense' and in the long term (2 years and 3–7 years later) voices sounded more 'rough' than the normal controls. She remarks, however, that in the very long term (7–10 years after radiotherapy) the voices were not rated differently from the normal controls. Summarizing her findings she concludes that 55% of 40 irradiated subjects' voices after radiotherapy were within normal limits and 45% were judged to have abnormal degrees of breathiness, roughness and/or tension.

A study by Stoicheff et al. (1983) showed significant differences in the degree of perceived 'dysphonia' between normal speakers and laryngeal cancer patients both before and after radiotherapy for T1 tumours. The treatment changed the voice quality of irradiated speakers from predominantly 'strained', 'hoarse' and 'breathy' to 'hoarse' and 'rough'.

The longitudinal retrospective study by Benninger et al. (1994b) reported 67 % of irradiated patients' voices rated as 'normal' or 'near normal', 25 % as 'raspy' or 'weak' and 12 % as having 'poor' voice quality. Forty of the 63 patients were rated by the researchers in the clinic and were also asked to rate their own voice quality using the same terms as above. There was found to be a 90% agreement between the ratings.

Lehman et al. (1988) found patients' self-perception of voice quality more favourable than objective measurements indicated. Their study concluded that the post-radiation voice is not normal. It seems, however, that patients perceive and experience a voice that is better than before radiotherapy. The fact that they have been cured of a potentially fatal disease may have made them more tolerant of residual hoarseness and limitations in function. This may explain both Mendonca's (1975) and Karim et al.'s (1983) observations regarding patients' more favourable opinions of their voice qualities than their clinicians'.

Stoicheff (1975) found that although patients rated their own voices more favourably with increasing time post radiotherapy, 80% reported persistent problems in vocal function and degrees of residual hoarseness. This was also found by Carlson (1995b). In the latter study there were wide individual variations in patients' self ratings between 2 and 63 months post radiotherapy, of residual 'hoarseness' and limitations in voice function, e.g. the voice fatiguing with use, ability to speak over noise, shout, sing and use the telephone. The most dramatic improvement was reported in the first two months. When asked to rate to what extent the voice was still a 'problem', the vast majority reported it as 'no problem'. However, at the same time they often reported significant limitations in function and degrees of hoarseness. Objective measures of regularity of vocal fold vibration and fundamental frequency parameters showed lower than normal values.

Effect of radiotherapy on aerodynamic and acoustic voice quality measurements

Over the years increasingly sophisticated instrumentation has been developed and used in studies of voice quality to try to reduce the inevitable subjectivity and range of terminology used in perceptual rating systems. Early systems were only able to measure sustained phonation of vowels, a few seconds in duration, as they required a stable signal for processing and analysis. In recent years, however, instruments have been developed that enable us to measure longer stretches of natural speech and reading. Some results of such studies of the post radiotherapy voice quality are reported below.

(a) Airflow measures

As a result of impaired vibration and closure of the vocal folds after radiotherapy, Werner-Kukuk et al. (1968) registered increased phonatory airflow values and a reduction in the patient's maximum phonation time. Aerodynamic measurements showed improvement in laryngeal function before recovery was observable through other means. This was confirmed by Murry et al. (1974) who measured mean airflow-rate during sustained vowel phonation in one subject, before, during and after radiotherapy. This was the only one of their measures which showed a constant reduction over four occasions at increasing intervals after radiotherapy.

However, Lehman et al. (1988) measured airflow in patients one year or more after radiotherapy and found wide variations in their subjects both at normal and loud intensity, but the airflow means fell within normal limits. The recent study by Verdonck-de Leeuw (1998) also failed to show any significant differences in aerodynamic measures between normal and irradiated speakers.

(b) Perturbation measures

Lehman et al. (1988) recorded subjects reading the 'Rainbow Passage' and in a two-minute conversation. Compared to the normal group, both jitter and shimmer, and the variability of these measures, were significantly higher in the post radiotherapy group. Signal to noise ratio was significantly lower. The vowel /a/ had the greatest degree of perturbation compared to /i/ and /u/. The latter showed the least.

Hoyt et al. (1992) analysed the voices of two groups of patients before radiotherapy and 6 months after completion. One group (N = 10) was irradiated for glottic carcinoma, the other (N = 25) for other head and neck lesions, but the radiation field included the larynx. They found that the patients with laryngeal lesions showed an improvement in perturbation measures post radiotherapy, the non-laryngeal group showed a deterioration in perturbation measures. The explanation lies in the beneficial effect of radiotherapy on the voice of a patient with a glottic tumour, but the detrimental effect on the presumably normal voices of patients with tumours in the naso- or oropharynx. The task consisted of sustained vowel /a/ phonation.

Carlson (1995a) found significantly more irregularity of vocal fold vibration measured by electrolaryngography (Fourcin, 1981; Carlson, 1995a,b) in a group of irradiated subjects compared to a group of age and sex matched normal speakers during conversational speech and reading aloud.

(c) Fundamental frequency measures

Murry (1978) extracted the third sentence from a reading of the first paragraph of the 'Rainbow Passage' and found that the mean speaking fundamental frequency, the standard deviation and the semitone range of the voices of patients with vocal fold palsy were significantly reduced compared to a sample of normal speakers. However, Mean Speaking Fundamental Frequency failed to separate normal speakers from the other two groups of pathological speakers, a group with benign mass lesions and a group with cancer of the larynx.

Stoicheff (1975) and Carlson (1995b) found a general trend for fundamental frequency central values, means and modes, to be lower, but not significantly so, among irradiated speakers compared to a group of normals. However, in the latter study was found a significantly lower maximum frequency range measure for irradiated speakers, indicating that radiotherapy affects the upper end of the phonatory range more than the lower end, and supports findings of reduced fundamental frequency ranges by Hecker and Kreul (1971) and Murry (1978). This also explains the trend towards lower mean change to fundamental frequency values.

Verdonck-de Leeuw (1998) found a significantly higher mean pitch for patients before radiotherapy compared to six months and two years post radiotherapy.

Lehman et al. (1988) recorded subjects reading the 'Rainbow Passage' and in a two-minute conversation. There was no significant difference in mean fundamental frequency. Nor were there any differences in these measures when different techniques of radiation, type or number of biopsies, location of tumour or time since the end of radiotherapy were compared. The reason for the lack of significance of differences in central measurements in most studies is likely to be wide variation within groups of both normal and irradiated speakers.

On the basis of their extensive measurements and comparisons of irradiated subjects with normal speakers, Lehman et al. (1988) conclude: 'radiation therapy of stage I glottic carcinoma results in an abnormal voice. It is produced with greater than normal effort. This appears to be the result of a diffuse process that affects more of the larynx than the area involved with tumour.'

The role of voice therapy in the rehabilitation of patients after radiotherapy

Increased mass and stiffness of vocal fold tissues resulting from oedema or the presence of a mass on one or both cords, leads to increased effort in the speaker's attempt at maintaining appropriate vocal pitch level, range and volume. This may be the case in the period before laryngeal cancer is diagnosed, when increasing hoarseness is the presenting symptom.

Radiotherapy to the larynx gives rise to vocal fold oedema and mucosal dryness, which develops during, and persists after, radiotherapy. Increased laryngeal effort is observed after radiotherapy (Lehman et al., 1988, Verdonck-de Leeuw, 1998) and hypertrophied ventricular folds are often observed on phonation (Carlson, 1995b). Lehmann et al. (1988) found abnormally high measures of subglottal pressure during phonation in their subjects compared to normal controls.

Carlson (1995b) and Verdonck-de Leeuw (1998) noted abnormal degrees of laryngeal tension in their perceptual voice quality ratings after radiotherapy. This is the likely result of the effort required to move the stiff vocal structures, leading to discomfort during speaking, the voice tiring with use and limitations in function, e.g. in shouting or speaking over noise and singing, reported by Stoicheff (1975) and Carlson (1995b). In the latter study a significant correlation was found between subjects' self-ratings of the degree of 'hoarseness' and the therapist's ratings of 'laryngeal tension'.

Based on their findings of great variability in patients' acoustic and aerodynamic measurements, which could not be explained by differences in radiotherapy treatment or demographic variables (some vowels in their study were produced with lower jitter and shimmer and higher signal to noise ratio), Lehman et al. (1988) suggest:

> there may be variable ability among patients to use a poor vibratory structure to maximum advantage through good vocal habits or compensatory vocal manoeuvres. The differences in vowel formants indicate that some compensation for glottic abnormalities is being attempted through vocal tract positioning (p.126).

This suggests that there may be potential benefits in offering voice therapy to improve irradiated patients' voice production.

An attempt at reducing the risk of secondary vocal abuse during and after radiotherapy by offering voice therapy in parallel with irradiation is reported by Fex and Henriksson (1969). Fifteen patients were examined and recorded before and after treatment. They were advised of the difficulties to come and instructed not to abuse or force the vocal mechanism while it was undergoing radiation treatment. They remark: 'while therapy is given the patient may have appreciable laryngeal trouble; dysphonia passing into aphonia for one or more weeks, pain on swallowing and occasionally a painful cough'.

Voice therapy consisted of instruction in vocal hygiene and practice of relaxation and breathing techniques and was aimed at teaching the patient to 'use the vocal cords as circumstances permit and to adapt to changed conditions in the larynx'. Most patients were aphonic immediately after radiotherapy. Three weeks later most of them reported having a useful voice. All patients except one 'had voice qualities well within normal limits'. The majority of the patients reported finding the voice treatment comfortable, and of good use also when the voice had returned. Fex and Henriksson concluded that their results support the assumption that the effect of radiation damage can be reduced by offering voice therapy.

The author offered voice therapy to a self-selected group of irradiated laryngeal cancer patients (Carlson, 1995b). The group consisted of two patients treated for T2 tumours of the glottis and seven treated for T1 tumours at a wide range of times post radiotherapy, 2–149 months. Their voices were compared to a group of eight patients who refused or did not feel the need for voice therapy, the 'no voice therapy' group (Table 15.2).

The 'voice therapy' group complained of vocal limitations and/or laryngeal discomfort irrespective of whether laryngeal examination revealed significant abnormalities. The subjects tended to be those who had gone back to work after radiotherapy (Table 15.2). Between 3 and 15 sessions of voice therapy, including advice on vocal hygiene, were given by the same therapist. The different amounts reflect the differing individual needs e.g. by a teacher (15 sessions) and by a retired diplomat (3 sessions).

Table 15.2 Comparisons of patients

Group		Voice therapy	No voice therapy
N		9	8
Age on last occasion	Mean	61.6	63.3
	Range	44–73	51–73
Smokers (n)		2	3
Workers (n)		5	2

Because of the wide range of times post radiotherapy, different tumour stages represented, the non-random sample of subjects and therapy sessions that varied according to each person's needs, no attempt was made to statistically prove the effect of voice therapy but only to describe a general trend in perceptual and instrumental voice quality measures.

To enable comparisons of voice quality by objective and perceptual means, before and after voice therapy, the patients were recorded in conversation and in reading aloud three paragraphs from the Rainbow Passage (Fairbanks, 1960), using Electrolaryngography (ELG) (Abberton et al., 1989). This is a non-invasive method for deriving fundamental frequency information straight from the voice source via two superficial electrodes placed either side of the thyroid cartilage.

Table 15.3 shows the fundamental frequency based measures derived from ELG, indicating an increased mean and range in the voice therapy group after completed therapy and also an increase in a measure of vocal fold regularity of vibration (%TS). They show a further increase in these measures on the last assessment occasion. A group of age and sex matched 'normal' speakers in the same study had a mean speaking Fx of 122 Hz and 37 %TS (Carlson, 1995b). The 'no voice therapy' group show overall

Table 15.3 Average fundamental frequency measurements: reading samples

GROUP	Median Months Post Radiotherapy	Mean (Hz)	90% Minimum Range limit (Hz)	90% Maximum Range limit (Hz)
With voice therapy				
Pre (N = 9)	9.0	113.4	87.7	163.6
16.2				
Post (N = 8)	12.5	118.6	88.0	183.1
21.5				
Last (N = 9)	50.0	120.5	87.0	187.8
21.9				
No voice therapy				
(N = 8)				
First	5.5	102.3	78.6	155.5
19.9				
Last	54.5	108.6	85.6	159.7
25.7				

lower pitch and range but slightly more regularity both on the first and the last occasion.

On the first assessment occasion the 'voice therapy' group had perceptually worse voice quality, both as rated by themselves and by the therapist, than the 'no therapy' group. All measures indicated improvement immediately after voice therapy. However, on the last assessment occasion, more than four years later, Vocal Profile Analysis ratings (Laver et al., 1981) showed a deterioration. However, 'laryngeal tension' remained less in the 'voice therapy' group than in the 'no therapy' group. Patients also reported the voice posing less of a problem than on the immediate post therapy occasion.

Conclusion

Irradiated laryngeal cancer patients benefit from explanation and advice on vocal structure and function, vocal hygiene and voice conservation measures. Abusive vocal habits may have been characteristic of many patients before cancer developed. What ultimately determines whether a patient will co-operate and benefit from voice therapy is his own perception of whether he has a problem or not and to what extent he experiences limitations in vocal function. Patients most likely to do so are those who use their voices for work purposes. Voice therapy may help such patients to make better use of a damaged mechanism, but many will experience some permanent limitations in quality and function.

CHAPTER 16

Voice care for the professional voice user

STEPHANIE MARTIN

Introduction

The generic term 'professional voice user' is often used for individuals whose professional role and employment is dependent on effective and efficient use of voice. In this group, for example, may be included teachers, actors, politicians, telephonists, radio announcers, vicars, barristers, dealers on the stock exchange, priests, salespeople and air traffic controllers. Undoubtedly, readers will be able to add to this list.

Koufman (1998) identifies four levels of vocal usage, which neatly illustrate the link between professional demands and vocal load. He suggests the following:

- *The Elite Vocal Performer (Level I)* is a person for whom even a slight aberration of voice may have dire consequences. Most singers and actors would fall into this group with the opera singer representing the quintessential level I performer.
- *The Professional Voice User (Level II)* is a person for whom a moderate vocal problem might prevent adequate job performance. Here would be included clergy, teachers, lecturers and receptionists.
- *The Non-Vocal Professional (Level III)* is categorized as a person for whom a severe vocal problem would prevent adequate job performance. This group includes lawyers, physicians, business men and women.
- *The Non-Vocal Non-professional (Level IV)* is a person for whom vocal quality is not a prerequisite for adequate job performance. In this group would be found, for example, clerks and labourers.

Ascribing the term 'professional voice user' carries with it an implicit expectation that the individual will have had the training to bring their vocal skills

283

up to a 'professional' level, and that he or she can therefore use these vocal skills effectively, in a variety of settings and to different numbers and groups of people. In many cases, however, the facts do not support this view. As we can see from Koufman's list above, people are potentially at risk because of the amount of time they spend talking during the working day, in jobs which require competent and reliable spoken communication.

Professional voice users and the incidence of vocal attrition

Teachers have been recognized as an at-risk group for voice disorders for a considerable time (Greene, 1964) and have traditionally had a high representation in voice therapy clinics. As an example, a small scale study of 40 clinics within the United Kingdom indicated that up to seven teachers per clinic were attending for treatment in any one month. There is also anecdotal evidence that many teachers with voice disorders do not seek help, perhaps fearing that formal recognition of a voice problem would label them as professionally vulnerable. If this is correct, it suggests that voice problems among teachers may be significantly more than we know.

A study by Herrington-Hall et al. (1988) explored the occurrence of laryngeal pathologies and their distribution across age, sex and occupation in several cities in the United States and concluded that teaching was one of the top ten occupations of those who presented with voice disorders; this confirms information from a previous study (Cooper, 1973). Sapir et al. (1990) have coined the term 'vocal attrition' to describe problems associated with 'wear and tear' on the larynx, due to inappropriate vocal use of heavy vocal demand. Surveys of symptoms of vocal attrition among teachers have been undertaken by Sapir et al. (1993), Martin (1994), Miller and Verdolini (1995), Smith et al. (1997, 1998a,b) and Koufman (1998); all of these have demonstrated a correlation between teaching activities and voice problems. Ramig and Verdolini (1998), in their summary of these studies, suggest that up to one third of teachers report that their voice problems interfered with their ability to teach effectively and that they had missed work because of these problems. A fifth of these teachers also reported that their voices had been a source of frustration and stress. In the United Kingdom, two ground-breaking cases within the past five years have highlighted the problems experienced by those in the teaching profession (Oldfield, 1995; Clowry, 1996a,b). These two teachers, whose voice loss effectively forced them into early retirement, were awarded compensation due to the vocal-occupational demands of their teaching role.

Studies with other professional groups whose work may be said to put their voice at risk show similar patterns of vocal attrition. For example, aerobic instructors (Heidel and Torgerson, 1993), dance teachers (Judd,

1995), army instructors, (Sapir et al., 1990) and military training instructors (Cantu 1997). Similar anecdotal evidence is available from as diverse a group as teachers of lip reading, aircraft controllers, dealers on the Stock Exchange, preachers and airport announcers.

These activities all place high demands on the vocal mechanism, because the activity is undertaken in situations which involve speaking over loud noise and for prolonged periods of time. In addition, many of these occupations include prolonged use of loud voice, which means that individuals are using extremes ranges of vocal performance (Ramig and Verdolini, 1998).

Ramig and Verdolini (1998) have estimated that just under 25% of the working population of the United States have jobs that critically require voice use and note that '3.29 % of the population (or 3,840,000 individuals) have occupations (e.g. air traffic controller, police, pilot) in which their voice is necessary for public safety' (p. S102). They agree with Laguaite (1972, p. 151) that the frequency of occurrence of voice problems is 'potentially one of great magnitude from a health, as well as an economic standpoint'.

Voice care and development

Because of increasing recognition that voice problems can be a direct consequence of an individual's professional role, and of the number of individuals involved, it is clear that professional voice users make up a particular clinical population which both deserves and requires greater attention. There is also increasing effort by some organizations to mitigate vocal abuse and misuse. Examples in the United Kingdom include British Airways, who have instigated training for their airport announcers, and the print industry, who have introduced noise havens or booths for their workers.

Despite the mounting evidence of need, however, there is still no official consistent support for voice care and development as a part of teacher training. The Teacher Training Agency handbook (TTA, 1997), which identifies teacher competencies, states that (among other things) all qualified teachers must be able to communicate clearly and effectively with pupils through questioning, instructing, explaining and feedback. However, few colleges of education in the UK offer voice courses for teachers as part of their training (Ormell, 1993). Paradoxically, although vocal quality is accepted as an essential parameter of the communication process and despite the awareness that vocal attrition can compromise the effectiveness of the message, voice care is not yet viewed as an essential component of training.

A similar lethargy seems to pervade other countries. In America, there is widespread concern at the number of teachers who suffer from voice problems but little evidence of any widespread preventative work (Ramig and Verdolini, 1998). In Sweden, an initiative in 1992 by the University of Gothenburg offered a voice course where university teachers were given weekly voice training in small groups (Ohlsson, 1993), but this is exceptional. Studies are certainly continuing apace into aspects of the teacher's voice but, as yet, little evidence is emerging to suggest that resources are available for preventative work.

Voice use and the professional voice user

It should perhaps be no surprise that 'so-called' professional voice users often present with voice problems. While it should be possible to use the voice without tiring, damaging or abusing it for prolonged periods of time, it might be said that this possibility exists only when optimum conditions prevail in the manner and place of production. The *manner of production* encompasses easy and relaxed onset of voice, well-balanced posture, good control of breath, minimal mental or emotional stress, a well-functioning and flexible vocal tract and healthy larynx. When considering *place*, this would be in acoustically balanced, warm but not over-heated and well-ventilated buildings, that do not add to the problems associated with dehydration.

It is clear that for most, if not all, professional voice users few if any of these conditions pertain, either in terms of physical space or production of voice. As a result there are limitless opportunities to precipitate and maintain poor vocal habits, leading inexorably to vocal abuse and misuse, and acute and chronic voice disorders.

It is axiomatic that in dealing with voice disorders we are dealing with an aspect of communication, voice, believed to be most natural of functions, whereas in the case of the professional voice user it can be a most unnatural process. Think of air traffic controllers who need to ensure that the pilot understands his instructions, the salesperson's need to make a sale, the preacher's need to get his message across, the lawyer's need to win his case, the teacher's need to maintain discipline, the actor's need to make his audience believe in the part he is playing. In all of these situations the 'need' to achieve a result can confer demand and stress on the voicing process, whether this is conscious or not. Tension, of course, is readily accepted as one of the most critical precipitating factors in vocal attrition.

It would be difficult within the confines of one chapter to offer a commentary on aspects of voice care for each of the many individual groups within the professional voice user category, so particular emphasis will be given to the teaching profession, as they are already identified as having well-documented voice problems. It is hoped that readers will draw parallels with other professional voice users and identify the similarities across professional boundaries in terms of diagnostic indicators, intervention, specific approaches and outcome measures.

The professional role as a factor in vocal abuse and misuse

The suggestion, within a professional voice text, that the vocal problems of the professional voice user are well documented is perhaps disingenuous, as there is still a widespread belief by many clients from the teaching profession that 'they' are the only teacher to experience such problems. In fact, many teachers appear to subscribe tacitly to the dictum that voice problems 'come with the territory'. Many of our clients attribute their voice loss to a virus or a cold, rather than a consequence of either their working environment or their pattern of voice use.

Teachers readily identify the importance of voice as an essential professional tool (Martin, 1994), yet, as has already been noted, a high proportion of teachers have had virtually no formal training and there does not appear to be any active demand from the profession's decision-makers for training. This discrepancy would seem to point to a conspiracy of silence about the extent of the problem. We have also noted earlier that there is anecdotal evidence that individual teachers hesitate to air concerns about their voice too openly. Presumably, highlighting a problem which may affect their ability to teach would make them feel professionally vulnerable. When questioned (Martin, 1994), teachers who had experienced voice problems reported that employing authorities had been supportive, but there is also anecdotal clinical evidence to suggest that many teachers ask for therapy appointments after school hours so that the school does not need to be informed.

The impact of voice loss

It is important not to underestimate the impact of voice loss on the professional voice user. In the World Health Organization International Classification of lmpairments, Disabilities and Handicaps in 1980 (WHO, 1980), the definition of the term *impairment* is defined as 'any loss or abnormality of psychological, physiological or anatomical structure of function'. Gordon and Lockhart (1995) suggest vocal cord palsy as an example of this, but vocal nodules and vocal attrition would also fall into this category. The term *disability* is defined as 'any restriction or lack (resulting from an impairment) of ability to perform an activity in the manner or within the range considered normal for a human being'. Gordon and Lockhart identify dysphonia as an example of this category. *Handicap* is defined as 'a disadvantage for a given individual resulting from an impairment or disability that limits or prevents the fulfilment of a role that is normal (depending an age, sex and social and cultural factors) for that individual'. Again, a teacher with voice impairment would fall into this category.

Smith et al. (1997) support the view that teachers are at high risk for disability from voice disorders and that this health problem may have significant work-related and economic effects. If we further consider the distress experienced by individual teachers and professional voice users to episodes of voice disorder, the fourth parameter, 'distress' which was added to the WHO definition by Enderby (1992), is particularly appropriate. Gordon and Lockhart (1995) suggest that all these factors should be included in the clinician's assessment of the dysphonic patient. This suggestion should be carefully considered when working with the professional voice user group of clients, as voice patients frequently report that the experience of voice loss includes a sense of isolation and distress with accompanying periods of depression. Clients also perceive that their voice problems impinge upon their working lives (Smith et al., 1996). Martin and Darnley (1996) report on a teacher whose episode of voice loss made her feel as though she was 'shut in a box without any means of escape'.

There are few standardized methods for assessing the psychosocial consequences of voice disorders. Llewellyn-Thomas et al. (1984) developed a linear analogue scale with patients with laryngeal cancer in an effort to quantify self-assessment of voice quality. More recently, Smith et al. (1996) designed a questionnaire to elicit information from patients to assess quality of life, or functional impact of voice disorders in various aspects of their lives. The Vocal Handicap Index or VHI developed by Jacobson et al. (1997) also gives a way to assess functional outcomes in behavioural, medical and surgical treatments of voice disorders, which may also be used to assess the patient's judgment about their perceptions of the impact of their voice disorder on daily activities.

Impetus for change

As we can see, the evidence suggests that the health care message is not getting through to the professional voice user. Why is this the case? In part, it may be due to the lack of visibility of the problem and indeed the somewhat dismissive reaction to voice disorders. If individuals could see the damage they are inflicting on their vocal folds, then perhaps they would consider them more carefully. It is unlikely that these same individuals would willingly repeatedly strike a badly bruised limb without questioning their sanity, yet this in effect is what happens when individuals determine to continue to speak with swollen and damaged vocal folds. Perhaps a voice disorder does not seem to be a 'proper' disorder to the general public (see Freeman, in Chapter 8), despite the fact that clinicians can clearly see that it completely fulfils the WHO criteria.

Intervention and management

Other chapters in this book illustrate best practice in terms of approach and management of voice disorders, while other texts detail aspects such as initial case history taking and assessment with dysphonic patients in general, for example Martin (1986), Greene and Mathieson (1989), Colton and Casper (1996). Sataloff (1997) gives a comprehensive account of the clinical evaluation and physical examination specific to the professional voice user. This chapter looks at aspects of intervention and management with the professional voice user, which will possibly differ from those offered to a dysphonic patient whose voice use does not have 'professional' status.

It is always critical to remember the level of anxiety that nearly all voice patients experience when they attend for their first appointment (Colton and Casper, 1996; Freeman, Chapter 8, this volume). For the professional voice user, this anxiety is compounded by the fact that, for many, their career and future working life may quite literally be 'on the line'.

The art of interviewing remains a skill which is difficult to specify in terms of training competencies. Inexperienced clinicians, when dealing with professional voice users, may underestimate the level of anxiety, seeing instead aggression and defensiveness on the part of the patient. It is important to recognize this as a defensive response to a feared situation, and to remember that attempts to instigate new techniques and approaches may well be jeopardized by the anxiety. Ley's (1988) work has emphasized that clients cannot recall information and advice when they are anxious, which means that wherever possible it is advisable to write down or record critical instructions or advice.

It is salutary to consider the advice of Aronson (1985b) when he stated: 'Any in-depth study of voice disorders forces us to conclude that so long as clinicians obtain privileged information from patients; so long as people have voice problems because of life stress and interpersonal conflict; so long as voice disorders produce anxiety, depression, embarrassment and self-consciousness; so long as patients need a sympathetic person with whom they can discuss their distress, will speech pathologists need to consider their training incomplete until they have learned the basic skills of psychologic interviewing and counselling' (p. 271).

Certainly for the clinician, the first interview with the professional voice user is critically important. There are specific issues in relation to the case history and voice use of the professional voice user that it may be useful to highlight here. The list below highlights aspects pertinent to the professional voice user that are *additional to, not instead of,* completion of a standard case history. Individual approaches differ in relation to the recording of case history information: it may be transcribed, memorized for future transcription or recorded. All of the above have particular benefits but remain very much a question of personal choice.

Case history information

Professional actors or singers usually demonstrate a very intimate and acute perceptual knowledge of their own voice, and can often identify with precision changes that occur in range and vocal quality. While these patients may not be able to identify or define the cause of the voice disorder, they will have little difficulty describing the resulting vocal changes. When we consider the broader category of professional voice user such as the teacher, salesperson, instructor, dance teacher, the chances are that they will give us far more vague descriptions of how their voice used to sound, although there may be a heightened awareness of vocal change, which reflects the importance of voice in their professional role.

The patient's perspective

An exploration of the patient's perception of the problem is very important. In eliciting a response, questions that are as open-ended as possible ('tell me about the problem...') will give a better outcome than 'I understand from my notes that you have...'. The initial response will provide some insight into the patient's true understanding of the problem and, through well-honed clinical skills of questioning, observation and listening, a more complete picture of the effect of the disorder on the patient can be gained.

Equally critical is the patient's information about the onset and development of the voice disorder, the length of time that the problem has existed and the consistency or inconsistency of the disorder. In addition, it is important to record any additional signs or symptoms that the patient experiences, that he or she identifies as being associated with the voice disorder, such as physical discomfort, vocal fatigue, the need to clear the throat and any other changes in sensation (Mathieson, 1993; Harris, 1998).

The vocal history must be closely aligned to the patient's life history, as the relationship between voice, emotion and physical state has been clearly established for many years. The information accessed from the voice history allows the clinician to build a more complete picture of the patients and to make a judgment, albeit rather superficial at that early stage, as to the extent that the voice disorder affects their life.

One of the difficulties associated with accurate reporting by patients regarding a voice disorder is the length of time that usually elapses between the patient noting the problem and actually seeing the clinician. Clinicians must therefore be particularly scrupulous in trying to elicit as much information as possible, while recognizing that reporting past events accurately is notoriously difficult (Morrison and Rammage, 1994; Harris, 1998; Freeman, Chapter 8). Describing voice quality is particularly difficult, even for the 'experts' (Perkins 1971; Wilson 1979; Johnson 1985b; Martin 1986), so it is often helpful if the patient can be encouraged to use a comparative scale such as higher/lower, louder/softer, more/less range, and to support this information with anecdotal evidence from family and friends.

It is often useful to provide patients with a written list of questions, which they can distribute to specific friends, relations and colleagues. Examples of these could be: In your opinion, is my voice: – higher, lower, more husky, less clear, than it was? Individual clinicians can supply their own questionnaires to patients and in that way build up a much more complete picture than the often rather one-dimensional picture obtained from the patient history. It is important to remember that the spread of responses should be from those who have daily contact with the patient, to those who have more intermittent contact. Vocal change is often imperceptible if you are listening to individuals on a daily basis.

The clinician will want to explore specific issues with the professional voice user. Of paramount importance is whether or not the patient has had any professional voice training and if so, the extent and depth of training received. This should encompass all aspects of training, from in-service training days on voice care and development for teachers (known as INSET days in the UK), to professional training for singers and actors as part of their college courses.

Training as part of continuing professional development should be noted, either undertaken on an individual basis or as part of their job. For example, some theatre companies will offer company voice work with voice coaches. At the other end of the spectrum are those professional voice users without any formal vocal training. Clinicians are frequently surprised by the way in which professional singers and actors can apparently 'separate out' vocal technique. Often, they will successfully use excellent vocal techniques on stage, but completely omit to do so once they are off stage, demonstrating the confusion that may well exist for many between voice 'in performance' and voice use in general.

This differentiation clearly underlines the need to look at voice use in its totality and to offer individuals a firm knowledge base from which to begin to work. Regrettably, many professional voice users have a very limited understanding of the structure and function of the larynx, even with professional training. Although there is evidence that increased cross-professional and multidisciplinary exchange has done much to disseminate information across traditional professional barriers, it is always important to review the patient's individual knowledge during the initial interview, as this will dictate the approach to future intervention. It is critically important that individuals are informed about the structure and function of the larynx and the processes that underpin vocalization. It goes without saying that the language used to inform patients should be patient appropriate and should respect the individual's level of understanding. Boone's (1991) book, *Is Your Voice Telling on You?* provides a useful model for explanation in everyday language.

Recognizing the dynamic link between voice, emotion and physical state, the clinician will want to look closely at the patient's physical, psychological and emotional health. Here, it is most important that the case history looks closely at elements within the patient's environment and life, which may contribute to their voice disorder.

Stress and the professional voice user

Stress is a recognized factor in illness. In the UK, there are indications that some teachers are ending their careers early as a result of various types of stress-related illness, according to statements in the press from the National Association of Head Teachers. It is also widely accepted that voice disorders can be exacerbated by stress responses (Brodnitz, 1971; Butcher et al., 1993; Morrison and Rammage, 1994). Stress is frequently seen as a negative phenomenon, but it should be remembered that stress can be both negative and positive, with individuals reacting very differently to similar amounts of stress (see Freeman, Chapter 8).

For some individuals, the demands they face in their professional or in their private life are challenging, but they can handle them well, so the ensuing stress is both stimulating and exciting. For other individuals, similar demands would be overly demanding. Their response might be one of fear and anxiety which creates negative stress, and as a result physiological changes would occur, particularly if the stressors continued over time. Prolonged periods of stress can result in, for example, vocal fatigue, palpitations, a dry mouth and sometimes allied digestive disorders, such as heartburn and gastro-oesophageal reflux (Morrison and Rammage 1994; Rosen and Sataloff, 1997a).

For the professional voice user, stress at work may well be compounded by environmental stressors such as noise, pollution and overcrowding. The effect of these additional stressors within their personal life may in effect 'tip the balance' and result in voice loss and almost certainly be implicated in vocal hyperfunction. Increased general muscle tension with specific neck and head tension has a devastating effect on the respiratory, phonatory and resonatory processes.

Perceptual effects of teaching on the voice

While it is always dangerous to predict voice problems within a specific client group, it is possible to offer commentary on reported subjective opinions by teachers describing their own voices (Martin, 1995). When asked about the effects of teaching on their voice they reported:

* dryness
* tiredness

- hoarseness
- a lack of power
- a lack of flexibility
- a tight and constricted feeling
- soreness
- a rasping quality
- monotony
- feeling that you are stuck on one note
- voice fading after a few hours

In reviewing these comments, it is not unreasonable to suggest that the physiological and psychological effect of stress may be implicated in many of the vocal features mentioned.

Occupational demands on the voice

Additional occupational demands which the professional voice user experiences must be assessed. These can include:

Postural effects

The effect on the voice of specific classroom postures, for example in the case of the teacher who has to spend prolonged periods of time leaning over when speaking to children or marking their work. The posture that telephone sales people have to maintain, often cradling the phone between shoulder and chin while keying in information on to a computer. The degree of ergonomic support offered by the seating provided for airport announcers, the positioning of material in the pulpit for the preacher, *vis-à-vis* the requirement to reach all of the congregation with the message. The difficulties that the actor has when working on a raked stage. The list is endless but should be considered very carefully by the clinician.

The effect of the environment

Here aspects such as dust, germs, pollution from smoke and industrial material must be considered. Teachers work in a variety of school buildings from the overly hermetically sealed new school premises to old pre-twentieth century buildings, where dust and poor ventilation add to the catalogue of germs and viruses that abound when many are gathered into a small space! Teachers within Information and Design Technology departments are particularly vulnerable. They work with a range of different unspecified materials, often shaping them with lathes and saws, working with paints and varnishes; all can irritate the larynx and upper respiratory tract. Actors and singers work in environments which are often dusty; dust and materials leaking from set designs and stage pyrotechnics should be carefully considered. Those who work with actors and singers are well aware that they will frequently evidence dust and pollution as contributing to voice disorders, but will also refer to the lack of importance given to this by theatre management. Dealers on the Stock Exchange work in areas where fumes from fax and photocopying machines and teleprinters pollute the atmosphere. The clergy may preach in damp, musty and poorly ventilated spaces.

The effect of ageing

The vocal changes associated with ageing are well documented but it is important for those working with professional voice users to consider the effects of ageing on the voice. With demographic changes, many professional voice users will be working until they are quite old in chrono-logical and physiological terms, even if they feel and look younger. A recent directive in the United Kingdom has effectively prevented teachers retiring early, whereas many were previously able to take advantage of an early retirement package. Now many teachers, unless retiring on the grounds of ill health, will work until they are 60 years old. A similar age profile exists for the clergy and salespeople, while several well-known actors and singers appear to rapturous applause, at an age far beyond that of statutory retirement. Providing of course that the voice remains flexible, and attention is paid to postural, respiratory and vocal health, then vocal quality can be maintained.

The effect of acoustics

Classrooms, lecture halls, theatres, drama studios, sales rooms, bond markets and churches vary enormously in size and design. Teachers often find that they may have to work in a variety of spaces throughout the day, endeavouring to compensate vocally for the different acoustics within each space. Similarly actors, singers, salespeople and the clergy are equally affected by the structure of buildings and the materials used inside them which determine the acoustic properties of the specific space. It is impor-tant to look at the space within which an individual is working and assess the demands that this will impose on their voice.

Achieving change

There is every reason to suggest that the professional voice training given to actors or singers should be, in some way, replicated for those profes-sional voice users already identified in this chapter, including teachers, the clergy, salespeople, lawyers. Regrettably, there appears to be little likelihood of this occurring. This means that the approach to working with this client group must in part be dictated by the client's own need, as has been discussed above, to identify:

- specific external environmental factors which may have contributed to the voice disorder;
- specific factors which may maintain poor vocal practice;
- specific changes which the individual may make to establish new and less abusive voice use.

In working with the professional voice user the clinician should at all times keep a very clear vision of the specific needs of the individual, but also the needs that differentiate this group from those patients who are not professional voice users. It is important to demonstrate to the patient an understanding of the specific requirements of their professional role and to recognize that these requirements are different from those required by a more general dysphonic population. There are cogent arguments on each side for clinicians to have additional specialist training before working with this client group; but currently the jury is still out on this issue.

Professional voice users, in the main, demonstrate a noticeable desire to 'get their voice back as quickly as possible'. The clinician needs to respond to this, by keeping in mind the clear agenda that professional voice users need voices which have both stamina and quality, in order to complete their professional roles. For many singers and actors this can be very difficult; many of the less 'high profile' professionals do not have the benefit of enlightened management companies, which allow them to take sufficient time off to effect permanent and consistent improvement. Teachers are equally conscious that any time off work during the term creates considerable financial pressure for the school, because of the need to employ a supply teacher at high cost.

The pressure to obtain results in a few sessions can also be considered in relation to the costing of voice therapy, either in terms of health insurance or in relation to the current limited provision by the NHS within the UK. This is not to suggest unwarranted speed is an essential component of all work with professional voice users, but simply to signal the implications of voice problems within this clinical group. Intervention with this group should, in the words of Morrison and Rammage (1994), 'address all the lifestyle, emotional and technical issues that are represented in a complex system of symptom formation'.

As we have seen above, work with professional voice users, as with other client groups, must begin with the sharing of information regarding the structure and function of the vocal tract, the physiology of voice and speech and the way in which this may be affected by physical and psychological stress. It is increasingly recognized that the way in which information is processed is highly individual (Ley, 1989; Ogden, 1996). Clinicians should try to maximize learning opportunities by offering information in a way that is most accessible to the individual. For example, some individuals learn best within a visual, rather than an aural modality; for some a mixture of both will prove most effective (see Freeman, Chapter 8). Clinicians are recommended to look at recent theories of learning, to ensure that they are delivering information in as appropriate a manner as possible (Verdolini et al., 1998). For some, too much information too soon will be confusing, so the educational aspect of intervention should be delivered in easily digestible amounts.

The impact of the external environmental factors

Specific external environmental factors may have contributed to the voice disorder. It is important to recognize that it may not be possible to change some of these environmental factors, but it is appropriate to look at ways in which to modify the environment. This can be much more successful than we first think, and the following strategies are offered.

1. Make sure that individuals are encouraged to think about the acoustics of the room in which they work. It is important to provide professional voice users with at least introductory information about the way the voice can be affected by the local acoustic environment, an area explored by Howard and Angus (1996).

    Teachers, for example, may be able to change the acoustic from one which is vocally hard work, to one which supports the voice and minimizes the effort needed to produce voice. Recommended and fairly low cost solutions are, for example: (a) changes to wall and floor coverings; (b) repositioning of the desks to allow the teacher to move to a different part of the room when teaching; (c) if necessary the teacher may have to use a microphone.

2. Working with the acoustic of the room, rather than against it, can be achieved by experimenting with different pitch levels. It is always important to encourage the teacher to do this with guidance as imposed alterations in pitch can be vocally abusive. Actors and singers tend to work instinctively with the acoustic of the stage or space in which they are performing. Again, it is important to highlight this aspect of potential vocal strain. Often, it is possible to discuss this with the producer or director and encourage them to restrict difficult positions on stage to movement only positions.

3. Working in well-ventilated and well-hydrated surroundings is particularly important and again comparatively simple low cost solutions are available; water containers placed near radiators, covering radiators with damp cloths, goldfish in bowls, flowers and plants can all be used to introduce moisture to a room. Damping down a stage before a performance is important to reduce dust, as is the need to restrict exposure by performers to the use of stage ice or pyrotechnics if possible. If actors or singers are going to have to perform in adverse conditions then it is important to encourage them to steam just before and just after their performance to mitigate some of the dehydrating and vocally irritating effects (Verdolini-Marston et al., 1994).

4. Masks and protective clothing must be worn, where possible, if individuals are working in, for example, laboratory or workshop conditions. Breathing in the fumes of fixatives, glues or some paint material is not helpful. While individuals are often not happy about making this change it is important and compliance can sometimes be achieved if one uses the 'setting a good example to students' approach.

5. Seating and postural changes can bring about quite dramatic changes which impact on vocal tract positioning and laryngeal setting. It is important to examine these aspects with the patient and to identify how postural changes may be achieved. This may be by instigating comparatively small changes, like altering the height of a chair in relation to the desk or indeed moving furniture to encourage, rather than detract from, effective vocalization.

Focus on these aspects often prompts the patient to look more carefully at all aspects of their environment. It can also have the effect of making connections for the individual between previously unrelated aspects of their life, encouraging the identification of potentially harmful environmental features. For example, actors may need to maintain voice in demanding physical positions, on a raked stage or in restricting costumes. If they also work part-time in a smoky pub, then the combination is potentially vocally lethal. Understanding the link, however, allows change to be incorporated.

Specific factors which maintain poor vocal practice

The clinician needs to be aware of factors readily identifiable from the case history which are potentially abusive, but also of less transparent factors, particularly those which are discussed in health psychology references as influencing *compliance* (following the advice and instructions of the practitioner – Ley, 1988) or *adherence* (accepting an active share in the decision making – and believing that one's own actions will make the change possible – Stanton, 1987). It can be uncomfortable for the clinician to recognize that the relationship between clinician and patient may actively prevent improvement and change. The intimate link between emotion and voice is recognized; so too is the 'Sharma' effect, often seen in voice work when an individual is convinced that it is the special gifts and skills of the master clinician that have effected change. The obverse of this is that for some, fortunately few, patients the relationship with the clinician prevents, rather than facilitates change. Recognizing that intervention with a specific patient may be maintaining rather than changing poor vocal practice is a critical element in our evaluation of therapy practice and outcomes.

Specific treatment regimes

In structuring a therapy task, it is important to remember that individuals have preferred thinking and preferred learning styles. Work on learning and memory (Rose, 1985; Buzan, 1989) suggests that if individuals can tap into their preferred modality for learning, then new information is absorbed and retained with much greater speed and consistency. For example, patients who are more visual learners may be more comfortable with therapy which relies on visual display from the Laryngograph (Fourcin, 1974; Carlson, 1993) or Visipitch (Kay Elometrics) while other patients may respond better to a more auditory or kinaesthetic approach (Filter, 1980).

Notwithstanding this, there are specific areas which form the bedrock of intervention with voice patients. Work on general relaxation is an essential starting position for work on voice and many professional voice users find that once they have been introduced to the principles of relaxation, they can very effectively continue to work on their own. Work either on a stretch and release method or an image-based method is recommended (Jacobson, 1938; Martin and Darnley, 1992, 1996). It is also important to look at relaxation exercises which address specific areas of tension, for example the jaw, the neck, the face (Martin and Darnley, 1992).

Work on posture and alignment can mitigate against some of the problems identified earlier as a result of fixed occupational postures. General exercises for posture and work utilizing the Alexander Technique (Barlow, 1973; MacDonald, 1994) are of considerable benefit and indeed it is important to review conditions within the working environment with colleagues as this can often identify previously overlooked bad practice. It is easy to become habituated to particular conditions and, in effect, no longer see them. It is also true that individuals became 'posturally entrenched', often failing to 'feel' a position which is, in fact, potentially vocally abusive: voice is a physical skill and there is a need to consider the whole body in intervention.

Breathing exercises are very much part of the voice therapists' repertoire and breath support and control are essential prerequisites, particularly with those who need to project their voices. Working with the professional singer or actor, it quickly becomes evident that for many, breathing exercises are utilized for their professional life, but there is little carry-over into offstage work. For the professional voice user, coordinating breath with voice onset is very important and so 'teaching' effective breath support and control can later be supplemented with work on what Morrison and Rammage (1994) term coordinated voice onset, thus optimizing the opportunity for easy voicing and the reduction of hard attack.

The mouth is the only truly moveable resonator and it is important for it to be as relaxed and flexible as possible. In order to maximize resonance, designated jaw exercises are very often a useful starting point for more detailed work on the articulators, and certainly work on the lips and tongue should be part of the repertoire of exercises for voice patients.

Specific vocal problems

When teachers were asked to specify the vocal problems they experience (Martin and Darnley, 1996) the range of responses was:

- insufficient volume;
- constant need to swallow;
- sounding strained at the end of the day;
- tight feeling in the throat;
- hoarse every time I have a cold;
- cuts out in the middle of sentences;
- husky voice;
- unable to sing;
- voice collapsed;
- complete voice loss.

These responses came from a random sample of teachers, many of whom had never sought any professional help for their voice problems. However, they emphasize the range and extent of the voice problems experienced by teachers and, indeed, these problems are symptomatic of those experienced by most professional voice users.

Generalization

The acid test of the success of any clinical intervention must be whether the individual acquires the ability to monitor their voice on an ongoing basis, learning to recognize and accurately predict situations which are potentially vocally abusive. The clinician must encourage this skill and also ensure that the patient is fully aware of the various factors which influence vocal performance. It is imperative that intervention offers professional voice users the skills to maintain voice, even when severely vocally challenged, and offers them strategies to monitor their own voice and recognize factors which may precipitate vocal abuse and misuse.

The success of any programme of intervention depends on the individuals' ability to incorporate therapy techniques into their working environment and to build on what has been learned within the supportive clinical environment, so that they can achieve effective voice at all times, and in a variety of different environmental conditions, to differing groups of people. The challenge of voice work with the professional voice user is precisely that intervention fulfils these criteria and allows the individuals to feel secure in their ability to maintain voice and thus their professional role at all times. It is therefore useful to put the voice under pressure to replicate situations which may challenge the voice and to monitor carefully how well the voice responds. Techniques such as easy safe shouting should be taught, while ways in which to protect and care for the voice must be incorporated into daily living.

As with many other treatment programmes, group work as part of a maintenance programme can be most successful. Indeed, group voice work with professional voice users can be particularly helpful once the individual's needs have been evaluated.

Summary

Working with professional voice users is both a challenging and a rewarding experience. Challenging because the professional voice users expect and deserve to achieve vocal skills which fully meet their professional requirements and rewarding because successful intervention allows the individual not only to retrieve their *modus vivendi* as far as their professional status is concerned, but also to reinstate that unique characteristic which gives us our identity – our voice.

CHAPTER 17

Phonosurgery

MARC BOUCHAYER AND GUY CORNUT

Introduction

Phonosurgery is the name given to a branch of laryngeal surgery whose primary aim is the best possible restoration of laryngeal function, rather than the simple removal of lesions to restore normal laryngeal appearance. The concept of phonosurgery emerged in the early 1970s with the introduction of suspension microlaryngoscopy and the operating microscope. Considerable advances in surgical technique became possible, because surgeons using these instruments could make finer, more precise hand movements.

Phonosurgery embraces the treatment of a considerable range of benign vocal fold lesions such as nodules, polyps, Reinke oedema, cysts, and sulcus vocalis. Within this domain we would also include incomplete vocal-fold closure and approximation problems secondary to recurrent laryngeal nerve paralysis, as these may be corrected by intrafold injection. Surgical procedures intended to change vocal pitch and the surgical treatment of spasmodic dysphonia will not be considered in this chapter for two reasons: first, the surgical principles are still very much open to debate and we have no personal experience of these procedures, and secondly, the phonosurgical approach is inappropriate in the management of dysplasias or malignancies of the vocal folds.

Genuine phonosurgery is simply not possible without close collaboration between a phoniatrician/speech pathologist and a phonosurgeon. Their respective skills are complementary, the one being responsible for preoperative assessment and voice re-education, while the other is responsible for the surgery. The authors have worked together as a team in this manner for about twenty years.

Preoperative assessment

Before any phonosurgical procedure the patient undergoes a complete phoniatric assessment. This consists of:

1. *A videolaryngostroboscopy recording.* This is made using a rigid endoscope coupled to a videocamera. The vocal folds are first filmed in normal light in order to study laryngeal morphology, and then in stroboscopic light in order to study alterations in the vibratory behaviour of the vocal folds (assessment of the significance of faults of closure, localized rigidity, modification of the mucosal wave, etc.). We prefer to use a rigid endoscope rather than a fibreoptic nasendoscope, as the latter produces a smaller, less well-defined image, which makes precise assessment of detail more difficult. A good quality videorecorder incorporating both a slow-motion mode and a good freeze-frame image is important in order to get the maximum information from the recording. Good quality still photographic prints may also be produced by downloading direct from the videotape to a videoprinter.
2. *A full vocal assessment.* First, a tape recording of the voice is made while the subject is reading, speaking spontaneously and singing. A phonetogram is then performed, and when practicable the examination is completed by a full instrumental study (electrolaryngography, frequency analysis, sonography, etc.) in order to provide data on the various voice parameters for subsequent detailed analysis.

Maintenance of good acoustic and visual records is important in order to make an objective assessment of any modifications produced by phonosurgery.

The operation

This is performed as a suspension microlaryngoscopy and is always carried out under general anaesthesia with endotracheal intubation and full muscle relaxation. Full laryngeal relaxation allows for optimum positioning of the laryngoscope and hence nearly always gives excellent exposure of the whole glottis. Under these conditions the surgeon can operate safely, performing whatever surgical manoeuvres may be necessary in an unhurried manner. Patients usually remain in hospital for 48 hours following operation.

The equipment comprises:

1. a binocular operating microscope with a focal length of 350 or 400 mm;

2. two operating laryngoscopes of different sizes, together with a suspension arm;
3. relatively few instruments, most of which are angled to right or left: curved forceps, microscissors, dissectors, fine microforceps, fenestrated heart-shaped tissue-holding forceps, an arrowhead knife, a needle for injection, and a point monopolar diathermy electrode. All these instruments are approximately 22 cm long;
4. finally, the CO_2 laser. Use of the laser is strongly advocated by some practitioners although we prefer to use micro-instruments, which are even more precise in practice and are better suited to the size of lesions to be treated.

Postoperative follow-up

In the immediate postoperative period the patient must maintain complete vocal silence for eight days until reviewed at the first postoperative follow-up appointment.

Medication is routinely prescribed postoperatively. The patient is given an injection of a depot preparation of steroids, a laryngeal steroid spray and mucolytics. In addition, antibiotic cover may also be supplied in cases where infection is thought to be a significant factor or when fibrin glue has been used during the operation. When the phoniatrician sees the patient for the first postoperative follow-up appointment the full preoperative workup is repeated. A period of intensive speech therapy then begins, and sessions continue throughout a month of convalescence. Subsequently the frequency of sessions is reduced and the patient returns to work between four and six weeks after operation. Going back to work is always a vulnerable time for patients when their work demands extensive voice use, teachers being particularly at risk. The phoniatrician makes a final assessment at the end of the course of speech therapy.

Indications for operation: techniques and results

Acquired benign lesions of the vocal folds

Nodules

A nodule is a mucosal thickening situated at the junction of the anterior and mid-third of the vocal fold, slightly under the free border. The thickening is of variable size and is usually elongated, although occasionally it may be rounded. A nodule may be pink or whitish in colour where there is old surface keratinization, and may on occasion also present as a small, pearly-white, pointed heap, this latter appearance being generally seen in singers. The lesion is normally bilateral.

Histological examination shows that the predominant changes are in the stratified squamous layer of the vocal fold cover, which is always thickened and which shows many epithelial pegs penetrating deeply into the superficial layer of the lamina propria (Reinke's space). This latter usually presents as hyaline degeneration. There are other lesions that may resemble this typical nodule.

The serous pseudo-cyst is a well-circumscribed lesion whose macroscopic appearance is that of a translucent, thin-walled cyst containing serum that runs out as soon as the cyst is incised. Histological examination, however, shows that this lesion is not a true cyst as there is no cyst wall. These anomalies are predominantly situated within the superficial layer of the lamina propria and essentially consist of an area of gross oedema over which the epithelium of the vocal-fold cover is thinned and atrophic.

Fusiform thickening of the mucosa differs from a nodule in both its extent and its elongated shape, and in the degree of associated inflammatory changes. It is like the typical nodule in that the thickening is usually bilateral. Histological sections show that the epithelium of the cover is thickened and hyperplastic, while the superficial layer of lamina propria is diffusely oedematous.

Nodules are most commonly seen in adult females. They are unusual in adult males and children, particularly boys.

Indications for surgery. The principal factors in deciding whether surgery is appropriate or not are as follows:

• The size and, most importantly, the age of the lesion (whether the surface is keratinized or not).
• Alteration of stroboscopic vibration (the 'hour-glass' glottic chink is more clearly visible under stroboscopic light).
• The objective and subjective importance of the voice problem to the patient. With singers, for example, one may occasionally suggest operating on a very small nodule that produces significant problems in singing despite the speaking voice remaining virtually unaffected.
• Failure of medical treatment or speech therapy.

Preferably, one should always begin treatment with speech therapy prior to any surgical procedure.

The operation. Avulsion of tissue by tearing it off the fold with cupped or plain forceps is best avoided as it may remove unnecessarily large fragments of mucosa. A much better technique is to remove the lesion as precisely as possible by gripping it with fenestrated heart-shaped tissue-holding forceps, and then using microscissors to divide the mucosa alongside the edge of the forceps in order to conserve as much healthy tissue as possible. This method minimizes the risk of producing a secondary notch when the mucosa heals. Two nodules may be removed at the same time, even in older children over the age of eight, so long as a zone of intact mucous membrane is preserved around the anterior commissure. This prevents the formation of adhesions by subsequent scarring.

In 22% of cases of nodules, a congenital mucosal micro-web may be found at the anterior commissure. This may be divided with an arrowhead knife if the web is of significant size.

Finally, after excision of the nodule, if associated inflammatory changes are present, cortisone is injected into the fold and any remaining dilated capillaries on the upper surfaces of the folds are sealed with diathermy.

Postoperative follow-up and results. The immediate postoperative results are generally excellent. At the end of the eight-day period of complete voice rest, the folds have resumed their normal shape with a good, straight, free border. Stroboscopy shows that the mucosa is vibrating well, albeit with slightly diminished amplitude. At this stage it also shows a persistent small longitudinal notch. Initially the voice is usually slightly higher in pitch, with a clearer though still slightly veiled quality. Voicing is still somewhat unstable and weak.

Postoperative speech therapy produces rapid stabilization of the results and normal voicing generally returns within a few weeks. During this period there is marked improvement in the stroboscopic appearance of the vibration and glottal closure. Nonetheless, speech therapy should be continued over several months in order to stabilize modified vocal habits and prevent recurrence.

Long-term results are on the whole excellent, and very much depend on the quality of the speech therapy. Recurrence of a nodule is rare when speech therapy has been regularly attended (3% of revision procedures in our personal series).

Capillary telangiectases

These present as small, dilated vessels situated on the superior aspect of the vocal folds. These vessels normally travel in a direction parallel to the free border but frequently terminate in angiomatous clusters of variable size; this appearance is often referred to as 'vascular corditis'. The term 'varices of the vocal cords' is sometimes used (incorrectly) and should be avoided.

Indications for surgery. The most important aspect of the diagnosis at indirect laryngoscopy is the elimination of intrafold lesions of which capillary telangiectases are simply the superficial manifestation. Stroboscopy may make one suspect the presence of cysts or a sulcus vocalis, both of which are associated with these vascular dilatations.

Capillary telangiectases are also frequently associated with nodular lesions. In this instance, vocal problems and indications for surgery are related more to the nodule than to the telangiectasis itself.

There are occasions, however, when a capillary telangiectasis alone may be solely responsible for all the laryngeal symptoms. Generally these lesions do not hamper stroboscopic vibration, nor do they produce much modification of vocal timbre. Patients mostly complain of vocal fatigue. Without doubt this is due to secondary vasomotor phenomena which appear after prolonged voice use. It is therefore the functional disability experienced by the patients (especially singers), rather than any visible change in vibration patterns, that suggests a surgical solution.

The operation. A series of point coagulations are made along the length of the vessel with a needle-point monopolar diathermy electrode. It is always wise to check that palpation of the fold does not show any localized areas of induration, which would make one suspect the presence of an underlying intrafold lesion. Where there is any uncertainty, one can perform an exploratory cordotomy.

As before, hydrocortisone suspension is injected into the fold at the end of the procedure.

Postoperative follow-up and results. Postoperative follow-up is straightforward. It is important to remember that cauterized vessels take many weeks to disappear completely. The final result is usually good from both the anatomical and vocal point of view, as long as the patient has pre- and postoperative speech therapy. Even so, from time to time there are patients who will relapse.

Polyps

The vocal fold polyp is an inflammatory laryngeal pseudotumour seen almost exclusively in males, and most common in the age group between 25 and 50 years. Vocal strain is a recognized factor in the production of polyps.

Histologically a polyp is composed of fibrinous exudates separated by proliferations of vascular clefts. They are described as being oedematous or haemangiomatous, depending on the predominant component.

Polyps nearly always arise anteriorly near the free border of the vocal fold. They may be sessible or pedunculated, and vary in size. Contralateral keratotic lesions with notching of the mucosal cover of the fold arise when the polyp has been present for a long time.

Indications for surgery. All polyps warrant microsurgical removal, as spontaneous regression is the exception rather than the rule. In addition, it is worth remembering that 15% of polyps represent a complication of an intrafold lesion – cyst or sulcus – which is often extremely difficult to demonstrate at preoperative assessment.

The operation. We are firmly of the opinion that polyps should not be removed at indirect laryngoscopy, regardless of the ability of the surgeon. Operating under direct vision using the microscope diminishes the likelihood of incomplete removal with subsequent recurrence, and more importantly, avoids production of a scarred notch where an over-enthusiastic avulsion has 'bitten' into the vocal ligament.

Resection of a polyp is simple and is performed by excising it at its attachment to the vocal fold. Because polyps are most commonly sessile, the excision will tend to produce a large raw area which may be initially rather haemorrhagic and thus may require the application of swabs of vasoconstrictor. However, when secondary healing of the mucosa has taken place, this area fills out without leaving a depression.

Postoperative follow-up and results. After excision of a polyp, the anatomical and vocal recovery is normally extremely rapid. Where the base of the polyp has been particularly broad and deeply implanted within the superficial layer of the lamina propria (Reinke's space), on stroboscopic examination at the first follow-up, one may periodically see a minimal depression at the site of excision. This always disappears rapidly and perfect anatomical resolution is the rule. The voice is usually changed in a spectacular manner by this simple surgical manoeuvre. Even so, we insist on pre- and postoperative speech therapy as standard clinical practice, and perhaps because of this we have only ever had a single recurrence.

Reinke oedema

This particular form of chronic laryngitis is principally associated with smoking and vocal abuse. These days females are almost as commonly affected as males. Typically this is a myxoid oedema that develops in the easily distended Reinke's space, usually on the superior surface of the fold spreading over the free border, thus making it extremely bulky. This process can continue to the point where the oedematous mucosa may obstruct the whole glottic orifice.

The gelatinous quality of the vocal folds in Reinke oedema explains the low-pitched guttural vocal characteristics associated with the condition.

Indications for surgery. Indications for surgery are governed not so much by the anatomical appearance but more by the patient's vocal requirements. Some moderate pseudomyxomas are well tolerated, particularly by males, and do not necessarily justify surgery.

The operation. The greatest possible care should be taken of the mucosa covering the free border of the vocal fold. Over-enthusiastic resection of mucosa that has been distended by pseudomyxomatous oedema produces perfect anatomical results which may nonetheless be vocally disastrous.

Beginning with a mucosal incision just medial to the ventricle, the pseudomyxoma is dissected off the vocal ligament and aspirated. The mucosa is then laid back on the superior surface of the vocal fold and any excess is removed with microscissors. After an intrafold injection of cortisone the mucosa is kept in place with a biological glue.

Usually both sides are operated on at the same time. An intact zone of mucosa is always left anteriorly. However, if it is difficult to expose the whole glottis properly (which is quite common with this type of lesion) or if the lesion is very bulky, it may be preferable to operate on one fold at a time, leaving four to six months between procedures in order to avoid producing adhesions.

Postoperative outcome and results. The postoperative outcome is excellent. As soon as the period of voice rest is finished the folds no longer appear thickened and are supple on stroboscopic examination. The voice is higher in pitch, clearer and distinctly less rough. This type of minimal surgery avoids too radical (and often inappropriate) modification of vocal characteristics and conserves the 'vocal personality' of the patient.

The results should remain stable if the patient has stopped smoking and cooperated fully with the speech therapy programme. If neither of these conditions is met, the Reinke oedema tends to recur.

Mucus retention cyst

These are true cysts found in the submucosa. They are of glandular origin, hence their mucinous contents. The origin of a retention cyst is due to an obstruction of the excretory canal and the resultant accumulation of mucoid secretions within the lumen of the mucus gland. The cyst wall consists of glandular epithelium made up of two layers of cells, an external layer of cuboidal cells, and an internal layer made up of cylindrical ciliated cells lying on a basement membrane. The lumen typically contains mucinous liquid. These cysts may be found in any age group including children. They are as common in adult females as they are in male subjects.

Indications for surgery. The prime indication for surgery is the diagnosis of a mucus cyst at indirect laryngoscopy. The diagnosis may be made because of a yellowish and occasionally very voluminous arching of the middle third of the vocal fold, which causes a bulging outwards of both the free border and the superior surface. Usually the fold distended by this cyst will not vibrate on stroboscopy.

More commonly the cyst presents as an elongated bulge slightly below the free border, and may quite easily be confused with a nodule, especially if a contact lesion has developed on the opposite fold, producing an appearance of kissing nodules. Stroboscopy leads one to suspect a cyst when one finds a loss of stroboscopic vibration localized to the area of the bulge. Occasionally the presence of a cyst is only revealed at operation: when ablating a lesion that was thought to be a simple nodule produces a characteristic flow of mucous liquid.

The operation. Ablation with microcups or microscissors is not recommended because removal of too much overlying mucosa risks the production of a significant notch postoperatively. Moreover, an incomplete excision is liable to produce recurrence. We recommend another technique: incising the mucosa on the superior aspect of the fold where it overlies the bulge and meticulously dissecting out the cystic pocket with microdissectors. The dissection is extremely delicate because the cyst wall is particularly thin and fragile and one rarely performs a complete exenteration without rupturing the cyst. It is nonetheless possible to progressively separate the cyst wall from the mucosal cover, and even from the vocal ligament, and remove it intact. Cysts are routinely sent for histopathological examination. The nidus from which the cyst was removed is checked and cleaned with a very small cotton-wool ball soaked in vasoconstrictors. The mucosa then collapses down in a normal position on to the fold without any loss of substance. The contralateral contact lesion is always removed.

Postoperative follow-up and results. The immediate result is usually good. At the first postoperative visit the vocal fold remains slightly pink, the volume of Reinke's space has returned to normal and it is unusual to find a notch in the mucosa. Stroboscopic vibrations, however, are usually diminished in amplitude with respect to the contralateral vocal fold. The voice is much improved although at this stage it remains a little veiled and unstable. Voice breaks still persist on quiet phonation.

The final result after speech therapy is excellent both anatomically and functionally. There is always a risk of recurrence, however, because of the difficulty of dissecting out the entire contents of the cystic pocket clearly.

Congenital lesions

Epidermoid cysts

Epidermoid cysts of the vocal fold are more or less rounded or flattened structures, limited by a wall, and are situated in the submucosal space. From time to time they may invaginate into the fibroelastic fibres of the vocal ligament, which are spread apart. The contents are generally liquid, and are white and opalescent due to accumulation of squamous debris in the cavity. Histologically, an epidermoid cyst is composed of a cavity bounded by stratified squamous epithelium of variable degrees of keratinization and thickness, which develops in a centripetal manner from a rest on a basement membrane. The cavity contains cornified desquamated material together with crystals of cholesterol. There is sometimes an inflammatory reaction in the tissue of Reinke's space around the cyst.

Some cysts may have an opening, most commonly slightly underneath the free border of the vocal fold, which allows intermittent spontaneous emptying of the cyst.

These cysts may be seen at any age, including childhood.

Indications for surgery. Diagnosis of this lesion is sometimes easy at indirect laryngoscopy. Some cysts, however, present as a whitish arching of the mucosa, which bulges out of the superior surface of the mid-third of the fold and produces stroboscopic absence of vibration over the whole fold.

In general the lesion is not clinically obvious and the indirect signs suggesting the probable diagnosis are as follows:

- localized swelling of the mid-third of the fold, where stroboscopic examination shows a reduced amplitude of the mucosal wave where it overruns the swelling;
- dilated capillaries converging on a precise point on the superior surface of the vocal fold in the mid-third; monocorditis;
- in children, a fusiform appearance of the vocal folds with loss of stroboscopic vibration;
- when the appearance is not absolutely pathognomonic, other factors suggest that surgery is still the appropriate management;
- the characteristic acoustic patterns: lesions that increase rigidity of the vocal fold produce rather irregular, weak laryngeal vibrations;
- the clinical history which often suggests a dysphonia beginning in childhood;
- failure of speech therapy.

The operation. An incision (cordotomy) a few millimetres in length, slightly longer than the diameter of the cyst and running parallel to the free border, is made in the mucosa of the superior aspect of the vocal fold. A blunt dissector is then used to modify the incision appropriately.

In general, mobilization is fairly easy underneath the cyst next to the vocal ligament and more delicate superficially in the plane between the epithelium of the vocal fold cover and the cyst. From time to time the inferior pole of the outer surface of the cyst wall may be embedded within a split in the elastic fibres of the vocal ligament. As with aural surgery for cholesteatoma, when the cyst is excised intact there is no risk of future recurrence.

Following the removal of a cyst, the pocket should always be meticulously checked to avoid missing a second, deeper cyst, which sometimes occurs concealed within the vocal ligament.

Commonly there are inflammatory changes associated with the lesion and so cortisone is injected into the body of the fold before replacing the mucosa. The mucosa is not trimmed, the incision edges are simply approximated edge to edge and are held in place with an application of fibrin glue.

Postoperative follow-up and results. There is generally a satisfactory appearance of the vocal fold at the first postoperative inspection; although modest inflammatory changes remain, the cordotomy incision is usually no longer visible. Sometimes there is a slight depression in the vocal fold cover over the area that previously contained the cyst. Stroboscopic vibration is usually weak at the outset but rapidly improves during the first examination. Initially, voice quality is often rather mediocre, being rather veiled and unstable and producing voice breaks on quiet phonation. Postoperative speech therapy is absolutely essential in order to produce a steady and entirely satisfactory improvement in voicing. It must be stressed that improvement is a progressive affair and that it will be necessary for the patient to undergo a protracted course of therapy.

Sulci. The term sulcus has been used since the turn of the century to define a lesion that at indirect laryngoscopy appears as a 'whitish furrow running parallel to the free border of the vocal cord giving the glottis an oval appearance'. In reality the sulcus thus defined corresponds to two quite different anatomical entities.

The term sulcus glottidis, when correctly used, describes an invagination of the epithelial cover of the fold into Reinke's space. This produces a pocket of variable depth that pushes downwards and inwards, often deeply enough to contact the vocal ligament to which it may be more or less adherent depending on the degree of inflammatory reaction in the surrounding tissue. Histological examination shows that the sulcus is a true blind-ended sac, bounded by walls of stratified squamous epithelium of variable thickness, keratinization being most marked around the base of the pocket. We think that these features show that a sulcus is actually an open epidermoid cyst.

A furrow-like appearance may also be produced by an entirely different type of lesion that we have entitled a 'stretch mark' (Bouchayer and Cornut, 1992). This lesion presents as an atrophic furrow of variable extent lying underneath the free border of the vocal fold, giving the border a bowed appearance. The inferior margin of the furrow often contains a tight, stiff, submucosal band whereas the superior margin is rather more supple. The mucosa lining the floor of the stretch mark is thin, atrophic, and intimately bound to the fibres of the vocal ligament. This prevents any sliding between the layers.

Both sulcus and stretch marks may be seen from adolescence onwards, and they appear slightly more common in males than females. It would seem most likely that they are both congenital in origin.

Indications for surgery. In some cases the furrow may be obvious, lying at the level of the free border in one or both vocal folds, producing an oval appearance of the glottis highly suggestive of a sulcus or stretch mark. Occasionally the appearance is less obvious and the furrow may only be visible in stroboscopic light. There may only be evidence of an absent closed phase over the entire length of the free borders of the vocal folds, perhaps associated with monocorditis or some capillary telangiectases.

The acoustic voice patterns are highly characteristic and support the diagnosis: the voice is often loud, and particularly in males, dull. It is also rather veiled, with frequent voice breaks. Patients usually present with significant vocal fatigue, paralaryngeal aches, or the need for further treatment when speech therapy has not improved things sufficiently.

The operation. For a sulcus glottidis or open epidermoid cyst it is essential not to remove too much mucosa in order to avoid producing a secondary puckered scar. To achieve this the superior and inferior crests circumscribing the epidermal pocket are precisely incised with a very sharp arrowhead knife. The floor of the pocket is then dissected off the vocal ligament with blunt elevators. Following this the sulcus may be removed intact after section of the remaining anterior and posterior attachments with microscissors. The subglottic mucosa is mobilized over a few millimetres in order to achieve approximation of the superior and inferior mucosal margins without loss of tissue thickness.

Surgery is extremely difficult to perform. It requires excellent instruments and considerable competence of the surgeon, but it does give good primary and secondary anatomical and functional results. The phoniatrician in charge of the postoperative care will be well aware of this.

For a stretch mark the aim of the surgery is to elevate the atrophic adherent section of mucosa after distending the fold with an injection of hydrocortisone suspension. An incision is made on the superior surface of the fold and a plane between the mucosa and the ligament is created using a blunt elevator. This is always an extremely difficult dissection because the mucosa is closely adherent to the ligament and cannot always be preserved. It is frequently necessary to detach fibres of connective tissue from the mucosal cover, and when freed these fibres should be laid back in place on the vocal ligament. This is particularly important for the inferior bar where these fibres may act like a bow-string, pulling a flange of mucosa over the inferior margin of the stretch mark.

This operation generally produces a satisfactory sliding plane under the mucosa of both the free border and the subglottic margins. The period of scarring and shrinkage then pulls both parts into the closest possible approximation.

These lesions are generally bilateral and may be operated on at the same time. Nevertheless, when the dissection of the first side has been particularly difficult, or where the larynx is small, as for instance in children, then it is preferable to operate on one side only and to leave an interval of approximately six months before operating on the second side.

Postoperative follow-up and results. After removal of a sulcus, the area of resection often appears as a small discrete dent which rapidly fills out and becomes supple with postoperative speech therapy.

Eight days after operating on a stretch mark, the furrowed appearance is still evident and the stroboscopic vibration remains feeble. The voice is usually mediocre, and is sometimes actually rather worse than it was prior to the operation. Frequent voice breaks and very veiled voicing are the norm. It is only with protracted postoperative speech therapy that one begins to clearly see a steady improvement in the suppleness of the vocal folds. In particular, the stroboscopic appearance of the hitherto rigid inferior border demonstrates greatly improved mucosal waves, and one often ends up with a considerably improved closure of the folds, given that it is never possible to achieve a perfect result. The pitch of the voice is generally lower and the timbre improves although retaining a rather veiled quality. The majority of patients are well satisfied even though the objective result is not perfect, because the combination of surgery and speech therapy completely removes both the pronounced laryngeal ache and the vocal fatigue, thus producing a significant improvement in the patient's vocal comfort.

Mucosal bridge

A mucosal bridge presents as a separate mucosal band running parallel to the free border, having anterior and posterior attachments to the fold. Structurally it is composed of everted stratified squamous epithelium and is always associated with one of the three lesions previously described. We think that the bridge arises from a cyst open sac with two (superior and inferior) ostia. Between these openings there remains a characteristic healthy band of mucosa of variable size and it is this that becomes the mucosal bridge.

The operation. Usually mucosal bridges are thin, and most of the time the appropriate technique is simply to excise the bridge using microscissors at its anterior and posterior attachments. From time to time, however, a mucosal bridge is large and thick, and simple resection would incur an excessive loss of mucosal bulk, resulting in the secondary production of a notch on the free border of the vocal fold. These thick bridges are fortunately uncommon, their surgical treatment being particularly difficult. An attempt is made to reduce the thickness of the bridge by removing the mucosa from the underside of the bridge while leaving the band and the overlying mucosa intact. The epidermoid pocket underneath the bridge is then dissected out and removed, thus allowing the band and remaining overlying mucosa to be replaced against the vocal ligament.

Unilateral recurrent laryngeal nerve paralysis

Indications for surgery. Surgical treatment of unilateral recurrent laryngeal nerve paralysis is appropriate where speech therapy rehabilitation alone has produced insufficient improvement, and inspection shows that the vocal fold remains atrophic and inadequately medialized or has remained in the intermediate position. Stroboscopic examination is essential in order to assess the vocal importance of any misalignment of the folds, atrophic change in vocal fold bulk, and the degree of failure of glottal closure, and is thus the single most important examination for assessing suitability for surgery. We normally wait for a year after the onset of the paralysis before injecting a paretic fold.

The operation. The aim of intrafold injection, be it with Teflon or with collagen, is to expand the paralysed fold in order to bring the free border back towards the midline without interfering with the vocal fold cover's capacity to generate waves.

Teflon paste is injected with a needle having a double-angle offset near the tip, and which is fitted to a pistol with a notched plunger. The needle has a wide diameter and should be inserted deeply and lateral to the vocalis muscle, which will then be displaced from within by the Teflon.

It is essential to avoid two things:

• superficial or submucosal injection;
• injection of too much paste.

Generally, injection into an anterior and a posterior site is adequate, although Teflon paste cannot be spread in the area adjacent to the arytenoid; hence there is always a persistent posterior interarytenoid gap.

Phonagel (GAX collagen), after many initial problems, is now freely available and offers several advantages over Teflon:

• it is highly biocompatible;
• the suspension is much more fluid than Teflon paste, which allows the use of a much finer needle for injection and can thus be spread much more easily within the fold, usually from a single posterior injection site.

In either case massaging the fold with the end of the sucker or some other suitable instrument produces a much more even spread of the paste throughout the length of the fold, making the free border as straight as possible.

Postoperative follow-up and results. Postoperative benefits are immediately apparent. There is no point in the patient's remaining silent for a period and we advise them to start speaking again the day after operation. Following the repositioning of the fold, the voice is stronger and frequently rather lower in pitch. Dyspnoea while speaking diminishes and may disappear completely, coughing becomes more forceful, and episodes of overspill/inhalation of liquids cease.

Laryngeal examination shows a somewhat over-inflated fold initially, which will retain a rather inflamed appearance for several weeks. There is an obvious improvement in glottal closure.

Speech therapy sessions should be started again so that the patient learns how to use his or her new voice. A few patients may find the initial experience of a new voice quite disorientating.

In the majority of cases anatomical and functional improvement is maintained in the long term. After collagen injection, the fold seems to appear progressively more normal, rather as if the collagen were being evenly distributed throughout the substance of the interior of the fold; the stroboscopic vibration meanwhile reappears in a reasonably satisfactory manner. In a few cases following either Teflon or collagen injection the vocal result is not stable and a further topping-up injection is necessary.

A final note about Teflon. There is a risk of occasional serious secondary complications due to a granulomatous inflammatory reaction in the vocal fold. This may present as a pseudotumour of the fold – sometimes years after the original injection (seven years in one of our cases).

Special problems

Iatrogenic scars

Under the general heading 'scars of the vocal folds' we include:

- notches in the vocal folds;
- adhesions between folds;
        between a fold and ventricular band;
- fibrous scars;
- stiffening of the fold following use of the laser.

Indications for surgical revision must be carefully assessed. It is not always easy to say whether a poor result from previous surgery is due to scarring or vocal dysfunction.

Laryngeal examination may sometimes show clear evidence of a notch in the fold producing air escape and an explanation of the veiled quality of the voice. In contrast, sometimes the anatomical appearance shows little abnormality, and only stroboscopy will produce evidence of localized or even very extensive scarring of the fold.

Revision surgery may be suggested when a prolonged trial of speech therapy has been manifestly unhelpful, and if the patient is sufficiently motivated and has been fully forewarned about the hazards and limitations of this type of repeat procedure.

The operative technique that we use most commonly is derived from the technique used to elevate mucosa off a stretch mark. Where there is a notch or area of fold rigidity, one always finds that the mucosal scar and the surface of the vocal ligament are intimately stuck together. Using the technique described above, we try to mobilize the mucosa in order to restore some flexibility to this rigid area: intrafold injection of hydrocortisone suspension, superior cordotomy, meticulous dissection, and elevation of the mucosa in an attempt to find a plane of cleavage between mucosa and vocal ligament.

The results are difficult to schematize because they depend on both the initial lesion and the extent and difficulty of the revision surgery. However, postoperative examinations have shown us that after this 'mucosal freeing', the vocal fold does regain a degree of suppleness, which is demonstrable by improved stroboscopic vibration patterns and better glottic closure. At the same time there is an undeniable improvement in voicing which continues *pari passu* with postoperative speech therapy.

Microsurgery in children

Until very recently, phonosurgery in children was only undertaken with the greatest reluctance. In addition to the usual constraints, there are other relative contraindications to surgery in children: the small size of the immature larynx, the virtual impossibility of insisting on a period of postoperative silence, and above all, the habitual vocally abusive speech patterns of children presenting with lesions amenable to surgery. Nonetheless, several factors are causing us to turn to surgery as a treatment option with increasing frequency. Appropriate surgical and anaesthetic procedure is now well characterized, congenital lesions (cysts) are being discovered with increasing frequency when previous indirect examination had suggested that the lesions were simple vocal nodules, and speech therapy may fail to improve the voices of even the most co-operative children. The final decision to opt for surgery is often made on the basis of the length of the history of dysphonia, which may suggest that the lesion is congenital, and the degree of handicap caused by the dysphonia, for instance in children studying music. Full preoperative preparation of both the child and the family is absolutely essential.

The operation itself is no different from the adult procedure, and generally one is struck by the ease and quality of the exposure in a child's larynx. The optimum age for surgery is between 9 and 11 years old.

The outcome following surgery is straightforward and depends to a great extent on family support and speech therapy. The final result depends largely on the type of lesion that was removed. It is excellent following nodule excision and rather slower after removal of a cyst. The aim of postoperative speech therapy is to maintain this improvement, and therapy should be continued over several months to prevent the child's returning to vocally abusive patterns. Nodules recur more frequently than in adults and are the direct result of continuing vocal abuse.

Microsurgery for singers

Lesions found on the vocal folds of singers are perfectly amenable to microsurgical treatment, provided that the operator is particularly cautious and meticulous in avoiding leaving a scar, no matter how small, which could be catastrophic for the singing voice. The lesions found in singers on whom we have operated are not solely varieties of nodule; there are also a significant number of epidermoid cysts and sulci. We thus conclude that small congenital anomalies of the larynx may be entirely compatible with a good quality singing voice, but that the passage of time may lead to a secondary 'decompensation'.

When faced with any singer who presents with chronic vocal difficulties, it is thus obligatory to perform a full laryngeal assessment using optical magnification and stroboscopy, which may suggest the presence of a cyst or a sulcus, before blaming the problem on poor technique. In a few cases where the diagnosis remains uncertain, it may be necessary to inspect or explore the folds at microlaryngoscopy. One should be aware at all times that any laryngeal microsurgery poses particular problems for the professional singer:

- the anxiety of the patients that they may lose the tool with which they make their living;
- the difficulty of coping with a lengthy interruption in their professional singing career; in our experience, that interruption should not be less than three months;

- delicate postoperative adjustments in vocal technique require the help
  of a therapist with personal knowledge of singing problems.

Conclusion

Within the realm of phonosurgery, we feel that collaboration between
phoniatrician and surgeon is absolutely indispensable. Such a collaboration is highly instructive to both parties, who as a result are able to make
increasingly accurate diagnoses as well as adapting and refining surgical
techniques required to improve vocal function. Improved microsurgical
technique has drastically altered the prognosis for a large number of
benign laryngeal lesions: nonetheless pre- and postoperative speech
therapy remain an essential adjunct to the surgery.

CHAPTER 18

The multidisciplinary voice clinic

SARA HARRIS, TOM HARRIS, JACOB LIEBERMAN AND DINAH HARRIS

Introduction

Since this book first appeared in 1986, the number of multidisciplinary voice clinics in the UK has increased dramatically and our understanding and approach to voice disorders have changed as a result. Improvements in the equipment commercially available to assess voice production have not only enabled more accurate diagnosis, but also provided better means of measuring the changes resulting from surgical intervention or voice therapy. At the same time, financial constraints on the National Health Service have led to an increase in the number of patients who seek private therapy financed by medical insurance companies. There is pressure on clinicians to provide evidence that therapy techniques are effective and can be carried out in a given number of sessions. In other words, voice clinicians now have to justify their existence as providers of cost-effective care. In some respects these changes have been necessary, stimulating and challenging to carry out, but in others, they have seriously limited effective and lasting treatment and the possibilities for research.

This chapter will discuss the advantages and disadvantages of a multi-disciplinary voice clinic; the personnel and their roles; equipment; what to assess; approaches to administration; outcome measures and audit. A summary of a study to investigate the validity of manual therapy techniques in the treatment of dysphonia, carried out by the Queen Mary's Hospital Voice Clinic team, is also presented.

The advantages of a voice clinic

There are a number of advantages, for both patients and clinicians, in running a voice clinic. The voice clinic setting is useful in resolving a number of problems that often occur where dysphonics are routinely treated in outpatient clinics. These advantages depend on the increased amount of time given to each patient, continuity of care and the variety of approaches that can be applied to the diagnosis and management of patients in a multidisciplinary setting.

Continuity of care

It is comparatively rare for voice clinics in the UK to be run by several different consultants. Usually, one consultant within an ENT team takes an interest in voice and takes on the voice clinic. Similarly, there is rarely more than one speech and language therapist specialized in voice who takes responsibility for the clinic, although others may sometimes be involved in the patient's treatment or attend on a training basis. If the clinic team includes singing teachers, osteopaths, or psychotherapists they also tend to be regular members of the clinic, particularly as few are prepared to give up a session of private work for very little or no financial reward.

Patients usually report a strong preference for seeing the same staff at each clinic visit. They build up good relationships with the team and feel at ease to discuss their problems. This allows the team a much better overall picture of the patient, within the context of their general health, work and social life. As a result, causative factors that are often considered to be peripheral by the patient can be spotted early and the appropriate treatment provided.

Continuity of care enables clinicians to develop a 'clinical memory' of patients with difficult vocal problems, including the usual appearance of their vocal folds. Fine differences of appearance which herald change are then more likely to be noted; this can be particularly helpful where the clinic has no Mavigraph to print downloaded pictures from video and the clinician is reliant on a drawing or verbal description of the larynx.

The importance of team decisions

In most ENT clinics, the surgeon sees dysphonic patients as a routine part of the outpatient caseload. Neither the time nor the equipment is available for detailed case histories or analysis of vocal function. Pathology may be diagnosed accurately, but the management decision lies in the hands of the surgeon who may offer surgery, speech therapy, review or discharge. Each surgeon's criteria for making these decisions can be different and, with pressure on the National Health Service, many patients who could have responded well to voice therapy techniques, advice, vocal hygiene or counselling may not be referred for voice therapy. Sometimes, of course, reassurance is all that is needed and the patient gradually recovers. Unfortunately, others fail to resolve and finally re-present to the surgeon at a later date with visible pathology as a result of the continuing vocal misuse. If the surgeon decides to operate, patients may have their surgery, be reviewed and discharged with the original causative factors still present in their voice production.

Contributory medical factors

Medical problems that may be either causative or contributory to dysphonia are often not addressed in a general ENT clinic because of the shortage of time available for each patient and because the mental set of both patient and clinician is restricted to the ENT symptoms. Much depends on the patient providing unfiltered information about their health, in a way that their medical problems can be identified by the surgeon, and referred on for appropriate assessment. Patients do not necessarily realize that their indigestion, whiplash injuries, chest troubles, medications, or emotional difficulties can be related to the voice or swallowing problems they are experiencing.

Much has been written about these concomitant medical factors in recent years, so that many surgeons do now ask the relevant questions. Even so, concomitant medical conditions may still be missed because patients fail to recognize their symptoms from the questions they are asked. A common example can be found in patients who fail to relate their night cough, dry, tetchy, irritable throat and morning hoarseness to the heartburn that the surgeon inquires about.

Recognizing and treating the common concomitant medical problems is important. Patients with these problems often fail to respond to vocal techniques until their medical problems have been resolved, with the risk that they will lose faith in voice therapy and leave their ENT follow-up appointments unattended. Their unrecognized medical problems and poor voice production may then create or mask developing pathology or produce relapse at a later date.

Inappropriate referrals for speech therapy

Adequate equipment for detailed examination and analysis of vocal function is essential (see equipment section, pp. 327–32). All too often in the past, patients have been labelled 'neurotic' and subjected to long courses of inappropriate voice therapy or psychotherapy because the equipment used to examine them has been inadequate for assessing vocal function.

Hard, fibrous nodules, vocal fold sulci, intra-cordal cysts and advanced cases of Reinke oedema are not amenable to conventional voice therapy.

However, cases like these are still being referred to voice therapy and it may take several sessions of frustration on behalf of patient and therapist before the referral is queried. In the past, patients like these may have been responsible for some surgeons feeling that speech therapy was ineffectual for the treatment of dysphonia. Lack of faith in a treatment soon communicates itself to the patients, who then fail to keep their therapy appointments. In the past, audit has shown that quite a high proportion of patients referred to speech therapists fail to keep their initial appointment (Donnelly and Kellow, 1989). Inappropriately referred patients who do take up the option of voice therapy may soon become discouraged by their lack of progress and will sometimes fail to return for ENT reassessment. This jeopardizes any chance of the correct diagnosis being reached and the necessary surgery provided.

The aetiology of vocal dysfunction is multifactorial and complex and even with the appropriate level of equipment, microscopic or occult lesions may take several examinations and a variety of phonatory assessment tasks to identify. For example, if the patient has insufficient airflow, mucosal waves cannot be efficiently driven and it is therefore impossible to exclude the possibility of an occult lesion (such as a sulcus or intracordal cyst) affecting phonation. These patients will need short-term voice therapy to develop sufficient airflow before any previously hidden lesions can be identified at reassessment. Where patients understand the need for voice therapy, compliance is greatly increased. In some clinics patients are asked to leave the room while the team members discuss the management plan. However, a multidisciplinary voice clinic setting can be used effectively to encourage patients to take responsibility for their treatment and they generally respond extremely well when included in the team discussion and management decisions.

Disadvantages of voice clinics

There is no doubt that voice clinics are expensive in terms of equipment and personnel. Videostrobolaryngoscopy is a basic requirement these days and involves a big capital outlay. Balanced against this is the decrease in the number of operations required simply to exclude pathology and the decrease in the number of clinic appointments necessary for each patient.

Voice clinics are efficient in terms of reducing the number of clinic appointments patients require (Harris et al., 1986). However, patients do need to be seen for longer periods, especially initially. An average initial appointment is 30 minutes and an average follow up is 10–15 minutes depending on the outcome of treatment.

Personnel are expensive. The ENT surgeon and voice therapist form the basic core of necessary personnel but where possible, other practitioners, either on a regular basis or for specially selected patient groups (such as performers), are extremely valuable additions. At Queen Mary's Hospital voice clinic in Sidcup, the regular team seeing patients in the voice clinic each week includes an osteopath and a singing advisor. Fortuitously, the osteopath is also a qualified psychotherapist, which has proved invaluable on many occasions. Patients who are seen from outside the district as extra contractual referrals (ECR) help to fund both the personnel and maintenance of the equipment, but funding for voice clinics has always been a problem and may become increasingly difficult within the National Health Service in the future.

The financial constraints imposed by (and on) the British National Health Service produce conditions that are specific to the UK. For a good overview of the North American experience the book by Deborah Koschkee and Linda Rammage, *Voice Care in the Medical Setting* (1997), is recommended.

Personnel

The laryngologist

In the UK, the laryngologist provides a thorough examination of each patient's ENT systems, with particular attention to the structure and function of the larynx. In other European countries this role would fall to the phoniatrician, a consultant specializing in communication disorders. The examination these days requires videostroboscopy to exclude structural defects that cannot be detected with a laryngeal mirror, as already discussed. The clinic team can then replay the recording in slow motion so that they can observe and discuss the patient's voice production patterns. The recording can then be used to provide an explanation of the problem for the patient.

The laryngologist will also be closely involved in taking the clinical history, in order to diagnose concomitant medical problems. This ensures that the patient receives any appropriate investigations which may be requested, either in clinic or by returning the patient to the GP, who will then take over and arrange appropriate investigation or medication.

The speech and language therapist

The speech and language therapist should always be present at the examination, and actively involved in the history taking and diagnosis of vocal function. Together with the laryngologist, the speech and language therapist is responsible for explaining the nature of the voice problem to the patient and working out a viable treatment programme.

The osteopath/physiotherapist

Most voice disorders involve some form of muscular compensation and/or musculoskeletal hyperfunction. While the laryngologist and speech therapist do address these issues, more specialized help is often needed. The osteopath/physiotherapist can be particularly helpful in assessing the postural contribution to vocal problems, particularly if the patient has suffered injury such as whiplash to the neck, or has long-term problems from injuries sustained in childhood. More specifically, they have an important role to play in assessing hyperfunction of the extrinsic laryngeal muscles and in some cases some of the intrinsic muscles as well. Research (Harris et al., 1992) has shown that laryngeal manipulation can be extremely effective in resolving hyperfunctional voice production. The physical examination of the larynx and related structures will be discussed later in this chapter in the 'What to assess' section.

The osteopath or physiotherapist can then treat the hyperfunctional muscle groups, with the appropriate soft tissue techniques that are central to manual therapy. Laryngeal manipulation, either on its own or in conjunction with voice therapy, appears to be extremely effective in relieving symptoms of laryngeal pain/discomfort and restoring normal vocal function (Harris and Lieberman, 1993). It is particularly effective for singers and actors whose vocal muscles remain habitually tense and who are suffering from vocal fatigue. This also applies to those suffering from the aftereffects of upper respiratory tract infections. Both groups require emergency treatment to get them back on stage to perform in the shortest possible time. Without this modality of treatment, all that is left for these patients is a short course of steroids, which inevitably carry side effects and should be avoided if at all possible (Harris, 1992). Laryngeal manipulation also appears to be particularly valuable in the treatment of patients suffering from symptoms of globus and those with arytenoid granulomata.

These patient groups may only need reassurance that they are healthy, and the restoration of a more relaxed laryngeal musculature, in order for the condition to resolve spontaneously. Others with more long-standing or serious hyperfunctional patterns will do better with vocal retraining in addition to manipulation. Clinical observation of these cases suggests that laryngeal manipulation increases the speed with which patients respond to vocal rehabilitation techniques.

At present, there are very few osteopaths/physiotherapists who are actively involved on a regular basis in voice clinics, or who are prepared to take a special interest in developing laryngeal manipulation. Speech and language therapists and surgeons may need to take on this role, but will require special training. While surgeons have well-developed palpatory skills and the required knowledge of anatomy and physiology, speech and language therapists do not, as yet, have experience of palpation in their training and may also need a refresher course on their anatomy and physiology, especially if they have been qualified for some years! Speech and language therapists may also have reservations that manipulation requires them to touch their clients regularly, as part of their treatment. Many speech and language therapists are trained in counselling skills, or even doubly qualified as counsellors or psychotherapists. These professions do not usually include physical contact with clients because they are working with the client's emotional system, with all the attendant projections, transferences and defence mechanisms. Physical contact provides a very direct path to the patient's emotional mechanisms and may break down defences that are necessary to protect both the patient and therapist. Without careful handling and understanding, emotional problems may arise.

The singing coach/teacher/advisor

The singing coach may be a regular member of the assessment team, or brought in at intervals for clinics aimed specifically at performers. Some prefer to take voice clinic referral for assessments and courses of remedial work and report back, attending only with specific clients. As there is no formal professional training for singing teachers, many will feel they benefit considerably from regular attendance at the voice clinic, as it offers them a unique opportunity to learn about both normal and disordered voice.

Many multidisciplinary voice clinics report increasing numbers of professional or semi-professional actors and singers who have special needs from a voice assessment. They may have acute problems and need guidance as to whether it is safe for them to perform that night or long-standing vocal problems of a more nebulous nature. The singing coach has a valuable role to play here, both as a joint decision-maker and as a 'vocal detective'.

Few speech and language therapists or surgeons have a great deal of knowledge of the world of performance, its demands on the voice or its environmental and physical stresses. Stereotypes abound, particularly with pop/rock singers, who are often assumed to know nothing about voice production or singing technique and to be likely to abuse their bodies with smoking, drugs and alcohol. In some cases this may be true, but there are many highly trained singers in this genre who have survived without vocal problems, do not smoke or take drugs and run well on herbal tea! These singers have much to teach us about voice use and survival.

The singing advisor can bring to the clinic a unique understanding of the problems that are specific to performers, and ask the right case history questions. Unless specialized in singers, most speech and language thera-pists or surgeons will not routinely ask about fold back, use of raked staging, marking in rehearsals or difficulties with company managers and agents, for example. Performance also brings with it another language. Suddenly, Spintos, Helden Tenors, Buffo basses and Lyric mezzos come out of the woodwork with problems of fach, register and specific and other incomprehensible symptoms, such as 'a damper seems to come on the folds on F sharp above the stave'. It is easy for the more medically based team to dismiss singers as neurotic and voice-obsessed at best – and mad at worst. One wonderful thing about singing advisors is that they speak this language and can act as interpreters from 'singer speak' into 'medical speak', thus saving time and frustration on both sides and allowing an accurate diagnosis to be made with the minimum of misunderstanding.

Accurate diagnoses for singers can be difficult. Frequently, at first glance the larynx looks healthy and normal, and yet the singer is unable to perform at certain pitches or with certain dynamics. Stroboscopy is essential for these patients. So often, when examined with a strobed light, the intracordal cyst, fibrous plaque or sulcus vocalis appears on what seemed to be a pristine vocal fold. It is essential therefore, during the endoscopy, to ask the singer to vocalize at the pitch or dynamic where they experience the problem.

Sometimes technique that looks flawless in chest register may suddenly become hyperfunctional, higher in the range. Structural problems such as ventricular cysts, which are totally unrelated to phonation at one pitch of volume may suddenly interfere with, or affect, technique at another. The singing coach can often identify the components of the voice faster and most effectively.

Where the singer in clinic is really having difficulties with vocal technique, the singing teacher will have practical advice for the short term and a coterie of experienced colleagues to refer on to, at his or her finger tips. The role of interpreter is also necessary to relay the clinic findings and recommendations to the patient's current or recommended teacher, or to their training establishment if they are students. Some singing coaches will provide an advice session or a few sessions of remedial work as part of the clinic services, but this is rare within the NHS, due to funding problems.

The psychologist/counsellor/psychotherapist

In ideal circumstances, every voice clinic needs access to a qualified and interested psychologist, counsellor or psychotherapist. The presence of emotional factors, as either a trigger or concomitant of voice problems, is almost universal and many patients would benefit from some form of counselling, either as the focus of their management or in conjunction with surgery or voice therapy. Where possible, the counsellor is most valuable as a regular member of the clinic assessment team, seeing each patient. Where patients recognize and accept the psychological nature of their symptoms, the management is clear and the counsellor can take over immediately, reducing the possibility of resistance developing to the idea of a 'psychological' diagnosis. Where patients are unable to accept the psychological nature of their voice disorder, or if the disorder is multifaceted, the counsellor's clinical observations can be pivotal to the team management plan and their role as a supervisor for others in the team, who may have to deal directly with the patient, is invaluable.

In reality, this ideal is hard to achieve. However, it is strongly advised that links are forged with the local psychiatry/psychology department in order that patients can be referred on for assessment and treatment. The importance of psychological supervision for clinicians treating voice patients, whether they are speech therapists, singing coaches or osteopaths/physiotherapists, cannot be overestimated. Voice patients often present with complex and confusing psychological symptoms and clinicians who work with them frequently experience strong emotions around these patients. They need support and counselling to protect themselves and the patients from collusion and/or dependencies that could affect their clinical judgement.

The phonetician/acoustics department

Where multidisciplinary voice clinic teams are involved in research or clinical audit, links with a university phonetics department may provide access to equipment and analysis that may not be available in an NHS setting. Each individual clinic will work out their own needs in this area, depending on the equipment they have available to them and their research/audit needs. Research projects may require patients to visit the university for some of their assessment, for example acoustic analysis, while audit may well be possible to achieve by sending tape-recorded clinical data for analysis. However, phonetics departments are likely to charge a fee for their services and will expect acceptable recording quality for any taped data.

Equipment

Equipment for the voice clinic is expensive and vital. The minimum requirement is stroboscopy, using either a rigid telescope or flexible fibre-endoscope to visualize the larynx. As previously stated, it is not possible to view the movement of the mucosa over the body of the vocal folds during phonation with continuous light, and therefore stroboscopy is essential in order to eliminate microscopic or occult lesions that could be responsible the patient's symptoms.

The stroboscope

Stroboscopes are available from a number of companies; those made by Storz, Kay Elemetrics and Richard Wolf appear to be reliable and the producers offer reasonable aftercare/maintenance service, which is essential. Stroboscopes cost in the region of £8000. This price includes a microphone but excludes the endoscope and necessary cables.

The endoscope/telescope

The larynx may be viewed using a rigid telescope introduced into the oral cavity and rested on the back of the tongue. A prism at the distal end allows visualization of the larynx. There are choices in the degree of angle used, the most common being 90 or 70 degrees. The view using a rigid telescope is excellent as it allows a good magnification of the vocal folds and is ideal combined with stroboscopy for identifying microscopic/occult lesions. It also has the advantage that it can be conveniently sterilized in the clinic with isopropyl alcohol, after which it is washed in water. The drawback of using rigid telescopes is that in order to view the larynx the tongue needs to be pulled forward, interfering with the supraglottic resonators. There is some evidence that this posture may also alter vocal fold closure patterns during the examination (Sodersten and Lindestadt, 1992). Good models are available from companies such as Storz, Wolf and Olympus and cost between £1800 and £2500. It may be difficult to acquire the excellent but rather more expensive Japanese models from Machida or Nagashima.

Fibreoptic nasendoscopy provides a good alternative method of viewing the larynx with stroboscopy. Most modern nasendoscopes have a diameter between 3.5 and 4.2 mm and the tip is vertically manoeuvrable. Recent improvements and the new generation of fused silicon fibreoptic bundles allow better picture definition and smaller bundle diameter. These advantages are somewhat offset by the increase in rigidity their construction requires. In the future nasendoscopy will be able to provide similar quality video images to rigid telescopes. Rhinolaryngeal video endoscopes are a recent innovation (Olympus and Pentax). A small monochrome camera chip is placed at the distal tip of the endoscope so that the picture is no longer dependent on the fibre bundles. The field under review is then rapidly illuminated by sequences of red, green and blue light flashes from a special stroboscopic light generator. The camera input is reconstructed into high definition full colour pictures in a dedicated video processor. At present, these systems are very expensive; the endoscopes are large in diameter and they are not yet capable of producing stroboscopically slowed down images of vocal fold vibration, but hopefully this will come in time.

The advantages of nasendoscopy are that the view of the larynx is minimally invasive, allowing the patient to use their habitual phonation pattern and giving a good view of the supraglottic resonators. It is also excellent for viewing patients who have a brisk gag reflex and are unable to tolerate a rigid telescope in the mouth. The disadvantage is that it requires either at least 20 minutes to sterilize the endoscope (by soaking in Cidex) between patients or disposable sheaths and fitting apparatus, inevitably adding to clinic running costs. Patients tolerate nasendoscopy well on the whole, particularly if topical anaesthesia is used. Application of Co-phenylcaine forte spray (Paedpharma) seems to be less irritating to the patient's nose than the more commonly used Xylocaine, which produces a marked stinging sensation when first introduced. Good fibreoptic nasopharyngoscopes are available from such companies as Olympus, Pentax and Storz and cost around £5000–£8000.

Video equipment

The most useful equipment to add to stroboscopy is a camera and video recorder to allow the laryngeal images to be studied in slow motion by the clinic team. Single and three chip cameras are available for this purpose and have their strengths and weaknesses. Single chip cameras are small, extremely light sensitive and relatively cheap, starting at approximately £2200. The three chip cameras give better colour and more lines, but tend to be less light sensitive and far more expensive at approximately £5000. Additionally, the reduction in light sensitivity may make it necessary to buy a more expensive laryngoscope in order to achieve adequate light values for good video recording. This is becoming less important, as some systems now incorporate image enhancement. Whether the camera is digital or analogue is not critically important.

Video recorders vary in price between approximately £1000 and £3500 depending on the format and number of special features such as high quality freeze-frame, frame by frame, slow motion, etc. The standard format for video recorders in the UK and Europe is VHS but this system is now ageing and many clinics have switched to S-VHS. S-VHS records light values (luminance) and colour (chrominance) separately, improving the picture definition, particularly for re-recordings made from edited video material. As most clinicians need to edit videos these days for various purposes, it is worth buying a recorder that is at the upper end of the price bracket, as the freeze-frame capability and time-coding are superior on the more expensive models.

In addition to the camera and video recorder, a medical grade high resolution TV monitor is required. They cost up to £1500 depending on the quality and number of lines required. A small tie-clip microphone costing approximately £200 is also necessary to record the patient's voice during the assessment. Cables and a C mount adaptor to connect the Laryngoscope or nasendoscope to the camera may further increase the cost. A character generator to add the patient's name and clinic date to the film will cost between £200 and £1000, depending on the facilities, but is not essential in an everyday clinic setting. VAT, as always, is extra on all these items of equipment.

Looking to the future, clinics that invest in a fairly powerful computer will be able to install a frame grabber card. Using this card, the video input is digitized and stored to disc or to a read-write CD or DVD ROM, allowing vast amounts of data to be economically and compactly stored and indexed. It also allows for colour 'stills' to be easily printed from the video and stored for reference in the patient's notes. With less sophisticated systems, a single memory grade video printer such as the Sony Mavigraph TM can be attached to the video recorder, which can download a selected freeze-frame image and print it out on PVC paper for the clinic notes. Recent models now include a red-green-blue facility. Polaroid offer a similar system, which while versatile, requires the top of the range version to provide adequate definition.

Audio-recording

The equipment described above is a priority for visualizing the larynx, but in order to analyse the patient's phonation pattern more broadly, other techniques can be used. Perceptual analysis, still the cheapest, easiest and yet valid measure of dysphonia, requires a good audio tape recorder (Laver et al., 1981; McAllister et al., 1994). Where possible, a digital audiotape recording system (DAT) is ideal, as it is excellent for both perceptual and computer analysis of dysphonic voices. It is also the best system for recording the patient's progress through therapy. However, a good analogue system is still necessary, as most clients do not have DAT recorders at home and their therapy practice tapes need to be made to a good standard. A good DAT audiotape recorder costs in the region of £1000.

Electroglottograph/electrolaryngograph

The electroglottograph or electrolaryngograph is another valuable method of analysing the vocal output and measuring vocal change in treatment, accurately but non-invasively. This system measures the length of time the vocal folds are in contact with each other during phonation. It is linked to a computer and monitor which displays a waveform that can be printed out for the patient notes. The system can also analyse and represent longer samples of connected speech in the form of a histogram. A recent development (Laryngograph Ltd.) links the EGG equipment with stroboscopy so that the EGG data on vocal fold contact is synchronized with the videostroboscopy.

Two systems are readily available, the Electrolaryngograph (Fourcin and Abberton, 1971) and the Electroglottograph (Rothenberg, 1992). The

Laryngograph workstation, which is most commonly used in the UK, costs approximately £5000. This includes a suitable personal computer (PC), the laryngograph processor, the interface card, and software programmes for spectrography and phonetograms. The computer may also be used to run the Aerophone software (see airflow equipment) if airflow measures are required. Where the clinic already possesses a suitable computer, the Laryngograph system alone costs £3000.

Spectrography

Speech spectrographic analysis provides another non-invasive method of analysing the vocal output. Spoken material, collected either in real time or on audiotape, can be analysed using the appropriate computer software and displayed as a spectrograph on the computer screen. The display allows the clinician to measure the fundamental frequency and the associated formants created by the vocal tract. When the data is collected and analysed in real time, it can be used as visual biofeedback to show patients when they successfully achieve the pattern of formants required for different vowels and for spoken phrases. The most commonly used spectrographic analyses are available either from Laryngograph (see above) or Kay Elemetrics Ltd. as part of their CSL Speech Laboratory. Laryngograph will supply the necessary software separately for both their spectrograph and phonetogram, together with the digital signal processing (DSP) card, which can be installed on most types of computer. The DSP card costs £1000 and the spectrograph and phonetogram software packages cost £1000 respectively. Other packages are commercially available and liaison with the nearest university phonetics department may prove valuable.

Airflow studies

Airflow measures may be possible to access via the physiotherapy or respiratory physiology department, or may come as separate software that can be installed on the clinic computer. Measurements such as vital capacity, resting respiration and forced respiration are available, but the most useful for the voice clinic team will be the airflow patterns that occur in continuous phonation and speech. The Aerophone, produced by F-J Electronics appears to be most commonly used and costs approximately £5000. Like the laryngograph, it requires a suitable PC for operation. It is also available as an add-on unit for the Kay system.

Phonetograms

A phonetometer maps a visual record of the patient's range of pitch and intensity. It is non-invasive and easily carried out, provided that the patients are able to match the frequency of a computer generated tone with a sustained vowel. The patient matches the tone as loudly, then as softly, as they can throughout their range. The intensity values are plotted on to a graph in decibels, showing the highest and lowest scores at each frequency. When the plotted values are connected they form an outline that represents the patient's vocal and dynamic range (see Carding, Chapter 5). Software for this analysis can be installed on the clinic computer, increasing the scope of assessments available to suit individual patient needs. Phonetograms are particularly useful for assessing the dynamic range of singers and performers.

What to assess

Stroboscopy

Stroboscopic visualization of the larynx is used to determine laryngeal health and function. First, a description of the vocal folds is necessary, reporting the presence of any obvious lesions, their relative size, shape and position on the folds or elsewhere in the larynx. Where no obvious lesions are present, the colour of the vocal folds, the presence of enlarged blood vessels and the quality and texture of the mucosa are noted. If videostroboscopy is available, a printout of an appropriate freeze-frame is recommended for inclusion in the notes.

Otherwise the surgeon may make a sketch of the vocal findings or fill in the relevant details on a schematic picture.

A description of the vocal fold movement during phonation is necessary. The symmetry of vocal fold movement is recorded, together with the degree of closure and closure pattern. The presence of any other muscular activity within the larynx is noted; for example, the partial adduction of one or both false folds, the position of the base of the epiglottis and the position of the arytenoid cartilages. It can be very useful to observe these features at different vocal pitches, particularly when the patient is a singer or actor. It is important to note whether the vocal folds lengthen and shorten appropriately when the patient is asked to glide up and down their pitch range.

Finally, observation of the mucosal waves is reported. Are the mucosal waves present over the entire surface of the free borders of both vocal folds or is there any sign of deep tethering where the wave disappears? Are there areas where the mucosa appears to rock, rather than allowing smooth passage of the waves? Do the vocal folds vibrate symmetrically, so that both waves emerge from the subglottis and roll over the folds at the same time and at the same rate?

Do the mucosal waves respond to changes in vocal pitch, being of greater amplitude in modal voice and smaller at higher frequencies? (Hirano and Bless, 1993). Stroboscopy smooths out irregular vibration, and therefore in clinics where there is adequate funding for instrumentation, an excellent technique known as Videokymography may be used graphically to document vibratory irregularity, subharmonic beating of the folds and antero-posterior and left-right asymmetry of vibration patterns (Svec and Schutte, 1996). Inevitably, it requires the acquisition of another specially adapted video camera and related hardware.

These observations all help to build up a picture of the type of vibratory pattern used by each patient. Any lesions or areas of concern are noted along with the habitual vocal fold posture. These can then be compared with the findings at follow up.

Palpation of the extrinsic laryngeal muscles is essential, along with a description of the patient's general and head and neck posture. Where possible a manual therapist, such as an osteopath, needs to work with the voice clinic team in order to help develop palpatory skills for those not trained in palpation (e.g. speech therapists and singing teachers) and also to help with the development of a suitable protocol. The most relevant areas to examine are:

- the patient's general symmetry, weight bearing, spinal curvature;
- the state of the cervical spine and any hyperlordotic segments;
- the quality and tone of the cervical musculature;
- the position in which the head is carried;
- symmetry of jaw opening and excessive activity in the jaw muscles;
- the quality and tone of the suprahyoid musculature;
- the quality and tone of the thyrohyoid muscles/membranes;
- the quality and tone of the cricothyroid muscles and appropriate opening and closing of the cricothyroid visor;
- the quality and tone of the strap muscles;
- the ease of lateral shift of the larynx;
- the areas that the patient reports as painful or tender, which should be noted.

Where the clinic has access to a manual therapist who is experienced in laryngeal manipulation, the state of the posterior cricoarytenoid muscles and the crico-arytenoid joint may also be assessed.

Each member of the assessing team can rate the degree of tension palpated in the extrinsic laryngeal muscles and place it on a 3–5 point scale; the majority consensus rating can then be recorded in the patient's notes, to ensure practitioner agreement. More detailed protocols can be developed such as the Lieberman protocol (Harris et al., 1998).

The muscle groups are initially examined statically, to assess their tone and quality. Fibrosis and permanent shortening associated with prolonged contraction will be noted. The musculature is then assessed dynamically to establish the range of joint movement and efficiency of their habitual use. Where there has been damage to the larynx or suspensory mechanism (e.g. through paralysis or surgical division from such operations as thyroidectomy), the compensatory patterns are assessed. Many patients who have normal laryngeal mechanisms and normal muscle tone in the extrinsic laryngeal muscles at rest, produce hypertonic muscle patterns as soon as they begin to phonate. These cases are usually associated with emotional difficulties that are expressed in increased musculo-skeletal tension.

Other important measurements can be carried out either at a session with the speech therapist prior to the voice clinic, or by a technician either before or after the clinic examination. These measures might include audio recording, EGG, Phonetograms, airflow studies and spectrography, as available and appropriate. If they can be carried out before the examination, the results are available to the clinic team. However, it may be more appropriate to decide on which will be the most useful for individual patients after the laryngeal examination. The results can then be reviewed and added to the patient notes at the end of the clinic.

Administrative issues

There is no right way to run a voice clinic, but there are two definite approaches. The first is to assess all voice patients coming through the ENT department in the voice clinic, and the second is to see only those who present with complex problems or who have failed in conventional therapy.

The first approach has the advantage of providing a full assessment at the initial interview, ensuring the most effective use of clinic time and maximizing patient co-operation. The disadvantages are that some patients do not require a multidisciplinary approach and therefore may be considered as wasting clinical time. Also, hoarse patients need to be given priority in order to exclude malignancies. Voice clinics running only once a month will not be able to provide this service quickly enough. Finally, this approach often requires close co-operation between the hospital consultants, and where the voice clinic is staffed by a registrar or senior registrar, this may not always be possible.

The second approach has the advantage that screening of hoarse patients is carried out prior to their referral to the voice clinic, eliminating those with malignancies or who require primary surgery and selecting patients most likely to benefit from a multidisciplinary approach. It also allows time to arrange for the relevant team members to be present or to select special patient groups for certain clinics. The disadvantages are that patients may be selected for surgery rather than voice therapy unnecessarily and concomitant medical or psychosocial factors may be missed, with the attendant problems discussed earlier in the chapter.

Number of patients per clinic

Once the referral style has been decided, it remains necessary to work out the probable case load so that the number of clinics per month can be agreed. Most departments seem to decide to run voice clinics once a month initially, increasing or decreasing the frequency according to the case load demand and financial constraints. Once the team is experienced, new patients seem to need a maximum of half an hour while repeat patients can be seen in 15–20 minutes. Most clinics may have to manage between 7 and 12 patients in a session. More than 12 patients per session becomes impracticable.

History taking and clinical records

Case history forms can either be sent to patients to fill in prior to their clinic visit, be given to patients to complete in the waiting room or dealt with in clinic. Collecting the information prior to the clinic examination saves time, but there is a danger that patients may fail to understand some questions, or fail to recognize and report symptoms accurately without careful questioning. Where information is collected by questionnaire, it is recommended that the history is briefly recapped in clinic to prevent misunderstandings or omissions. The case history questionnaires can be kept in the notes along with the assessment check lists for stroboscopy and laryngeal palpation. They have the advantage that they are in the patient's own hand and confirm agreement of the case history facts that may be useful in the event of medico-legal disputes.

Video and audiotapes are usually stored in the clinic in date order. It is imperative that the dates of the patients' attendance at clinic are carefully recorded, in order to be able to access their previous recording(s) quickly. Ideally, long standing patients should have their own tapes, but this tends to be costly and increases the need for storage space. Once recordings are kept on CD or DVD ROMs it will be easier to access past recordings as it will be possible to file them under the patient's name.

Explanations

A significant part of the time allowed for clinical assessment is spent on explanation to the patient. It is very important that the patient understands the diagnosis and the proposed management plan and takes part in the decision-making process. It ensures that they take responsibility for the voice problem and for carrying out the voice therapy.

Support staff

Voice clinics require the usual administrative support and staff need to be clear about who is responsible for booking appointments, finding notes, typing the letters and reports and keeping the necessary statistics. Inevitably there are cost implications. If the clinic is run in the ENT department, it is usually the case that the voice clinic can be treated as another ENT clinic and the same support staff can be used for both. Where the clinic runs in the Speech Therapy department, it may be more difficult to negotiate and sometimes the speech therapist or speech therapy secretary will need either to collect notes from the ENT administrative staff or organize the appointments and typing themselves.

The voice clinic that runs in the ENT department will often be provided with a clinic nurse and allowed to share the receptionist. If it is run in speech therapy, sometimes a volunteer can be trained to act as receptionist. It is important that someone is responsible for welcoming patients, checking that their personal details are correctly recorded in the notes and making sure they know where to find other departments for tests when required.

Outcome and audit

In these days of financial restrictions, it is more important than ever that clinicians measure the outcomes of therapy and the clinic keeps accurate statistics. Records need to be kept of how many patients were seen per clinic, the number of new patients versus follow-up patients, how many failed to attend and the referral source. It is also useful to record the diagnosis and management for each patient, together with the number of clinic and therapy visits before discharge. The patient's age, sex and occupation may also be useful for research purposes.

It is up to each member of the voice clinic team to take their own measures of the patient's voice pre- and post-therapy. Usually, one good tape recording will be made at the beginning, at certain points during treatment (for example, before and after surgery, or after certain aims have been achieved, and at the end of the treatment period). The speech therapist may wish to carry out EGG, airflow measures or spectrography, while the singing teacher may decide to record the patient singing and carry out a phonetogram, depending on the technology available to the clinic. The clinic osteopath may have an assessment sheet grading muscle tone levels across a number of scalar degrees.

Questionnaires of patient satisfaction with the service they received in the voice clinic, together with their rating of their original problem and the final result, are also helpful (Harris et al., 1986). Recent work carried out by Enderby (1997) and Carding (2000) suggests that a valid way to measure outcome for the speech, language and voice impaired population is to rate the impairment (i.e. the severity of the hoarseness); the disability (how much the hoarseness prevents the patient from communicating effectively); the amount of handicap this creates (how much impact the hoarseness has on the patient's work and social activities) and the patient's own rating of the degree of distress the problem is causing. This seems a valid way of measuring the more subtle effects of voice therapy, such as psychological or attitude change, and the use of compensatory communication techniques.

Finally, it is important that one of the team collates the outcome measures either on to a computer spreadsheet or on to a single sheet to be included in the patient's discharge report.

Voice clinic research

Between 1990 and 1992 research was undertaken at the Voice Clinic at Queen Mary's Hospital, Sidcup into the association between head, neck and shoulder girdle dysfunction and dysphonia. The project was funded by Guy's Hospital Primary Care and Development Fund with the aim of establishing:

1. whether manual therapy/osteopathic techniques provide an effective alternative to speech therapy for dysphonic patients;
2. whether speech therapy, manual therapy or a combination of both is most effective in resolving dysphonia;
3. the existence of specific patient characteristics that could be used to determine the therapy mode most likely to benefit individual patients.

Dysphonic patients identified at their voice clinic assessment as needing voice therapy were offered the opportunity to take part in the research. Patients requiring surgery prior to their voice therapy and patients whose dysphonia/aphonia was judged to be predominantly emotional in aetiology were excluded. Sixty patients agreed to take part in the study and were randomly allocated to one of two therapy conditions: a six-session course of speech therapy, carried out by one of the two voice clinic speech therapists, or a six session course of manual therapy carried out by the voice clinic osteopath.

At the end of the six sessions, the assessment procedure was repeated, following which the patients completed six sessions of the alternative treatment before a final re-assessment. At the end of the study 39 patients had completed six sessions of speech therapy, six sessions of osteopathy and had been assessed three times – prior to therapy, after the first therapy condition and after the alternative therapy condition. The analysis was based on the data provided by these patients and carried out at Nottingham University Psychology Department by Dr David Clarke and Ms Louise Maskill.

The following measures were used for the initial and re-assessments.

1. Videostrobolaryngoscopy to monitor the patient's pre-therapy vocal fold posture, symmetry and vocal health. The videos for each subject were then edited randomly by the speech therapist and rated blind by the voice clinic surgeon, using a protocol designed for the study. An independent surgeon experienced in voice work also rated 10% of the subjects, chosen at random, using the same protocol, to act as a reliability check.

2. A digital tape recording of the patient reading a phonetically balanced passage was analysed, using pitch extraction techniques, by Dr David Howard, Lecturer in Music Acoustics at York University.

3. Vocal Profile Analysis (Laver, 1980) was carried out by an independent speech therapist experienced with the technique from the DAT tape recordings of the reading passage. A random 10% of the subjects were re-rated by a second speech therapist experienced in the same technique to act as a reliability check.

4. A phonetogram was carried out by the clinic therapists in order to provide an assessment of the patient's pre-therapy vocal frequency and intensity ranges. The loudest and softest notes and the frequency ranges were used to represent changes produced in the therapy conditions, ensuring that the analysis could be presented in a simple way compatible with the other measures.

5. A five-point rating scale was completed by each patient in order to assess his or her perception of their own vocal pitch, volume, quality, comfort and stamina prior to the onset of the dysphonia and prior to therapy. In this way patients who reported themselves as always having hoarse or weak voices could be identified. The same scales were repeated after each therapy condition.

6. A series of 17 neck and laryngeal variables were palpated and rated for position/muscular tension by yes/no answers on 3–5 point scales (as appropriate) by the clinic ENT surgeon, osteopath and speech therapist. The three independent ratings were then averaged together for the statistical analysis. This also allowed for practitioner agreement to be monitored.

7. A photo profile was made of each patient standing against a grid with a complex arrangement of mirrors allowing simultaneous views of the patient's posture from above, front, behind and side. The grid measurements were recorded to monitor changes in the patient's physical posture with treatment.

Analysis of variance carried out on the data found over half of the variables measured show statistically significant differences between the pre- and post-therapy mean scores. Where statistically significant differences were found for the treatment sequence (in three cases), all instances favoured the sequence: osteopathy followed by speech therapy. Although the number of cases analysed is quite small and needs to be interpreted with caution, the data appear to lend support to the hypothesis that osteopathy does provide an effective form of treatment for dysphonic patients. This does not, however, provide sufficient evidence that either speech therapy or osteopathy is the preferred mode of treatment for dysphonics. If anything the data seem to suggest that both forms of treatment produce similar improvements in the symptoms and the possibility that they may work in different ways on the same variables needs further research.

This pilot study has broken some new ground and as a result, a new perspective on voice production is beginning to emerge, particularly in the way we regard the significance of vocal postures and the importance of the vocal tensioning mechanism (cricothyroid visor) (Harris and Lieberman, 1993; Harris et al., 1998). It will hopefully pave the way for further research into the efficacy of manual therapy/osteopathic techniques for the treatment of dysphonia and the development of new tools to provide accurate measurements of variables such as laryngeal position, height and visor opening, which are, at present, only possible to assess subjectively with palpation.

References

Abberton EA, Fourcin AJ (1984) Electrolaryngography. In Code C, Ball M (eds) Experimental Clinical Phonetics. London: Croom Helm.

Abberton EA et al. (1984) Speech perceptual and productive rehabilitation in electro-cochlear stimulation. Tenth Anniversary Conference on Cochlear Implants Proceedings. New York: Raven Press.

Abberton EA, Howard DM, Fourcin AJ (1989) Laryngographic assessment of normal voice; a tutorial. Clinical Linguistics and Phonetics 3(3): 281–96.

Abitbol J, deBrux J, Millot G, Masson M, Mimoun OL, Pau H, Abitbol B (1989) Does a hormonal voice cord cycle exist in women? Study of vocal premenstrual syndrome in voice performers by videostroboscopy, glottography and cytology on 38 women. Journal of Voice 2: 151–62.

Akerlund L, Gramming P, Sundberg J (1992) Phonetogram and averages of sound pressure levels and fundamental frequencies of speech in relation to phonetograms: comparison of non-organic dysphonia patients before and after therapy. Journal of Voice 6: 55–63.

Allan CM, Turner JW, Gadea-Ciria M (1966) Investigations into speech disturbances following stereotaxic surgery for Parkinsonism. British Journal of Speech Communication Disorders 1: 55–9.

Altman JS, Benninger MS (1997) The evaluation of unilateral vocal fold immobility: is chest X-ray enough? Journal of Voice 11: 364–7.

Andrews ML (1982) Frequency characteristics of voices of 470 Australian school children. Unpublished doctoral thesis: Indiana University, Bloomington, Indiana.

Andrews ML (1991) Voice Therapy for Children: The elementary school years. San Diego, CA: Singular Publishing Group.

Andrews ML (1994) Your Best Voice. Tucson, Arizona: Communication Skill Builders.

Andrews ML (1995) Manual of Voice Treatment: Pediatrics Through Geriatrics. San Diego, CA: Singular Publishing Group.

Andrews ML, Champley EH (1993) The Elicitation of Vocal Responses from Preschool Children. Language, Speech and Hearing Services in Schools July: 156–7.

Andrews ML, Madiera S (1977) The Assessment of Pitch Discrimination in Young Children. Journal of Speech & Hearing Disorders 42: 279–86.

Andrews ML, Schmidt CP (1997) Gender presentation: perceptual and acoustical analyses of voice. Journal of Voice 11: 307–13.

Andrews ML, Summers A (1991) Voice Therapy for Adolescents. San Diego, CA: Singular Publishing Group.

Andrews S, Warner J, Stewart R (1986) EMG biofeedback and relaxation in the treatment of hyperfunctional dysphonia. British Journal of Disorders of Communication. 21: 353–69.

Ardran G, Kinsbourne M, Rushworth G (1966) Dysphonia due to tremor. Journal of Neurology, Neurosurgery and Psychiatry 29: 219–23.

Argov Z, Mastaglia FL (1979) Drug therapy – disorders of neuromuscular transmission caused by drugs. New England Journal of Medicine 301(8): 409–13.

Aring C (1965) Supranuclear (pseudobulbar) palsy. Archives of International Medicine 115: 198–9.

Arnold GE (1961) Physiology and pathology of the cricothyroid muscle. Laryngoscope 71: 658–65.

Arnold GE (1962) Vocal nodules and polyps: laryngeal tissue reaction to habitual hyperkinetic dysphonia. Journal of Speech and Hearing Disorders. 27: 205–17.

Aronson AE (1971) Early motor unit disease masquerading as psychogenic breathy dysphonia: a clinical case presentation. Journal of Speech and Hearing Disorders 36: 116–24.

Aronson AE (1980) Clinical Voice Disorders: An Interdisciplinary Approach. New York: Thieme-Stratton.

Aronson AE (1985a) Adductor spastic dysphonia: abductor spastic dysphonia. In Aronson AE (ed.) Clinical Voice Disorders: An Interdisciplinary Approach 2nd edn. New York: Thieme-Stratton.

Aronson AE (1985b) Clinical Voice Disorders: An Interdisciplinary Approach 2nd edn. New York: Thieme-Stratton.

Aronson AE (1990) Clinical Voice Disorders: An Interdisciplinary Approach 3rd edn. New York: Thieme-Stratton.

Aronson AE, DeSanto L (1983) Adductor spastic dysphonia; three years after recurrent laryngeal nerve resection. Laryngoscope 36: 116–24.

Aronson AE, Hartman DE (1981) Adductor spastic dysphonia as a sign of essential (voice) tremor. Journal of Speech and Hearing Disorders 46: 52–8.

Aronson AE, Brown JR, Litin EM, Pearson JS (1968a) Spastic dysphonia I: voice, neurologic and psychiatric aspects. Journal of Speech and Hearing Disorders 33: 203–18.

Aronson AE, Brown JR, Litin EM, Pearson JS (1968b) Spastic dysphonia II: Comparison with essential (voice) tremor and other neurologic and psychogenic dysphonias. Journal of Speech and Hearing Disorders 33: 220–31.

Aronson AE, Ramig L, Winholtz W, Silber S (1992). Rapid voice tremor or 'flutter' in amyotrophic lateral sclerosis. Annals of Otology, Rhinology and Laryngology 101: 511–18.

Asbury A, McKhann G, McDonald W (1992) Diseases of the Nervous System. Clinical Neurobiology. Philadelphia, PA: WB Saunders.

Aten J (1983) Treatment of spastic dysarthria. In Perkins WH (ed.) Current Therapy of Communication Disorders: Dysarthria and Apraxia (pp. 69–78). New York: Thieme-Stratton.

Audelman JU, Hoel RL, Lassman FF (1970) The effect of L-dopa treatment on the speech of subjects with Parkinson's disease. Neurology 20(4): 410–11.

Austin SF, Titze IC (1997) The effects of subglottal resonance upon vocal fold vibration. Journal of Voice 11: 391–402.

Bagnall A (1995) 'Yell Well'. (Videocassette) North Adelaide, South Australia: AB Voice International.

Bakal DJ (1979) Psychology and Medicine. London: Tavistock.

Baken RJ (1987) Clinical Measurement of Speech and Voice. San Diego, CA: College Hill Press.

Baken RJ, Cavallo SA (1981) Pre-phonatory chest wall posturing. Folia Phoniatrica 33: 193–202.

Baker J (1997) Psychogenic dysphonia: peeling back the layers. Journal of Voice 12: 527–35.

Baker DC, Savetsky L (1966) Congenital partial atresia of the larynx. Laryngoscope 77.

Baker K, Ramig L, Freed C, Johnson A (1997) Preliminary voice and speech analysis following fetal dopamine transplants in 5 individuals with Parkinson disease. Journal of Speech and Hearing Research 40: 615–26.

Bamford KA, Caine ED, Kiddo KK et al. (1989) Clinical pathological correlation in Huntington's disease: a neuropsychological and computed tomography study. Neurology 39: 796–801.

Barchi R, Furman RE (1992) Pathophysiology of myotonia and periodic paralysis. In Ashbury AK, McKhan GM, McDonald WI (eds) Diseases of the Nervous System: Clinical Neurobiology 2nd edn (pp. 146–63). Philadelphia, PA: WB Saunders.

Barlow W (1973) The Alexander Technique. New York: Warner Books.

Barnes C (1992) Evaluating the efficiency of Botox in the treatment of spasmodic dysphonia. Metropolitan University of Manchester 1992. Unpublished BSc thesis.

Bassich CJ, Ludlow CL (1986) The use of perceptual methods by clinicians for assessing voice quality. Journal of Speech and Hearing Disorders 51: 133–41.

Bastian RW, Keidar AK, Verdolini-Marston K (1990) Simple vocal tasks for detecting vocal fold swelling. Journal of Voice 4: 172–83.

Bastian RW, Nagorsky MJ (1987) Laryngeal image biofeedback. Laryngoscope 97: 1346–9.

Beck K (1918) Uber Erfahrungen mit Stimmstoerungen bei Kriegsteilnehmen. Passow-Schaefer Beitrage. Annat Ohjres Usw 11: 130.

Beck AT (1970) Depression: causes and treatment. Philadelphia, PA: University of Pennsylvania Press.

Beery QC (1991) Psychosocial aspects of adolescent dysphonia: an approach to treatment. Language, Speech, and Hearing Services in Schools 22: 163–7.

Belisle GM, Morrison MD (1983) Anatomic correlation for muscle tension dysphonia. Journal of Otolaryngology 12: 319–21.

Benjamin H (1966) The Transsexual Phenomenon. Julian Press: New York.

Bennett S, Bishop S, Lumpkin S (1987) Phonatory characteristics associated with bilateral diffuse polypoid degeneration. Laryngoscope 97: 446–50.

Benninger MS, Schwimmer C (1995) Functional neurophysiology and vocal fold paralysis. In Rubin JS, Sataloff RT, Korovin GS, Gould WJ (eds) Diagnosis and Treatment of Voice Disorders (pp. 105-21). Tokyo: Igaku-Shoin.

Benninger MS, Crumley RL, Ford CN, Gould WJ, Hanson DG, Ossoff RH, Sataloff RT (1994a) Evaluation and treatment of the unilateral paralyzed vocal fold. Otolaryngology Head and Neck Surgery 111: 497–508.

Benninger MS, Gillen J, Thieme P, Jacobson B, Dragovich J (1994b) Factors associated with recurrence and voice quality following radiation therapy for T1 and T2 glottic carcinomas. Laryngoscope 104 (March): 294–8.

Berendes J (1938) Zur Enstehung und Behandlung der Dysphonia Spastica. Z Hals. Usw Heilk 44: 78–84.

Bernstein DA, Borkovec TD (1973) Progressive Relaxation Training: A manual for the helping professions. Illinois: Research Press.

Berry WR (1983) (ed.) Clinical Dysarthria. San Diego: College-Hill.

Bielamowicz S, Kreiman J, Gerratt B, Dauer M, Berke G (1996) Comparison of voice analysis systems for perturbation measurement. Journal of Speech & Hearing Research 39: 126–34.

Biever DM, Bless DM (1989) Vibratory characteristics of the vocal folds in young adult and geriatric women. Journal of Voice 3(2): 120–31.

Blair RG (1965) Vagitis Uterinus: Crying in Utero. Lancet 11: 1164–5.

Bless DM (1991) Measurement of Vocal Function. Otolaryngologic Clinics of North America 24: 1023–33.

Bless DM, Hirano M, Feder, R (1987) Videostroboscopic evaluation of the larynx. Ear, Nose and Throat Journal. 66: 289–96.

Blitzer A, Brin M (1991) Laryngeal Dystonia: a series with botulinum toxin therapy. Annals of Otology, Rhinology and Laryngology 100: 85–9.

Blitzer A, Brin M (1992) The dystonic larynx. Journal of Voice 6: 294–7.

Blitzer A, Lovelace RE, Brin MF, Fahn S, Fink ME (1985) Electromyographic findings in focal laryngeal dystonia (Spastic Dysphonia). Annals of Otology, Rhinology and Laryngology 94: 591–4.

Blitzer A, Brin MF, Fahn S, Lovelace RE (1988) Clinical and laboratory characteristics of laryngeal dystonia: a study of 110 cases. Laryngoscope 98: 636–40.

Blitzer A, Brin MF, Stewart C et al. (1992) Abductor laryngeal dystonia: a series treated with botulinum toxin. Laryngoscope 102: 163–7.

Bloch P (1965) Neuro-psychiatric aspects of spastic dysphonia. Folia Phoniatrica 17: 301–64.

Boliek CA, Hixon TJ, Watson PJ, Morgan WJ (1996) Vocalisation and breathing during the first year of life. Journal of Voice 10: 1–22.

Boliek CA, Hixon TJ, Watson PJ, Morgan WJ (1997) Vocalisation and breathing during the second and third years of life. Journal of Voice 11: 373–90.

Boltezar IH, Burger ZR, Zargi M (1997) Instability of voice in adolescence: pathologic condition or normal developmental variation? Journal of Paediatrics 130(2): 185–90.

Bonduelle M (1975) Amyotrophic lateral sclerosis. In Vinten PJ, Gruyn GW (eds) Handbook of Clinical Neurology (pp. 281–338). Amsterdam: North Holland.

Boone DR (1966) Modification of the voices of deaf children. Volta Review. 68: 686–92.

Boone DR (1971) The Voice and Voice Therapy. Englewood Cliffs, NJ: Prentice Hall.

Boone DR (1977) The Voice and Voice Therapy 2nd edn. Englewood Cliffs, NJ: Prentice-Hall.

Boone DR (1983) The Voice and Voice Therapy 3rd edn. Englewood Cliffs, NJ: Prentice Hall

Boone DR (1991) Is Your Voice telling on You? San Diego, CA: Singular Publishing Group.

Boone DR (1993) The Boone Voice Program for Children 2nd edn. Austin, TX: Pro-Ed.

Boone DR (1997) The three ages of voice: the singing/acting voice in the mature adult. Journal of Voice 11(2): 161–4.

Boone DR, McFarlane SC (1988) The Voice and Voice Therapy. Englewood Cliffs, NJ: Prentice Hall.

Boone DR, McFarlane SC (1993) A critical view of the yawn-sigh as a voice therapy technique. Journal of Voice 7: 75–80.

Boone DR, McFarlane SC (1994) The Voice and Voice Therapy 6th edn. Englewood Cliffs, NJ: Prentice Hall.

Bootle C, McGlashan J, Robinson F (1998) Larynx synchronised stroboscopy – a new tool for outcome measures in the voice clinic. International Journal of Language and Communication Disorders, 33 Suppl: 296–303.

Botnik LE, Rose CM, Goldberg I, Recht A (1984) The role of radiation therapy in the treatment of laryngeal cancer. Otolaryngologic Clinics of North America 17(1).

Bouchayer M, Cornut G (1992) Microsurgical treatment of benign vocal fold lesions: indications, technique, results. Folia Phoniatrica (Basel) 44: 155–84.

Bowler NW (1964) A fundamental frequency analysis of harsh vocal quality. Speech Monograph 31.

Boysson-Bardies BD, Halle P, Sagart L, Durand C (1989) A cross-linguistic investigation of vowel formants in babbling. Journal of Child Language 16: 1–8.

Boysson-Bardies BD, Vihman MM, Roug-Hellichius L, Durand C, Landberg I, Arao F (1992) Maternal evidence of infant selection from the target language: a cross-linguistic phonetic study. In Fergusson C, Menn L, Stoel-Gammon C (eds) Phonological Development: Models, Research, Implications. Parkton, MD: York Press.

Brackett IP (1971) Parameters of voice quality. In Travis LE (ed.) Handbook of Speech Pathology and Audiology. New York: Appleton-Century-Crofts.

Brin MF, Fahn S, Moskowitz et al. (1987) Localized injections of botulinum toxin for the treatment of focal dystonia and hemifacial spasm. Movement Disorders 2: 237–54.

Brin MF, Blitzer A, Fahn S, Gould W, Lovelace RE (1989) Adductor Laryngeal Dystonia (Spastic Dysphonia): Treatment with local injections of Botulinum Toxin (Botox). Movement Disorders 4(4): 287–96.

Brin MF, Fahn S, Blitzer A, Ramig L, Stewart C (1992) Movement disorders of the larynx. In Blitzer A, Brin MF, Sasaki CT, Harris K (eds) Neurologic Disorders of the Larynx (pp. 248–78). New York: Thieme Medical.

Brin MF, Blitzer A, Stewart C (1998) Laryngeal dystonia (spasmodic dysphonia): observations of 901 patients and treatment with Botulinum Toxin. In Dystonia 3: Advances in Neurology. Vol. 78. Philadelphia, PA: Lippincott-Raven.

Brodnitz FS (1958) Vocal rehabilitation in benign lesions of the vocal cords. Journal of Speech and Hearing Disorders. 23 112–17.

Brodnitz FS (1959) Vocal Rehabilitation 4th edn. Rochester, Minnesota: American Academy of Opthalmology and Otolaryngology.

Brodnitz FS (1965) Vocal Rehabilitation 5th edn. Rochester, Minnesota: American Academy of Opthalmology and Otolaryngology.

Brodnitz FS (1971) Hormones and the human voice. Bulletin of the New York Academy of Medicine 47:183–91

Brodnitz FS (1976) Spastic dysphonia. Annals of Otology, Rhinology and Laryngology 85: 210–14.

Brodnitz FS (1981) Psychological considerations in vocal rehabilitation. Journal of Speech and Hearing Disorders 46: 22–6.

Brookes G (1995) Treatment of spasmodic dysphonia. In Moore PA (ed.) Handbook of Botulinum Toxin. Oxford: Blackwell.

Brown JR, Simonson I (1963) Organic voice tremor. Neurology 13: 520–5.

Brown WS, Vinson BP, Crary MA (eds) (1996) Organic Voice Disorders: Assessment and Treatment. San Diego, CA: Singular Publishing Group.

Bryan-Smith P (1986) Transsexual voice therapy. Speech Therapy in Practice 2(3), 28–9.

Bunch MA (1982) Dynamics of the Singing Voice. Wien: Springer Verlag.

Butcher P (1995) Psychological processes in psychogenic voice disorder. European Journal of Disorders of Communication 30: 467–74.

Butcher P, Cavalli L (1998) Fran: understanding and treating psychogenic dysphonia from a cognitive-behavioural perspective. In Syder D (ed.) Wanting to Talk: Counselling case studies in communication disorders. London: Whurr.

Butcher P, Elias A (1995) Redefining the Hysterical Conversion Model of Psychogenic Voice Disorder. Voice and Laryngectomy Special Interest Group Study Day. 2 December. London: St Thomas's Hospital.

Butcher P, Elias A, Raven R, Yeatman J, Littlejohns D (1987) Psychogenic voice disorders unresponsive to speech therapy: pychological characteristics and cognitive-behaviour therapy. British Journal of Disorders of Communication 22: 81–92.

Butcher P, Elias A, Raven R (1993) Psychogenic Voice Disorders and Cognitive Behaviour Therapy. London: Whurr.

Butterworth B (1980) Language Production I. London: Academic Press.

Buzan T (1989) Use Your Memory (revised edn). London: BBC Books.

Calas M, Verhuist J, Lecoq M, Dalleas B, Seilhean M (1989) Vocal pathology of teachers. Revue de Laryngologie, 110, 397–406.

Calvert DR (1962) Deaf voice quality – a preliminary investigation. Volta Rev 62: 402–3.

Cann CI, Fried MP (1984) Determinants and Prognosis of Laryngeal Cancer. Otolaryngologic Clinics of North America 17(1).

Cannito M (1989) Vocal tract steadiness in spasmodic dysphonia. In Yorkston K, Beukelman D (eds) Recent Advances in Clinical Dysarthria. San Diego, CA: College Hill Press.

Cannito M (1991) Emotional considerations in spasmodic dysphonia: psychometric quantification. Journal of Commuication Disorders 24: 313–29.

Cannito M, Murry T, Woodson G (1994) Attitudes toward communication in adductor spasmodic dysphonia before and after treatment with botulinum toxin injection. Journal of Medical Speech-Language Pathology 2: 125–33.

Cannon WB (1932) The Wisdom of the Body. New York: Norton.

Cantu F (1997) Extent of Vocal Pathology in a Group of Military Training Instructors. Paper presented at ASMA, Boston, MA, November.

Carding PN (2000) Measuring the Effectiveness of Voice Therapy. London: Whurr.

Carding PN, Horsley IA (1992) An evaluation study of voice therapy in non-organic dysphonia. European Journal of Disorders of Communication 27: 137–58.

Carlson EI (1993) Accent method plus direct visual feedback of electroglottographic signals. In Stemple JC : Voice Therapy: Clinical Studies. St Louis, Baltimore, MD: Mosby Year Book.

Carlson EI (1995a) Electrolaryngography in the assessment and treatment of incomplete mutation (Puberphonia) in adults. European Journal of Disorders of Communication 30(2): 140–9.

Carlson EI (1995b) A study of voice quality in a group of irradiated laryngeal cancer patients, tumour stages T1 and T2. University of London: Unpublished PhD thesis.

Carpenter RJ III, McDonald TJ, Howard FM Jr (1979) The otolaryngologic presentation of mysathenia gravis. Laryngoscope 89(6): 922–8.

Carrow E, Rivera V, Mauldin M, Shamblin L (1974) Deviant speech characteristics in motor neuron disease. Archives of Otolaryngology 100: 212–18.

Casper JK, Colton RH, Brewer DW (1985) Selected therapy techniques and laryngeal physiological changes in patients with unilateral vocal fold immobility. In Van Lawrence M (ed.) Transcripts of the 14th Symposium: Care of the Professional Voice (pp.318-23). New York: The Voice Foundation.

Casper JK, Colton RH, Brewer DW, Woo P (1989) Investigation of selected voice therapy techniques. Paper presented at the 18th Symposium of the Voice Foundation, Care of the Professional Voice: New York.

Casper JK, Woo P, Colton RH, Brewer DW, Griffin B (1996) Therapy vs. surgical augmentation: Voice after vocal fold paralysis. Presented at Pacific Voice Conference San Francisco, CA.

Chaloner J (1991) Gender identity problems. In Gravell R, France J (eds) Speech and Communication Problems in Psychiatry: Therapy in Practice 22. London: Chapman & Hall.

Champley EH, Andrews ML (1993) The elicitation of vocal responses from preschool children. Language, Speech and Hearing Services in Schools 24: 121–8.

Chatani M, Matayoshi Y, Masaki N (1993) Radiation therapy for larynx carcinoma: long term results of stage I glottic carcinoma. Strahlenterapie und Onkologie 169(2): 102–6.

Chernobelsky S (1998) Effect of the menstrual cycle on laryngeal muscle tension of singers and non-singers. Logopedics, Phoniatrics, Vocology 23: 128–32.

Chevrie-Muller C, Arabia-Guiden C, Pfaundel M (1987) Can one recover from spasmodic dysphonia? British Journal of Disorderts of Communication 22(2): 117–28.

Child DR, Johnson TS (1991) Preventable and nonpreventable causes of voice disorders. Seminars in Speech and Language. 12: 1–13.

Clowry J (1996a) Letter to The Times 30/12/96.

Clowry J (1996b) Letter to Guardian, 31/12/96.

Cohen LG, Ludlow CL, Warden BS (1989) Blink reflex excitability recovery curves in patients with spasmodic dysphonia. Neurology 39: 527–77.

Coleman RD (1983) Acoustic correlates of speaker sex identification: implications for the transsexual voice. Journal of Sex Research 19: 193–295.

Collins M, Rosenbek J, Donahue E (1982) The effects of posture on speech in ataxic dysarthria. Journal of the American Speech and Hearing Association 24: 767.

Colton RH, Casper J (1990) Understanding Voice Problems. Baltimore, MD: Williams & Wilkins.

Colton RH, Casper JK (1996) Understanding Voice Problems: A Physiological Perspective for Diagnosis and Treatment 2nd edn. Baltimore, MD: Williams & Wilkins.

Colton RH, Woo P, Casper JK, Brewer DW (1992) An objective comparison of treatment alternatives for vocal fold paralysis. Presented at the ASHA annual meeting.

Colton RH, Casper JK, Kelley RT, Friedberg B, Brewer DW (1998) Stroboscopic Signs of Unilateral Vocal Fold Immobility. Paper presented at 27th Symposium: Care of the Professional Voice. Philadelphia, PA.

Cooper M (1973) Modern Techniques of Vocal Rehabilitation 2nd edn. Springfield, Illinois: Charles C Thomas.

Cooper M (1984) Change Your Voice, Change Your Life. New York, NY: Macmillan.

Cooper M, Cooper MH (eds) (1977) Modern Techniques of Vocal Rehabilitation. Springfield, IL: Charles C. Thomas.

Cooper CL, Cooper RD, Eaker LH (1988) Living with Stress. London: Penguin.

Countryman S, Ramig L (1993) Effects of intensive voice therapy on speech deficits associated with bilateral thalamotomy in Parkinson disease: a case study. Journal of Medical Speech-Language Pathology 1: 233–50.

Cragle SP, Brandenburg JH (1993) Laser cordectomy or radiotherapy; cure rates, communication and cost. Otolaryngology Head and Neck Surgery 108(6): 648–54.

Crary MA, Kotzur IM, Gauger J, Gorham M, Burton S (1996) Dynamic Magnetic Resonance Imaging in the Study of Vocal Tract Configuration Journal of Voice 10(4): 376–88.

Critchley M (1939) Spastic Dysphonia (Inspiratory Speech). Brain 62: 95–103.

Crown S, Crisp A (1966) A short clinical diagnostic self-rating for psychoneurotic patients. Br J Psychiatry 112: 917–23.

Crumley RL (1990) Repair of the recurrent laryngeal nerve. Otolaryngologic Clinics of North America 23: 553–63.

Crumley RL (1991) Muscle transfer for laryngeal paralysis. Restoration of inspiratory vocal cord abduction by phrenic-omohyoid transfer. Archives of Otolaryngology 117: 1113–17.

Crystal D (1981) Clinical Linguistics New York: Springer-Verlag.

Crystal D (1987) The Cambridge Encyclopedia of Language Cambridge: Cambridge University Press.

Dalton P (1994) Counselling People with Communication Problems. London: Sage.

Dalton P, Hardcastle WJ (1977) Disorders of Fluency and their Effects on Communication. London: Edward Arnold.

Damasio AR (1994) Descartes' Error: Emotion, Reason and the Human Brain. London: Papermac.

Damste PH (1967) Voice change in adult women caused by virilising agents. Journal of Speech and Hearing Disorders 32(2).

Damste PH (1983) Diagnostic behaviour patterns with communicative abilities. In Bless DM, Abbs JH (eds) Vocal Fold Physiology. San Diego, CA: College Hill Press.

Damste PH (1987) Disorder of voice. In Stell J (ed.) Otolaryngology, Vol. 5. London: Butterworths.

Daniloff R, Schuckers G, Feth L (1980) The Physiology of Speech and Hearing, Englewood Cliffs, NJ: Prentice Hall.

Darley FL, Aronson AE, Brown JR (1969a) Clusters of deviant speech dimensions in the dysarthrias. Journal of Speech and Hearing Research 12: 462-96.

Darley FL, Aronson AE, Brown JR (1969b) Differential diagnostic patterns of dysarthria. Journal of Speech and Hearing Research 12: 246–69.

Darley FL, Brown JR, Goldstein N (1972) Dysarthria in multiple sclerosis. Journal of Speech and Hearing Research 15: 229–45.

Darley FL, Aronson AE, Brown JR (1975) Motor Speech Disorders. Philadelphia, PA: WB Saunders.

De Langen (1996) A Case of Spasmodic Dysphonia Restricted to Propositional Language Tasks. Paper presented at the Fifth Annual Conference of the

International Clinical Phonetics and Linguistics Association, Munich, 16–18 September 1996.

de Pinto O, Hollien H (1982) Speaking fundamental frequency characteristics of Australian women: then and now. Journal of Phonetics 10: 367–75.

Deal RE, Emanuel FW (1978) Some waveform and spectral features of vowel roughness. Journal of Speech and Hearing Research 21: 250–64.

DeCasper A, Spence M (1986) Prenatal maternal speech influences new-borns' perception of speech sounds. Infant Behaviour and Development 9: 133–50.

Dedo HH (1976) Recurrent laryngeal nerve section for spastic dysphonia. Annals of Otology, Rhinology and Laryngology 85: 875–80.

Dedo HH, Izdebski K (1983) Problems with surgical (RLN section) treatment of spasmodic dysphonia. Laryngoscope 93: 268–71.

Dedo HH, Urrea RD, Lawson L (1973) Intracordal injection of Teflon in the treatment of 135 patients with dysphonia. Ann Otolaryng 82: 661–6.

deGaudemar I, Roudaire M, Francois M, Marcy P (1996) Outcome of laryngeal paralysis in neonates: a long-term retrospective study of 113 cases. Internat J Ped Otorhinolaryngol 34: 101–10.

Dejonckere PH, Obbens C, Demoor GM, Wieneke GH (1993) Perceptual evaluation of dysphonia: reliability and relevance. Folia Phoniatrica 45: 76–83.

Delack JB (1976) Aspects of infant speech development in the first year of life. Canadian Journal of Linguistics 21.

Dennis DP and Kashima H (1989) Carbon dioxide laser posterior-cordectomy for treatment of bilateral vocal cord paralysis. Annals of Otology, Rhinology and Laryngology 98: 930.

Descartes R (1664) Traite de l'homme. Paris.

Deuster CV (1977) Irreveresible Stimmestrung in der Schwangerschaft. HNO 25: 430–2.

DiClemente CC, Prochaska JO, Fairhurst SK, Velicer WF, Valsquez MM, Rossi JS (1991) The process of smoking cessation: an analysis or precontemplation, contemplation and preparation stages of change. Journal of Consulting and Clinical Psychology 59: 295–304.

Dikkers FG, Hulsteart CE, Oosterbaan JA, Cervera-Paz FJ (1993) Ultrastructural changes of the basement membrane zone in benign lesions of the vocal folds. Acta Otolaryngologica (Stockholm) 113: 98–101.

D'Odorico L (1984) Nonsegmental features in prelinguistic communication: an analysis of some types of infant cry and noncry vocalisations. Journal of Child Language 11: 17–27.

Donnelly P, Kellow B (1989) An experience in setting up a joint voice clinic. Voice Research Society Newsletter, March:18–21.

Draper MH, Ladefoged P, Whitteridge D (1960) Expiratory pressures and air flow during speech. British Medical Journal, 18: 1837–43.

Dromey C, Ramig LO, Johnson AB (1995) Phonatory and articulatory changes associated with increased vocal intensity in Parkinson disease: a case study. Journal of Speech and Hearing Research 38: 751–64.

Duffy J (1995) Motor Speech Disorders. St Louis, MO: Mosby.

Dworkin J, Hartman D (1979) Progressive speech deterioration and dysphagia in patients with amyotrophic lateral sclerosis: a case report. Archives of Physical Medicine & Rehabilitation 60: 423–5.

Dworkin JP, Melecca RJ (1997) Vocal Pathologies: Diagnosis, Treatment, and Case Studies. San Diego, CA: Singular Publishing Group.

Eckel F, Boone DK (1981) The s/z ratio as an indicator of laryngeal pathology. Journal of Speech and Hearing Disorders 46: 147–9.

Eimas PD, Siqueland ER, Jusczuk P, Vigorito J (1971) Speech perception in infants. Science 171: 303–6.

Elble RJ, Koller WC (1990) Tremor. Baltimore, MD: John Hopkins University Press.

Elston JS (1988) The clinical use of Botulinum Toxin. Seminars in Ophthalmology 3 (4): 249–60.

Enderby P (1992) Outcome measures in speech therapy: impairment, disability, handicap and distress. Health Trends 24: 2–7.

Enderby P (1997) Therapy Outcome Measures in Speech and Language Therapy: Technical Manual. San Diego, CA: Singular Publishing Group.

Enderby P, Emerson P (1995) Does Speech and Language Therapy Work? A Review of the Literature. London: Whurr.

Engel GL (1977) The need for a new medical model: a challenge for biomedicine. Science 196: 129–35.

Epstein R (1996) Anxiety associated with botulinum toxin injections. Journal of Logopedics, Phonology and Vocology 21: 131–6.

Epstein R (1997) The short term impact of botulinum toxin injections on speech variables in adductor spasmodic dysphonia. Journal of Disability and Rehabilitation 19(21): 20–5.

Erikson E (1963) Childhood and Society. New York: Norton.

Eskenazi L, Childers DG, Hicks DM (1990) Acoustic correlates of vocal quality. Journal of Speech and Hearing Research 33: 298–306.

Estill J (1988) Belting and classic voice quality: some physiological differences. Medical Problems of Performing Artists. 3:37–43.

Estill J (1997) Compulsory Figures for Voice: A User's Guide to Voice Quality. Santa Rosa, CA: Estill Voice Training Systems.

Estill J, Yanigisawa E (1991) Laryngeal constriction and its retraction. (Videocassette)

Faaborg-Anderson K (1957) Electromyographic investigation of intrinsic laryngeal muscles in humans. Acta Physiologica Scandinavica 41 (suppl.140): 1–148.

Fabre P (1957) Un procédé électrique percutane d'inscription de l'accolement glottique au cours de la phonation: glottographie de haute fréquence; premiers resultats. Bull. Acad.Nat. Med 141: 66–9.

Fahn S, Marsden C, DeLong M (eds) (1998) Dystonia 3: Advances in Neurology. Vol. 78. Philadelphia, PA: Lippincott-Raven.

Fairbanks G (1960) Voice and Articulation Drillbook. New York: Harper & Row.

Farmakides MN, Boone DR (1960) Speech problems of patients with multiple sclerosis. Journal of Speech and Hearing Disorders 25: 385–90.

Fawcus R (1980) The treatment of phonological disorders. In Jones FM (ed.) Language Disabilities in Children. Lancaster: MTP Press.

Fawcus R (1986) Persistant Puberphonia. In Fawcus M (ed.) Voice Disorders and their Management. London: Croom Helm.

Fawcus, R (1991) The physiology of phonation. In Fawcus M (ed.) Voice Disorders and their Management 2nd edn (Ch. 1). London: Croom Helm.

Feldman M, Nixon JY, Finitzo-Hieber T, Freeman FJ (1984) Abnormal parasympathetic vagal function in patients with spasmodic dysphonia. Ann Inter Med 100: 491–5.

Ferrand CT, Bloom RL (1996) Gender differences in children's intonational patterns. Journal of Voice 10: 284–91.

Fex B, Fex S, Shiromoto O, Hirano M (1994) Acoustic analysis of functional dysphonia before and after voice therapy (Accent Method). Journal of Voice 7: 163–7.

Fex B, Henriksson B (1969) Phoniatric treatment combined with radiotherapy of laryngeal cancer for the avoidance of radiation damage. Acta Otolaryngologica Supplement 263.

Fifer W, Moon C (1989) Early Voice Discrimination. In Von Euler C, Forssberg H, Lagercrantz H (eds) The Neurobiology of Early Infant Behavior. New York: Stockton Press.

Filter MD (1980) Proprioceptive-tactile-kinaesthetic approach to voice disorders. Proceedings of the 19th Congress, International Association of Logopaedics and Phoniatrics. August 1983, Edinburgh.

Findley LJ, Gresty M (1988) Head, facial and voice tremor. Advances in Neurology 49: 239–53.

Finitzo T, Freeman F (1989) Spasmodic dysphonia, whither and where: results of seven years of research. Journal of Speech and Hearing Research 32: 541–55.

Fink BR, Demarest RJ (1978) Laryngeal Mechanics. Cambridge, MA: Harvard University Press.

Fitch JL, Holbrook A (1970) Modal vocal fundamental frequency of young adults. Archives of Otolaryngology 92: 379–82.

Flach M, Schwickardi H, Simen R (1968) Welchen Einfluss haben Menstruation und Schwangerschaft auf die ausgebildete Gesangsstimme? Folia Phoniatrica 21: 199–210.

Flanders WD, Rothman KJ (1982) Interaction of alcohol and tobacco in laryngeal cancer. American Journal of Epidemiology 115: 371–9.

Flint PW, Cummings CW (1998) Phonosurgical Procedures. In Cummings CW et al. (eds) Otolaryngology Head and Neck Surgery 3rd edn. New York: Mosby.

Flynn P, Andrews ML (1990) Using Your Voice Wisely and Well. Tucson, AZ: Communication Skill Builders.

Ford CN (1998) Laryngeal EMG in clinical neurolaryngology. Arch Otolaryngol Head and Neck Surg 124: 476–7.

Ford CN, Bless DM, Lowery JD (1990) Indirect laryngoscopic approach for injection of botulinum toxin in spasmodic dysphonia. Otolaryngology Head and Neck Surgery 103(5): 752–8.

Ford CN, Bless DM, Loftus JM (1992a) Role of injectable collagen in the treatment of glottic insufficiency: a study of 119 patients. Annals of Otology, Rhinology and Laryngology 101: 237–47.

Ford CN, Bless DM, Prehn RB (1992b) Thyroplasty as primary and adjunctive treatment of glottic insufficiency. Journal of Voice 6: 277–85.

Fourcin AJ (1974) Laryngographic examination of vocal fold vibration. In Wyke B (ed.) Ventilatory and Phonatory Control Mechanisms. London: Oxford University Press.

Fourcin AJ (1981) Laryngographic assessment of phonatory function. In Ludlow CL, Hart MO (eds) Proceedings of the Conference of the Assessment of Vocal Pathology, Maryland.

Fourcin AJ (1989) An aspect of voice quality in speech pathology. Speech Hearing and Language – work in progress. University College London, 3: 255.

Fourcin AJ, Abberton EA (1971) First applications of a new laryngograph. Medicine and Biology 21: 172–82.

Freed C, Breeze R, Rosenberg N, Schneck S, Kriek E, Qi J, Lone T, Zhang Y, Snyder J, Wells T, Ramig L, Thompson L, Mazziotta J, Juang S, Grafton S, Brooks D, Sawle G, Schroter G, Ansari A (1993) Survival of implanted fetal dopamine cells and neurologic improvement 12 to 46 months after transplantation for Parkinson's disease. The New England Journal of Medicine 327: 1549–55.

Freeman FJ, Schaefer SD (1988) Voice Disorders: Diagnosis and treatment. Eleventh Symposium. Care of the Professional Voice. Part Two. 78-88. The Voice Foundation

Freeman F, Ushijama T (1978) Laryngeal muscle activity during stuttering. Journal of Speech Hearing Research 21: 538–62.

Freeman F, Cannitto M, Finitzo-Heiber T (1984) Classification of spasmodic dysphonia by perceptual acoustic visual means. In Gates G (ed.) The Care of the Professional Voice. New York Voice Foundation, pp. 44.

Freeman FJ, Schaefer S, Cannito MP, Finitzo T (1987) Episodic reactive dysphonia: A case study. Journal of Communication Disorders. 20: 259-63.

Freud S (1905) Fragment of an Analysis of a Case of Hysteria. Standard Edition Vol. 7 (pp. 1-122). London: Hogarth Press.

Friedl W, Friedrich G, Eggar J, Fitzek I (1993) Psychogenic aspects of functional dysphonia. Folia Phoniatrica 45: 10–13.

Fritzell B (1996) Voice disorders and occupations. Logopedics, Phoniatrics, Vocology. 21: 7–12.

Fritzell B, Fuer E, Haglund S, Knutsson E, Schiratzki H (1982) Experiences with Recurrent Laryngeal Nerve Section for Spastic Dysphonia. Folio Phoniatrica 34: 1220–5.

Froeschels E (1952) Chewing method as therapy: a discussion with some philosophical conclusions. Archives of Otolaryngology, 56: 427–34.

Froeschels E, Kastein S, Weiss DA (1955) A method of therapy for paralytic conditions of the mechanisms of phonation, respiration, and glutination. Journal of Speech and Hearing Disorders 20: 365–70.

Fu KK, Woodhouse RJ, Quivey JM, Philips TL, Dedo HH (1982) The significance of laryngeal oedema following radiotherapy of carcinoma of the vocal cord. Cancer 15: 655–8.

Gandour J, Petty SH, Dardarananda R (1989) Tonal disruption in the speech of a language-delayed Thai adult. Clinical Linguistics and Phonetics 3(2): 191–202.

Garcia M (1855) Physiological observations on the human voice. Proceedings of the Royal Society, London 7: 399.

Garfield Davies D, Dhillon RS, Epstein R (1989) Treatment of spastic dysphonia using botulinum toxin. Paper presented at the 18th annual symposium: Care of the Professional Voice, June 1989, Philadelphia.

Garfinkle TJ, Kimmelman CP (1982) Neurologic disorders: Amyotrophic lateral sclerosis, myasthenia gravis, multiple sclerosis, poliomyelitis. American Journal of Otolaryngology 3: 204–12.

Gelfer MP, Andrews ML, Schmidt CP (1991) Effects of prolonged loud reading on selected measures of vocal function in trained and untrained singers. Journal of Voice 5:158–67.

Gereau SA, LeBlanc EM, Rubin RJ (1995) Congenital anomalies of the larynx. In Rubin RJ, Sataloff RT, Korovin GS, Gould, WJ (eds) Diagnosis and Treatment of Voice Disorders. Tokyo: Igaku-Shoin.

Gerratt BR, Kreiman J, Antonanzas-Barroso N, Berke GS (1993) Comparing internal and external standards in voice quality judgements. Journal of Speech and Hearing Research 36: 14–20.

Gerritsen GJ, Snow GB (1991) The patterns of growth and spread of laryngeal cancer. Chapter 2 in Castelijns JA, Snow GB, Valk J (eds) MR Imaging of Laryngeal Cancer. The Netherlands: Kluver Academic.

Gerritsima EJ (1991) An investigation into some personality characteristics of patients with psychogenic aphonia and dysphonia. Folia Phoniatrica 43: 13–20.

Gilbert H, Campbell M (1980) Speaking fundamental frequency in three groups of hearing impaired individuals. Journal of Communication Disorders 13: 195–205.

Gilmore SI, Guidera AM, Hutchins SI, van Steenbrugge W (1992) Intrasubject variability and the effect of speech task on vocal fundamental frequency of young Australian males and females. Australian Journal of Human Communication Disorders 20: 65–73.

Ginsberg VI, Wallach JJ, Svain JJ, Biller JF (1988) Defining the psychiatric role in spastic dysphonia. General Hospital Psychiatry 10: 132–7.

Glass L (1992) He Says, She Says. London: Piatkus.

Goetzinger C (1966) Study of Rorschach with deaf and hearing adolescents. Am Ann Deaf 3.

Goldberg DP, Williams P (1988). A User's Guide to the General Health Questionnaire. Windsor: NFER-Nelson.

Goldman SL, Hargrave J, Hillman RE, Holmberg E, Gress C (1996) Stress, anxiety, somatic complaints, and voice use in women with vocal nodules: Preliminary findings. American Journal of Speech-Language Pathology 5: 44–54.

Golper L, Nutt JG, Rau MT, Coleman RO (1983) Focal cranial dystonia. Journal of Speech and Hearing Disorders 48: 128-134.

Gordon M (1986) Assessment of the dysphonic patient. In Fawcus M (ed.) Voice Disorders and their Management. London: Croom Helm.

Gordon M, Lockhart M (1995) Efficacy for speech and language therapy for dysphonia. In Caring to Communicate: Proceedings of the Golden Jubilee Conference of the Royal College of Speech and Language Therapists, York, October 1995.

Gould W, Korovin S (1994) Laboratory advances for voice measurement. Journal of Voice 8 : 8–17.

Gowers WR (1893) A Manual of Diseases of the Nervous System 2nd edn. London: Churchill.

Gramming P (1988) The phonetogram: an experimental and clinical study. Academic dissertation. Malmo: University of Lund, Department of Otolaryngology.

Gramming P, Akerlund L (1988) Non-organic dysphonia. II. Phonetograms for normal and pathological voices. Acta Otolaryngolica (Stockholm) 106(5–6), Nov.–Dec.: 468–76.

Gramming P, Sundberg J, Ternstrom S (1988) Relationship between changes in voice pitch and loudness. Journal of Voice 6: 224–34.

Gravell R, France J (1991) Mental Disorders and Speech Therapy: an introduction. In Gravell R, France J (eds) Speech and Communication Problems in Psychiatry. London: Chapman & Hall.

Gray SD (1991) Basement membrane zone injury in vocal nodules. In Gauffin J, Hammarberg B (eds) Vocal Fold Physiology: Acoustic, perceptual and physiological aspects of voice mechanisms. San Diego: Singular Publishing Group: 21–8.

Gray SD, Titze I (1988) Histologic investigation of hyperphonated canine vocal cords. Annals of Otology, Rhinology and Laryngology 97: 381–8.

Gray SD, Barkmeier J, Jones D, Titze IR, Druker BS (1992) Vocal evaluation of thyroplastic surgery in the treatment of unilateral vocal fold paralysis. Laryngoscope 102: 415–22.

Gray SD, Hirano M, Sato K (1993) Molecular and cellular structure of vocal fold tissue. In Titze IR (ed.) Vocal Fold Physiology: Frontiers in basic science. San Diego, CA: Singular Publishing Group.

Green G (1988) Personal communication.

Green G (1989) Psycho-behavioural characteristics of children with vocal nodules: WPBIC ratings. Journal of Speech and Hearing Disorders 54: 306–12.

Greene MCL (1957) The Voice and Its Disorders. Edinburgh: Churchill Livingstone.

Greene MCL (1961) Problems involved in the speech and language training of the partially deaf child. Speech Pathology and Therapy 4: 22.

Greene MCL (1964) The Voice and Its Disorders 2nd edn. Edinburgh: Churchill Livingstone.

Greene MCL (1972) The Voice and Its Disorders 3rd edn. London: Pitman Medical.

Greene MCL (1980) The Voice and Its Disorders 4th edn. London: Pitman.

Greene MCL, Mathieson L (1989) The Voice and its Disorders. 5th edn. London: Whurr.

Grob D (1981) Myasthenia gravis – retrospect and prospect. Annals of the New York Academy of Sciences 377: xiii–xvi.

Grob D, Brunner NG, Namba T (1981) The natural course of myasthenia gravis and effect of therapeutic measures. Annals of the New York Academy of Sciences: 377: 652–69.

Groves J, Gray RF (1985) A Synopsis of Otolaryngology 4th edn. Bristol: Wright.

Guenel P, Chastang JF, Luce D, Leclerc A, Bougere J (1988) A study of the interaction of alcohol drinking and tobacco smoking among French cases of laryngeal cancer. Journal of Epidemiology and Community Health 42: 350–54.

Gutzmann H. Sr. (1897) Ein Beitrag zur Frage der Eunuchenaehnlichen Stimme. Med. Padagog. Monatsschr 33.

Haerer AF, Anderson DW, Schoenberg BS (1982) Prevalence of essential tremor: Results from the Coplah County Study. Archives of Neurology 39(12): 750–1.

Hagg U, Tarranger J (1980) Menarche and voice change as indications of the pubertal growth spurt. Acta Odontal Scan 38: 179–86.

Hallberg L, Carlsson S (1993) A Qualitative Study of Situations: turning a hearing disability into a handicap. Disability Handicap and Society 8(1): 71–86.

Hallet J (1995) Is dystonia a sensory disorder? Ann Neurol 38: 139–40.

Hammarberg B (1987) Pitch and quality characteristics of mutational voice disorders before and after therapy. Folia Phoniatrica 39: 204–16.

Hammarberg B, Fritzell B, Gauffin J, Sundberg J (1986) Acoustic and perceptual analysis of vocal dysfunction. Journal of Phonetics 14: 72–82.

Hammond TH, Zhou RX, Hammond EH, Pawlak A, Gray SD (1997) The intermediate layer: a morphological study of the elastin and hyaluronic acid constituents of normal human vocal folds. Journal of Voice 11(1) 59–66.

Hanson DG, Ludlow CL, Bassich CJ (1983) Vocal fold paresis in Shy-Drager syndrome. Annals of Otology, Rhinology and Laryngology 92: 85–90.

Hanson DG, Gerratt BR, Ward PH (1984) Cinegraphic observations of laryngeal function in Parkinson's disease. Laryngoscope 94: 348–53.

Hardcastle WJ (1976) Physiology of Speech Production. London: Academic Press.

Harding AE (1983) Classification of the hereditary ataxias and paraplegias. Lancet 1: 8334: 1151–5.

Harding AE (1984). The hereditary ataxias and related disorders. Edinburgh: Churchill Livingstone.

Harris TM (1992) The pharmacological treatment of voice disorders. Main report to World Congress XXII of IALP, Folia Phoniatrica 44(3–4): 143–54.

Harris S (1998) Speech therapy for dysphonia. In Harris TM, Harris SRC, Rubin JS, Howard DM (eds) The Voice Clinic Handbook. London: Whurr.

Harris TM, Lieberman J (1993) The crico-thyroid mechanism, its relation to vocal fatigue and vocal dysfunction. Voice 2: 89–96.

Harris TM, Collins SRC, Clarke DD (1986) The Oxford voice clinic: preliminary research results. In Harris TM, Collins SRC, Clarke DD (eds) Developments in Voice Conservation. London: Bruel & Kjaer.

Harris TM, Harris SRC, Lieberman J (1992) The association between head, neck and shoulder girdle dysfunction and dysphonia. Final report for the Primary Care Development Fund, Guy's Hospital.

Harris TM, Harris SRC, Rubin JS, Howard DM (1998) The Voice Clinic Handbook. London: Whurr.

Hartman DE (1984) Neurogenic Dysphonia. Annals of Otology, Rhinology and Laryngology 93: 57–64.

Hartman DE, Aronson AE (1981) Clinical investigations of intermittent breathy dysphonia. Journal of Speech and Hearing Disorders 46: 428–32.

Hartman E, von Cramon D (1984) Acoustic measurement of voice quality in central dysphonia. Journal of Communication Disorders 15: 21–9.

Harvey GL (1996) Treatment of Voice Disorders in Medically Complex Children. Language, Speech and Hearing Services in Schools 27: 282–91.

Harvey PL (1997) The three ages of man: the young adult patient. Journal of Voice 11 (2): 144–52.

Haynes WO, Pindzola RH (1998) Laryngeal Voice Disorders. In Haynes WO, Pindzola RH (eds) Diagnosis and Evaluation in Speech Pathology 5th edn. Boston, MA: Allyn & Bacon.

Heaver L (1958) Psychiatric observations on the personality structure of patients with habitual dysphonia. Logos. 1: 21–6.

Heaver L (1959) Spastic Dysphonia: Psychiatric considerations. Logos 2: 15–24.

Heck AF (1964) A study of neural and extra-neural findings in a large family with Friedreich's ataxia. Journal of the Neurological Sciences 1: 226–55.

Hecker MHL, Kreul EJ (1971) Descriptions of the speech of patients with cancer of the vocal folds. Part 1: Measures of fundamental frequency. Journal of the Acoustical Society of America 49: 1275–82.

Heidel SE, Torgerson JK (1993) Vocal problems among aerobic instructors and aerobic participants. Journal of Communication Disorders 26(3), September, 179–91.

Herrington-Hall BL, Lee L, Stemple JC, Niemi KR, McHone MM (1988) Description of laryngeal pathologies by age, sex, and occupation in a treatment-seeking sample. Journal of Speech and Hearing Disorders 53: 57–64.

Heuer RJ, Sataloff RT, Emerick K, Rulnick R, Baroody M, Spiegel JR, Durson G, Butler J (1997) The importance of preoperative voice therapy. Journal of Voice 11: 88–94.

Hicks DM, Bless DM (1996) Principles of treatment. In Brown WS, Vinson BP, Crary MA (eds) Organic Voice Disorders. Assessment and Treatment. San Diego, CA: Singular Publishing Group.

Hillman RE, Holmberg EB, Perkell JS, Walsh M, Vaughan C (1989) Objective assessment of vocal hyperfunction: an experimental framework and initial results. Journal of Speech and Hearing Research. 32: 373–92.

Hillman RE, DeLassus Gress C, Hargrave J, Walsh M, Bunting G (1990) The efficacy of speech-language pathology intervention: Voice disorders. Seminars in Speech and Language 11: 297–309.

Hirano M (1975) Phonosurgery: basic and clinical investigations. Otologia (Fukuoka) 21: 239–40.

Hirano M (1977) Structure and vibratory behaviour of the vocal folds. In Sawashima M, Cooper F (ed.) Dynamic Aspects of Speech Production. Tokyo: University of Tokyo Press.

Hirano M (1981) Clinical Examination of Voice. Wien: Springer-Verlag.

Hirano M (1982) The role of the layer structure of the vocal fold in register control. In Hurme P (ed.) Vox Humana. Jyvaeskylae: University of Jyvaeskylae.

Hirano M (1989) Objective Evaluation of the Human Voice: clinical aspects. Folia Phoniatrica 41(92–3): 89–144.

Hirano M, Bless DM (1993) Videostroboscopic examination of the larynx. San Diego, CA: Singular Publishing Group.

Hirano M, Ohala J (1967) Use of hooked wire electrodes for electromyography of the intrinsic laryngeal muscles. Working Papers in Phonetics UCLA, 7: 35–45.

Hirano M, Koike Y, von Leden H (1968) Maximum phonation time and air usage during phonation: clinical study. Folia Phoniatrica. 20: 185–201.

Hirano M, Vennard W, Ohala J (1970) Regulation of register, pitch and intensity of voice – an electromyographic investigation of intrinsic laryngeal muscles. Folia Phoniatrica 22: 1–20.

Hirano M, Nozoel, Shin T, Maeyama T (1974) Electromyographic findings in recurrent laryngeal nerve paralysis. Pract. Otol Kyoto 67: 231–42.

Hirano M, Matsuo K, Kakita Y, Kawasaki H, Kurita S (1983) Vibratory behaviour versus the structure of the vocal fold. In Titze IR, Scherer RC (eds) Vocal Fold Physiology: Biomechanics, acoustics and phonatory control. Denver, CO: Denver Center for the Performing Arts.

Hirano M, Kiyokawa K, Kurita S (1988) Laryngeal muscles and glottic shaping. In Fujimura O (ed.) Vocal Fold Physiology Vol. 2. New York: Raven Press.

Hiraoka N , Kitazoe Y, Ueta H, Tanaka S, Tanabe M (1984) Harmonic intensity analysis of normal and hoarse voices. Journal of the Acoustical Society of America 76: 1648–51.

Hirose H (1971) Electromyography of the articulatory muscles: current instrumentation and technique. Status Report on Speech Research (Haskins Laboratory) 25126: 73–86.

Hiroto I, Hirano M, Toyozumi Y, Shin T (1962) A new method of placement of a needle electrode in the intrinsic laryngeal muscles for electromyography: insertion through the skin. Pract. Otol (Kyoto) S5: 499–504.

Hixon TJ, Weismer G (1995) Perspectives on the Edinburgh study of speech breathing. Journal of Speech and Hearing Research 38: 42–60.

Hixon TJ, Mead J, Goldman M (1976) Dynamics of the chest wall during speech production: function of the thorax, rib cage, diaphragm and abdomen. Journal of Speech and Hearing Research 19: 297–356.

Hoit JD (1995) Influence of body position on breathing and its implications for the evaluation and treatment of speech and voice disorders. Journal of Voice 9: 341–7.

Hollien H (1974) On vocal registers. Journal of Phonetics 2: 125–43.

Hollien H (1983) In search of frequency control mechanisms. In Bless DM, Abbs JH (eds) Vocal Fold Physiology. San Diego, CA: College Hill Press.

Hollien H (1987) Old voices: what do we really know about them? Journal of Voice 1(1): 2–17.

Hollien H, Michel J, Doherty ET (1973) A method for analysing vocal jitter in sustained phonation. Journal of Phonetics 1: 85–91.

Hollien H, Paul P (1969) A second evaluation of the speaking fundamental frequency characteristics of post-adolescent girls. Language and Speech 12: 119–24.

Hollien H, Shipp T (1972) Speaking Fundamental Frequency and chronological age in males. Journal of Speech and Hearing Research 15: 155–69.

Hollien H, Jackson B (1973) Normative data on the speaking fundamental characteristics of young adult males. Journal of Phonetics 1: 117–20.

Holmes TH, Rahe RH (1967) The social readjustment rating scale. Journal of Psychosomatic Research 11: 213–18.

Horii Y (1975) Some statistical characteristics of voice fundamental frequency. Journal of Speech and Hearing Research 22: 5–19.

Horii Y (1979) Fundamental frequency perturbation observed in sustained phonation. Journal of Speech and Hearing Research 25: 12–14.

Horii Y (1980) Vocal shimmer in sustained phonation. Journal of Speech and Hearing Research 25: 202–9.

House AO, Andrews HB (1987) The psychological and social characteristics of patients with functional dysphonia. Journal of Psychosomatic Research 31: 483–90.

House AO, Andrews HB (1988) Life events and difficulties preceding the onset of functional dysphonia. Journal of Psychosomatic Research 32: 311–19.

Howard PM, Angus JA (1996) Acoustics and Psychoacoustics. Oxford: Focal Press.

Hoyt DJ, Lettinga JW, Leopold KA, Fisher SR (1992) The Effect of Head and Neck Radiation Therapy on Voice Quality. Laryngoscope 102(5): 477–80.

Hubble JP, Busenbark KL, Koller WC (1989) Essential tremor. Clinical Neuropharmacology 12(6): 453–82.

Hudgins CV (1934) A comparative study of the speech co-ordination of deaf and normal subjects. J Genet Psychol 44: 1–34.

Hudgins CV (1937) Voice production and breath control in the speech of the deaf. Am Ann Deaf 82: 338–63.

Hughes RG, Gibbin KP, Lowe J (1998) Vocal fold abductor paralysis as a solitary and fatal manifestation of multiple system atrophy. Journal of Laryngology and Otology 112: 177–8.

Husson R (1953) Theorie de la vibration des cordes vocales. C.R. Acad. Sci. (Paris) 236: 1697.

Husson R (1957) Comment vibrent nos cordes vocales. Nature, Dunod, Paris: 3262.

Husson R (1962) Physiologie de la Phonation. Paris: Masson.

Iacono RP, Lonser RR, Morenski JD (1994) Stereotactic surgery for Parkinson's disease. Movement Disorders 9: 470–3.

Ingrisano D, Weismer G, Shuckers GH (1980) Sex identification of preschool children's voices. Folia Phoniatrica 32: 61–9.

Inoue T, Inoue T, Chatani M, Teshima T (1992) Irradiated volume and arytenoid oedema after radiotherapy for T1 glottic carcinoma. Strahlentherapie-Onkologie 168(1): 23–6.

Ishizaka K (1981) Equivalent lumped-mass models of vocal fold vibration. In Stevens KN, Hirano M (eds) Vocal Fold Physiology. Tokyo: University of Tokyo Press.

Isselbacher KJ, Braunwald E, Wilson JD, Martin JB, Fauci AS, Kasper DL (eds) (1994) Harrison's Principles of Internal Medicine 13th edn. New York: McGraw-Hill.

Isshiki N, Okamura H, Tanabe M, Morimoto M (1969) Differential diagnosis of hoarseness. Folia Phoniatrica 21: 9–19.

Isshiki N, Okamura H, Ishikawa T (1975) Thyroplasty Type I (lateral compression) for dysphonia due to vocal cord paralysis or atrophy. Acta Otolaryngologica 80: 465–73.

Isshiki N, Tanabe M, Sawada M (1978) Arytenoid adduction for unilateral vocal cord paralysis. Archives of Otolaryngology 104: 555–7.

Izdebski K (1993) Adductor Spasmodic Dysphonia Symptomatology. Journal of Voice 6: 306–19.

Jacobson F (1938) Progressive Relaxation 2nd edn. Chicago: University of Chicago.

Jacobson E (1976) You Must Relax 5th edn. New York: McGraw-Hill.

Jacobson BH, Johnson A, Grywalski C, Silbergleit A, Jacobsen G, Benninger MS, Newman CW (1997) The Voice Handicap Index (VHI): Development and Validation. American Journal of Speech-Language Pathology 6: 66–9.

Jacome DE, Yanez GF (1980) Spastic dysphonia and Meige's Disease. Neurology 30: 349.

Jankovic J, Brin M (1991) Therapeutic uses of botulinum toxin. New England Journal of Medicine 324(17): 1186–94.

Joanette Y, Dudley JG (1980) Dysarthric symptomatology of Friedreich's ataxia. Brain and Language 10(10): 39–50.

Johnson TS (1985a) Vocal abuse reduction program. Philadelphia, PA: Taylor & Francis.

Johnson TS (1985b) Voice disorders: the measurement of clinical progress. In Costello J (ed.) Speech Disorders in Adults: recent advances. San Diego, CA: College Hill Press.

Jones C (1967) Deaf voice – a description derived from a survey of the literature. Volta Review 69(507–8): 39–40.

Jones LJ (1994) The Social Context of Health and Health Work. Basingstoke: Macmillan.

Judd GBM (1995) A comparison of vocal problems experienced by aerobics instructors and dance teachers. Unpublished Bsc (Hons) project: The Central School of Speech and Drama London.

Kahane J (1987) Connective tissue changes in the larynx and their effects on voice. Journal of Voice 1: 31–7.

Karim ABMF, Snow GB, Diek HTH, Hanjo KH (1983) The quality of voice in patients irradiated for laryngeal carcinoma. Cancer 51(1): 47–9.

Kashima HK (1991) Bilateral vocal fold motion impairment: pathophysiology and management by transverse cordotomy. Annals of Otology, Rhinology and Laryngology 100: 717.

Kent R (1976) Anatomical and neuromuscular maturation of the speech mechanism: evidence from acoustic studies. Journal of Speech and Hearing Research 19: 421–7.

Kent RD, Kent J, Rosenbek J (1987) Maximum performance tests of speech production. Journal of Speech and Hearing Research 52: 367–87.

Kereiakas TJ (1996) Clinical evaluation and treatment of vocal disorders. Language Speech and Hearing Services in Schools 27: 240–3.

Kieff DA, Zeitels SM (1996) Phonosurgery. Comprehensive Therapy 22: 222–30.

Kim KM, Kakita Y, Hirano M (1982) Sound spectrographic analysis of the voice of patients with recurrent laryngeal nerve paralysis. Folia Phoniatrica 34: 124–33.

Kiml FJ (1965) Recherches experimentales de la dysphonia spastique. Folia Phoniatrica 17: 241–301.

Kinzl J, Bieble W, Raucchegger H (1988) Functional aphonia: psychosomatic aspects of diagnosis and therapy. Folia Phoniatrica 40: 131–7.

Kirchener JA (1988) Functional evolution of the human larynx: variations among the vertebrates. In Fujimura O (ed.) Vocal Fold Physiology. New York: Raven Press.

Kitzing P (1985) Stroboscopy: a pertinent laryngological examination. Journal of Otolaryngology 14(3): 151–7.

Kjellèn G, Brudin L (1994) Gastroesophageal reflux disease and laryngeal symptoms. Journal for Oto-Rhino-Laryngology and Its Related Specialities 56: 287–90.

Klatt DH, Klatt LC (1990) Analysis, synthesis, and perception of voice quality variations among female and male talkers. Journal of the Acoustical Society of America 87: 820–57.

Klingholz F (1987) The measurement of signal to noise ratio in connected speech. Speech Communication. 6: 15–26.

Koda J, Ludlow C (1992) An evaluation of laryngeal muscle activation in patients with voice tremor. Otolaryngology Head and Neck Surgery 107(5): 684–96.

Koike Y (1973) Application of some acoustic measures for the evaluation of vocal function. Studia Phonologica 7: 17–23

Koller W, Biary N, Cone S (1986) Disability in essential tremor: effect of treatment. Neurology 36: 1001–4.

Koller WC, Busenbark K, Miner K (1994) The relationship of essential tremor: effect of treatment. Neurology 36: 1001–4.

Koschkee DL, Rammage L (1997) Voice Care in the Medical Setting. San Diego, CA: Singular Publishing Group.

Kotby MN (1995) The Accent Method of Voice Therapy. San Diego, CA: Singular Publishing Group.

Kotby MN, El-Sady SR, Basiouny S, Abou-Rass YA, Hegazi MA (1991) Efficacy of the accent method of voice therapy. Journal of Voice 5: 316–20.

Koufman JA (1998) What are Voice Disorders and Who Gets Them? Website: http://www.bgsm.edu/voice/voice_disorders.html.

Koufman JA, Blalock PD (1982) Classification and approach to patients with functional voice disorders. Annals of Otology, Rhinology and Laryngology 91: 372–7.

Koufman JA, Blalock PD (1988) Vocal fatigue and dysphonia in the professional voice user: Bogart–Bacall syndrome. Laryngoscope 98: 493–8.

Koufman JA, Blalock PD (1991) Functional Voice Disorders. Otolaryngologic Clinics of North America 24: 1059–73.

Koufman JA, Sataloff RT, Toohill R (1996) Laryngopharyngeal reflux: Consensus conference report. Journal of Voice 10: 215–16.

Kreiman J, Gerratt BR, Kempster GB, Erman A, Berke GS (1993) Perceptual evaluation of voice quality: review, tutorial, and a framework for future research. Journal of Speech and Hearing Research 36: 21–40.

Kuhl PK, Meltzoff AN (1988) Speech as an intermodal object of perception. In Yonas A: Perceptual Development in Infancy: Minnesota Symposia on Child Psychology. Hillsdale, N.J: Erlbaum.

Kummer AW, Lee L (1996) Evaluation and treatment of resonance disorders. Language Speech and Hearing Services in Schools 27: 271–81.

LaBlance GR, Maves MD (1993) Acoustic characteristics of post-thyroplasty patients. Otolaryngology Head and Neck Surgery 107: 558–63.

Ladefoged P (1983) The linguistic use of different phonation types. In Bless DM, Abbs JH (eds) Vocal Fold Physiology. San Diego, CA: College Hill Press.

Ladefoged P, Maddieson I, Jackson M (1988) Investigating phonation types in different languages. In Fujimura O (ed.) Vocal Fold Physiology, Vol. 2. New York: Raven Press.

Laguaite JK (1972) Adult voice screening. Journal of Speech and Hearing Disorders 37(2), May, 147–51.

Laitman JT, Crelin ES, Conlogue GJ (1977) The function of the epiglottis in monkey and man. Yale Journal of Biology and Medicine 50: 43–8.

Lancer JM, Syder D, Jones AS (1988) Vocal cord nodules: a review. Clinical Otolaryngology 13: 43–51.

Lange DJ, Brin MF, Fahn S, Lovelace RE (1988) Distant effects of locally injected botulinum toxin: incidence and course. In Fahn S, Marsden CD, Calne DE (eds) Advances in Neurology, Vol. 50, Dystonia 2. New York: Raven Press.

Larson CR (1992) Brain mechanisms involved in the control of vocalisation. Journal of Voice 2: 301–11.

Larson K, Ramig L, Scherer R (1994) Acoustic and glottographic voice analysis during drug-related fluctuation in Parkinson disease. Journal of Medical Speech-Language Pathology 2: 227–39.

Laver JD (1968) Voice quality indexical information. British Journal of Disorders of Communication 3: 43–54.

Laver JD (1980) A Phonetic Description of Voice Quality. Cambridge: Cambridge University Press.

Laver JD, Wirz SL, Mackenzie J, Miller S (1981) A perceptual protocol for the analysis of vocal profiles. University of Edinburgh Work in Progress, 14. Edinburgh: University Linguistics Department.

Laver JD, Hiller S, Mackenzie Beck J (1992) Acoustic waveform perturbations and voice disorders. Journal of Voice 6: 115–26.

Lazarus RS (1975) A cognitively oriented psychologist looks at biofeedback. American Psychologist 30: 553–61

Lecluse FLE (1977) Elektroglottografie. Utrecht: Drukkerij Elinkwijk.

Leder SB, Sasaki CT (1994) Long-term changes in vocal quality following Isshiki thyroplasty type 1. Laryngoscope 104: 275–7.

Legerstee M (1990) Infants use multimodal information to imitate speech sounds. Infant Behaviour and Development 13: 343–54.

Lehman JJ, Bless DM, Brandenburg JH (1988) An objective assessment of voice production after radiation therapy for stage I squamous cell carcinoma of the glottis. Otolaryngology Head and Neck Surgery 98:121–9.

Lenneberg EH (1967) Biological Foundations of Language. New York :Wiley.

Lessac A (1967) The Use and Training of the Human Voice: A Practical Approach to Speech and Voice Dynamics. New York: Drama Book Specialist Publications.

Leventhal H, Prochaska TR, Hirschman RS (1985) Preventive health behaviour across the life span. In Rosen JC, Solomon LJ (eds) Prevention in Health Psychology. Hanover NH: University Press of New England.

Levine HL, Wood BG, Batza E, Rusnov M, Tucker HM (1979) Recurrent laryngeal nerve section for spasmodic dysphonia. Annals of Otology, Rhinology and Laryngology 88: 527–30.

Levitt H (1971) Speech production and the deaf child. In Corner LE (ed.) Speech of the Deaf Child. Washington: Alex Graham Bell.

Lewis MM (1936) Infant Speech: A study of the beginnings of language. New York: Harcourt Brace.

Lewis M (1969) Infants' responses to facial stimuli during the first year of life. Developmental Psychology 1: 75–86.

Ley P (1988) Communicating with Patients. New York: Croom Helm.

Ley P (1989) Improving patients' understanding, recall, satisfaction and compliance. In Broome A (ed.) Health Psychology. London: Chapman & Hall.

Li CN, Thompson SA (1978) The acquisition of tone. In Fromkin VA (ed.) Tone: A Linguistic Survey. New York : Academic Press.

Liberman P (1961) Perturbations in vocal pitch. Journal of the Acoustical Society of America 33: 597–603.

Lidsky T, Manetto C, Schneider J (1985) A consideration of sensory factors involved in motor functions of the basal ganglia. Brain Research Reviews 19: 133–46.

Lieberman P (1984) The biology and evolution of language. Cambridge, MA: Harvard University Press.

Link DT, McCaffrey TV, Krauss WE, Link MJ, Ferguson MT (1998) Cervicomedullary compression: an unrecognized cause of vocal cord paralysis in rheumatoid arthritis. Annals of Otology, Rhinology and Laryngology 107: 462–71.

Linke CE (1973) A study of pitch characteristics of female voices and their relationship to vocal effectiveness. Folia Phoniatrica 25: 173–85.

Linville SE (1996) The sound of senescence. Journal of Voice 10: 190–200.

Liss JM, Weismer G (1992) Qualitative acoustic analysis in the study of motor speech disorders. Journal of the Acoustical Society of America 92: 2984–7.

Llewellyn-Thomas HA, Sutherland HJ, Hogg SA, Ciampi A, Harwood AR, Keane TJ, Till JE, Boyd NE (1984) Linear analogue self-assessment of voice quality in laryngeal cancer. Journal of Chronic Diseases 37: 917–24.

Lo TCM, Salzman FA, Schwartz MR (1985) Radiotherapy for Cancer of the Head and Neck. Otolaryngologic Clinics of North America 18(3): 521–31.

Locke JL (1995) The Child's Path to Spoken Language. Paperback edition. Cambridge, MA: Harvard University Press.

Logemann JA, Fisher HB, Boshes B, Blonsky ER (1978) Frequency and occurrence of vocal tract dysfunctions in the speech of a large sample of Parkinson's patients. Journal of Speech and Hearing Disorders 42: 47–57.

Luchsinger R, Arnold GE (1965) Voice, Speech and Language. London: Constable.

Ludlow CL (1981) Research needs for the assessment of phonatory function. ASHA Reports 11: 3–8.

Ludlow CL (1994) The spasmodic dysphonias: speech, movement and physiological characteristics. In Tseu J, Caine D (eds) Handbook of Dystonia. New York: Dekker.

Ludlow CL (1995) Management of spasmodic dysphonias. In Rubin J, Sataloff R, Korovin G, Gould W (eds) Diagnosis and Treatment of Voice Disorders. New York: Igaku-Shoin.

Ludlow CL, Bassich CJ, Connor NP, Coulter DC (1986) Phonatory characteristics of vocal fold tremor. Journal of Phonetics 14: 509–15.

Ludlow CL, Bassich CJ, Connor N, Coulter D, Lee Y (1987) The validity of using phonatory jitter and shimmer to detect laryngeal pathology. In Baer T, Sasakic, Harris K Laryngeal Function in Phonation and Respiration (pp. 492–508). Boston, MA: Brown & Co.

Ludlow CL, Naunton RF, Sedory SE, Schulz GM, Hallet M (1988) Effects of botulinum toxin injections on speech in adductor spasmodic dysphonia. Neurology 38: 1220–5.

Ludlow CL, Yeh J, Cohen LG, Van Pelt F, Rhew K, Hallett M (1994) Limitations of electromyography and magnetic stimulation for assessing laryngeal muscle control. Annals of Otology, Rhinology and Laryngology 103: 16–27.

McAllister A, Sederholm E, Sundberg J, Gramming P (1994) Relations between vocal range profiles and physiological and perceptual voice characteristics in 10 year old children. Journal of Voice 8(3): 230–9.

McCall GN, Skolnick ML, Brewer DW (1971) A preliminary report of some atypical movement patterns in the tongue, palate, hypopharynx and larynx of patients with spasmodic dysphonia. Journal of Speech and Hearing Disorders 36: 466–70.

McClosky DG (1977) General techniques and specific procedures for certain voice problems. In Cooper M, Cooper MH (eds) Approaches to Vocal Rehabilitation (pp. 138–52). Springfield, IL: Charles C. Thomas.

MacCurtain F (1990) Dynamic Displays of Voice Disorders by Magnetic Resonance Imaging. Conference on Care of the Professional Voice. London: Ferens Institute, Middlesex Hospital.

MacCurtain F, Fourcin AJ (1982) Applications of the electroglottograph waveform display. In Van Lawrence M (ed.) Transcripts of the 10th symposium: care of the professional voice: 51–7. New York: Voice Foundation.

MacDonald G (1994) The Alexander Technique. London: Hodder.

McGlone RE (1967) Air flow during vocal fry phonation. Journal of Speech and Hearing Research 10: 299–304.

McGlone RE (1970) Air flow in the upper register. Folia Phoniatrica 22: 231–8.

McGlone R, Hollien H (1963) Vocal pitch characteristics of aged women. Journal of Speech and Hearing Research 6: 164–70.

McGuirt WF, Koufman JA, Blalock D (1992) Voice analysis of patients with endoscopically treated early laryngeal carcinoma. Annals of Otology, Rhinology and Laryngology 101: 142–6.

McHenry MA, Kuna ST, Minton JT, Vanoye CR (1996) Comparison of Direct and Indirect Calculations of Laryngeal Airway Resistance in Connected Speech. Journal of Voice 10: 236–44.

McHugh-Munier C, Scherer KR, Lehmann W, Scherer U (1997) Coping strategies, personality and vocal nodules in patients with vocal fold nodules and polyps. Journal of Voice 4: 452–61.

MacIntyre JM (1980) An evaluation of the incidences, causes and types of dysphonia observed over a period of ten years in one district of an industrial city. Proceedings of the 19th Congress, International Association of Logopaedics and Phoniatrics. August 1983, Edinburgh.

McNair D, Lorr M (1964) An analysis of mood in neurotics. Journal of Abnormal Psychology 69: 620–7.

Maki J (1980) Visual feedback as an aid to speech therapy. In Subtelny J (ed.) Speech Assessment for Hearing Impaired. Washington, DC: Alex Graham Bell.

Makuen GH (1899) Falsetto voice in the male. Journal of American Medical Association 32: 474.

Manaligod JM, Smith RJ (1998) Familial laryngeal paralysis. American Journal of Medical Genetics 77: 277–80.

Manen J, van Speelman JD, Tans RJ (1984) Indications for surgical treatment of Parkinson's disease after levodopa therapy. Clinical Neurology and Neurosurgery 86: 207–12.

Mantravadi RVP, Liebner EJ, Haas RE, Skolnik EM, Applebaum EL (1983) Cancer of the glottis: prognostic factors in radiation therapy. Radiation 149: 311–14.

Marion M, Sheehy M, Sangla S, Soulayrol S (1995) Dose standardisation of botulinum toxin. Journal of Neurology, Neurosurgery and Psychiatry 59(1): 102–3.

Markides A (1983) The Speech of Hearing Impaired Children. Manchester: Manchester University Press.

Marsden CD, Quinn N (1990) The Dystonias. British Medical Journal 300: 139–44.

Marsden CD, Sheehy MP (1982) Spastic Dysphonia, Meige's Disease and Torsion Dystonia. Neurology 32: 1202–3.

Martin S (1986) Working with Dysphonics. Bicester: Winslow Press.

Martin FG (1988) Drugs and vocal function. Journal of Voice 2: 338–44.

Martin S (1994) Voice care and development for teachers: survey report. Voice 3: 92.

Martin S (1995) Do similarities and differences exist between voice teachers and speech and language therapists in their description of voice quality? Unpublished MA Thesis: The Central School of Speech and Drama London.

Martin GB, Clark RD (1982) Distress crying in neonates: species and peer specificity. Developmental Psychology 18: 3–9.

Martin S, Darnley L (1992) The Voice Sourcebook. Bicester, Oxon: Winslow

Martin S, Darnley L (1996) The Teaching Voice. London: Whurr.

Martony J (1966) Studies on the speech of the deaf. Progress Report, Speech Transmission Lab. Stockholm: Royal Institute of Technology.

Masuda T, Ikeda Y, Manako H, Komiyama S (1993) Analysis of vocal abuse: fluctuations in phonation time and intensity in four groups of speakers. Acta Otolaryngologica (Stockholm) 113: 547–52.

Mathieson L (1993) Vocal tract discomfort in hyperfunctional dysphonia. Voice 2(1): 40–8.

Mathieson L (1997) The effect of the menopause on voice. Paper presented at the Effectiveness in Voice Therapy Conference. Freeman Hospital, Newcastle upon Tyne, UK.

Mawdsley C, Gamsu CV (1971) Periodicity of speech in parkinsonism. Nature 231: 315–16.

Max L, Mueller PB (1996) Speaking F_0 and cepstral periodicity analysis of conversational speech in a 105-year-old woman: variability of aging effects. Journal of Voice 10 : 245–51.

Mayer EA (1996) Breaking down the functional and organic paradigm: Review article. Current Opinion in Gastroenterology 12: 3–7

Mayeux R, Williams J, Stern Y, Cote L (1986) Depression and Parkinson's disease. In Yahr MD, Bergmann KJ (eds) Advances in Neurology (pp. 241–50). New York: Raven Press.

Medini E, Medini A, Gapany M, Levitt SH (1996) Radiation therapy in early carcinoma of the glottic larynx. International Journal of Radiology, Oncology, Biology and Physics 36(5): 1211–13.

Mendenhall WM, Parsons JT, Stringer SP (1988) T1-T2 vocal cord carcinoma: a basis for comparing the results of irradiation and surgery. Head and Neck Surgery 10: 373–7.

Mendonca DR (1975) State of the patient after successful irradiation for laryngeal cancer. Laryngoscope 85 (1): 534–9.

Michel JF (1968) Fundamental frequency investigation of vocal fry and harshness. Journal of Speech and Hearing Research 11: 590–4.

Michel JF et al. (1966) Speaking fundamental frequency characteristics of 15, 16, 17 year old girls. Lang Speech 9: 46–51.

Miles B, Hollien H (1990) Whither belting? Journal of Voice 4: 64–70.

Miller MA (1968) Speech and voice patterns: association with hearing impairment. Audecibel 17: 162–7.

Miller MK, Verdolini K (1995) Frequency and risk factors for voice problems in teachers of singing and control subjects. Journal of Voice 9(4): 348–62.

Miller RH, Woodson GE, Jankovic J (1987) Botulinum toxin injection of the vocal fold for spasmodic dysphonia. Archives of Otolaryngology Head and Neck Surgery 113: 603–5.

Moncur JP, Brackett IP (1974) Modifying Vocal Behaviour. New York: Harper & Row.

Money JM, Erhardt A (1972) Boy and Girl. Baltimore, MD: Johns Hopkins University Press.

Monsen R (1978) Towards measuring how well hearing impaired children speak. Journal of Speech and Hearing Research 21: 197–219.

Montague JC Jnr., Hollien H, Hollien PA, Wold DC (1978) Perceived pitch and fundamental frequency comparisons of institutionalised Down's syndrome children. Folia Phoniatrica 30: 245–56

Moon C, Fifer WP (1990) Syllables as signals for two-day-old infants. Infant Behaviour and Development 10: 477–91.

Moore GP (1971) Voice disorders organically based. In Travis LE (ed.) Handbook of Speech Pathology and Audiology. New York: Appleton-Century-Crofts.

Moore GP (1977) Have the major issues in voice disorders been answered by research in speech science? A fifty year perspective. Journal of Speech and Hearing Disorders 42: 152–60.

Moos RH, Swindle RW (1990) Stressful life circumstances: concepts and measures. Stress Medicine 6: 171–8.

Morris J (1974) Conundrum. London: Faber.

Morris J (1991) Pride against Prejudice: Transforming Attitudes to Disability. London: The Women's Press.

Morrison, M (1997) Pattern recognition in muscle misuse voice disorders: How I do it. Journal of Voice 11: 108–14.

Morrison MD, Rammage L (1994) The Management of Voice Disorders. London: Chapman & Hall Medical.

Morrison MD, Rammage LA, Belisle G, Pullan CB, Nichol H (1983) Muscular tension dysphonia. Journal of Otolaryngology 12: 302–6.

Mosby DP (1970) Psychotherapy versus voice therapy for a child with a deviant voice: a case study. Perceptual Motor Skills 30: 887–91.

Mosby DP (1972) Appraising psychotherapeutic change in voice-deviant children with the Rorschach index of repressive style. Perceptual Motor Skills 34: 701–2.

Motta G, Cesari U, Iengo M, Motta G (1990) Clinical application of electroglottography. Folia Phoniatrica 42: 111–17.

Mount KH, Salmon S (1988) Changing the vocal characteristics of a postoperative transsexual patient: a longitudinal study. American Journal of Communication Disorders 21: 229–38.

Mueller PB, Wilcox JC (1980) Effects of marijuana smoking on vocal pitch and quality. Ear, Nose and Throat Journal 59: 506–9.

Mulder DS (1980) The diagnosis and treatment of amyotrophic lateral sclerosis. Boston, MA: Houghton-Mifflin.

Murphy AT (1964) Functional Voice Disorders. Englewood Cliffs, NJ: Prentice-Hall.

Murphy AT (1965) Functional Voice Disorders 2nd edn. Englewood Cliffs, NJ: Prentice-Hall.

Murray E, Tiffin J (1934) An analysis of some basic aspects of effective speech. Arch Speech 1: 61–83.

Murry T (1978) Speaking fundamental frequency characteristics associated with voice pathologies. Journal of Speech and Hearing Disorders 43(3): 374–9.

Murry T, Bone RC, von Essen C (1974) Changes in voice production during radiotherapy for laryngeal cancer. Journal of Speech and Hearing Disorders 39: 194–9.

Mysack ED (1959) Pitch and duration characteristics of older males. Journal of Speech and Hearing Research 2: 46–54.

Negus VE (1949) The Comparative Anatomy and Physiology of the Larynx. London: Heinemann.

Neiman RF, Mountjoy JR, Allen EL (1975) Myasthenia gravis focal to the larynx. Archives of Otolaryngology 101: 56–570.

Netsell R (1981) The acquisition of speech motor control: a perspective with directions for research. In Stark R (ed.) Language Behaviour in Infancy and Early Childhood. New York: Elsevier.

Netsell R, Daniel B (1979) Dysarthria in adults: physiologic approach to rehabilitation. Archives of Physical Medicine and Rehabilitation 60: 502–8.

Netsell R , Hixon T (1978) A noninvasive method for clinically estimating subglottal air pressure. Journal of Speech and Hearing Disorders 43: 326–30.

Netterville JL, Stone RE, Luken ES, Civantos FJ, Ossoff RH (1993) Silastic medialization and arytenoid adduction: the Vanderbilt experience. Annals of Otology, Rhinology and Laryngology 102: 413–25.

Newsome-Davis, J (1992) Diseases of the neuromuscular junction. In Ashbury AK, McKhann GM, McDonald WW (eds) Diseases of the Nervous System. Clinical Neurobiology 2nd edn (pp. 197–212). Philadelphia, PA: WB Saunders.

Nichol H, Morrison MD, Rammage LA (1993) Interdisciplinary approach to functional voice disorders: the psychiatrist's role. Otolaryngology Head and Neck Surgery 108: 643–7.

Nickerson RS (1975) Characteristics of the speech of deaf persons. Volta Review 77: 342–62.

Nunn JF (1987) Applied Respiratory Physiology. London: Butterworths.

Oates JM, Dacarkis G (1983) Speech pathology considerations in the management of transsexualism – a review. British Journal of Disorders of Communication 18: 139–51.

Ogden J (1996) Health Psychology: A Textbook. Buckingham: Open University Press.

Ohlsson AC (1993) Preventative voice care for teachers. Voice:2(2): 112–15.

Oldfield P (1995) Fact Sheet: Professional Association of Teachers. UK.

Oppenheim H (1911) Uber Eine Eigenartige Krampfkrankheit des Kindlichen und Jugenlichen Alters (Dysbasia Lordotica Progressiva, Dystonia Muselform Deformans) Neurologic Centralblatt 30: 1090–1107.

Ormell C (1993) Down to a whisper. Times Educational Supplement, 8 Oct.

Papathanasiou I, MacDonald L, Whurr R, Brookes G, Jahanshahi M (1997) Perceived stigma among patients with spasmodic dysphonia. Journal of Medical Speech-Language Pathology 5: 251–62.

Parker A, Irlam S (1995) Speech intelligibility and deafness: skills of listener and speaker. In Wirz (ed.) Perceptual Approaches to Communication Disorders. London: Whurr.

Parnes SM, Lavorato AS, Myers EN (1978) Study of spastic dysphonia using video-fiberoptic laryngoscopy. Ann Otol 87: 322–6.

Paty D, Ebers C (1998) Multiple Sclerosis. Philadelphia, PA: FA Davis.

Pawlas A, Ramig L (in review). Perceptual characteristics of speech and voice in idiopathic Parkinson disease. Neurology.

Pawlby SJ (1977) Imitative interaction. In Schaffer HR Studies in Mother–Infant Interaction. New York: Academic Press.

Peacher WG (1949) Neurological factors in the aetiology of delayed speech. Journal of Speech and Hearing Disorders 14: 137–42.

Pemberton C, McCormack P, Russell A (1998) Have women's voices lowered across time? A cross sectional study of Australian women's voices. Journal of Voice 12: 208–13.

Perello J (1962) Dysphonies fonctionelles: phonopose et phononevrose. Folia Phoniatrica 14: 150–205.

Perez K, Ramig LO, Smith ME, Dromey C (1996) The Parkinson larynx: tremor and videolaryngostroboscopic findings. Journal of Voice 10(4): 354–61.

Perkins T (1971) Vocal function: a behavioural analysis. In Travis LE (ed.) Handbook of Speech Pathology and Audiology. New York: Appleton-Century-Crofts.

Perkins WH (1983) Quantification of vocal behaviour: a foundation for clinical management. In Bless DM, Abbs JH (eds) Vocal Fold Physiology: contemporary research and clinical issues. San Diego, CA: College Hill Press.

Pershall KE, Boone DR (1986) A videoendoscopic and computerized tomographic study of hypopharyngeal and supraglottic activity during assorted vocal tasks. Transcripts of the Fourteenth Symposium: Care of the Professional Voice (pp. 276–82). New York: The Voice Foundation.

Pinker S (1994) The Language Instinct. New York: Harper Collins.

Pope CE (1994) Acid Reflux Disorders. New England Journal of Medicine 331: 656–60.

Posner MI, Raichle ME (1997) Images of the Mind. New York: Scientific American Library.

Postma GN, Shockley WW (1998) Transient Vocal Fold Immobility. Annals of Otology, Rhinology and Laryngology 107: 236–40.

Pou AM, Carrau RL, Eibling DE, Murry T (1998) Laryngeal framework surgery for the management of aspiration in high vagal lesions. American Journal of Otolaryngology 19: 1–17.

Prater RJ, Swift RW (1984) Manual of Voice Therapy. Boston, MA: Little, Brown.

Prevelic GM (1996) Changes in the female voice with the menopause. Performing Arts Medicine News 4: 19–20.

Prosek R, Montgomery AA, Walden BE, Schwartz DM (1978) EMG biofeedback in the treatment of hyperfunctional voice disorders. Journal of Speech and Hearing Disorders 43: 282–94.

Putnam AHB (1988) Respiratory dysfunction management. In Yoder DE, Kent RD (eds) Decision making in speech-language pathology (pp. 121–31). Philadelphia, PA: Decker.

Ramig, LA (1986) Acoustic analyses of phonation in patients with Huntington's Disease: Preliminary report. Annals of Otology, Rhinology and Laryngology 95: 288–93.

Ramig LA (1995a) Speech therapy for patients with Parkinson's disease. In Koller W, Paulson G. (eds) Therapy of Parkinson's Disease (pp. 539–48). New York: Marcel Dekker.

Ramig, L. (1995b) Voice treatment for neurological disorders of the larynx. Current Opinion in Otolaryngology Head and Neck Surgery 3: 174–82.

Ramig LA, Ringel R (1983) Effects of physiological aging on selected acoustic characteristics of voice. Journal of Speech and Hearing Research 26: 22–30.

Ramig LA, Scherer RC, Titze IR, Ringel SP (1988) Acoustic analysis of voices of patients with neurologic diseases: rationale and preliminary data. Annals of Otology, Rhinology and Laryngology 97: 164–72.

Ramig LA, Countryman S, Thompson L, Horii Y (1995a) A comparison of two forms of intensive speech treatment for Parkinson disease. Journal of Speech and Hearing Research 38(6): 1232–51.

Ramig LA, Pawlas A, Countryman S (1995b) The Lee Silverman Voice Treatment: A practical guide for treating the voice and speech disorders in Parkinson disease. Iowa City, IA: National Center for Voice and Speech, University of Iowa.

Ramig LA, Countryman S, O'Brien C, Hoehn M, Thompson L (1996) Intensive speech treatment for Parkinson Disease. Journal of Speech and Hearing Research 38: 1232–51.

Ramig LO, Scherer RC (1992) Speech therapy for neurologic disorders of the larynx. In Blitzer A, Bri MF, Sasaki CT, Fahn S, Harris KS (eds) Neurologic Disorders of the Larynx (pp. 163–81). New York: Thieme Medical.

Ramig LO, Verdolini K (1998) Treatment efficacy: voice disorders. Journal of Speech Language and Hearing Research 41: S101–16.

Ramig LO, Wood R (1983) Personal notes.

Rammage LA (1992) Acoustic, aerodynamic and vibratory characteristics of phonation with variable posterior glottis postures. Unpublished doctoral dissertation, University of Wisconsin-Madison.

Rao SM (1990) Neurobehavioral Aspects of Multiple Sclerosis. New York: Oxford University Press.

Rawlings CG (1935) A comparative study of the movements and breathing muscles in speech of deaf and normal subjects. Am Ann Deaf 80: 136–50.

Reed CG (1980) Voice therapy: a need for research. Journal of Speech and Hearing Disorders 45: 157–69.

Reed Thompson A (1995) Pharmacologic agents with effects on voice. American Journal of Otolaryngology 16: 12–18.

Reich A, Till J (1983) Phonatory and manual reaction times of women with idiopathic spasmodic dysphonia. Journal of Speech and Hearing Research 26: 10–18.

Ringel R (1987) Vocal indices of biological age. Journal of Voice 1: 31–8.

Riska TB, Lauerma S (1966) Die stimmfunktion nach der Behandlung von Stimmbandskarzinan im Stadium I. Acta Otolaryngologica Supplement 224: 501–14.

Ritchie J (1996) Vocology: the psychological underpinning of voice. British Journal of Therapy and Rehabilitation 3: 75–81

Robe E, Brumlick J, Moore P (1960) A study of spastic dysphonia. Neurologic and Electroencephalographic Abnormalities. Laryngoscope 50: 219–45.

Robertson S, Thompson F (1984) Speech therapy in Parkinson's disease: a study of the efficacy and long-term effect of intensive treatment. British Journal of Disorders of Communication 19: 213–24.

Robertson AG, Robertson C, Boyle P, Symonds RP, Wheldon TE (1993) The effect of differing radiotherapeutic schedules on the response of glottic carcinoma of the larynx. European Journal of Cancer 29a(4): 501–10.

Rollin WJ (1987) Psychological considerations of voice disordered people and their families. In Rollin WJ (ed.) The Psychology of Communication Disorders in Individuals and Their Families. Englewood Cliffs, NJ: Prentice-Hall, 188–229.

Rontal M, Rontal E, Leuchter W (1978) Voice spectrography in the evaluation of myasthenia gravis of the larynx. Annals of Otology, Rhinology and Laryngology. 87: 722–8.

Rontal E, Rontal M, Silversman B, Kileny PR (1993) The clinical differentiation between vocal cord paralysis and vocal cord fixation using EMG. Laryngoscope 103: 133–7.

Rose C (1985) Accelerated Learning. Aylesbury, Bucks: Accelerated Learning Systems.

Rosen DC, Sataloff RT (1997a) The Psychology of Voice Disorders. San Diego, CA: Singular Publishing Group.

Rosen DC, Sataloff RT (1997b) Psychological aspects of voice disorders. In Sataloff RT (ed.) Professional Voice Care: The Science and Art of Voice Care. San Diego, CA: Singular Publishing Group.

Rosen M, Malmgreen LT, Jacek RR (1983) Three dimensional computer reconstruction in the distribution of the neuromuscular junctions in the thyroarytenoid muscle. Annals of Otology, Rhinology and Laryngology 92: 424–9.

Rosenbek J, LaPointe LL (1985) The dysarthrias: description, diagnosis, and treatment. In Johns DF (ed.) Clinical Management of Neurogenic Communicative Disorders 2nd edn (pp. 97–152). Boston, MA: Little, Brown.

Rosenfield DB, Donovan DT, Sulek M, Viswanath NH, Inbody GP, Nuedlman HB (1990) Neurologic aspects of spasmodic dysphonia. Journal of Otolaryngology 19: 231–6.

Rothman KJ, Cann CI, Flanders (1980) Epidemiology of laryngeal cancer. Epidemiological Review 2: 195–209.

Rowland L (ed.) (1991) Amyotrophic lateral sclerosis and other motor neuron diseases: Advances in Neurology, Vol. 56. Philadelphia, PA: Lippincott-Raven.

Roy N, Leeper HA (1993) Effects of the manual laryngeal musculoskeletal tension reduction technique as a treatment for functional voice disorders: perceptual and acoustic measures. Journal of Voice 7: 242–9.

Roy N, Tasko SM (1994) Speaking fundamental frequency (SFF) changes following successful management of functional dysphonia. Journal of American Speech Language Pathology Association, 18, 115–20.

Roy N, Bless DM, Heisey D, Ford CN (1997a) Manual circumlaryngeal therapy for functional dysphonia: an evaluation of short- and long-term treatment outcomes. Journal of Voice 11: 321–31.

Roy N, McGrory JJ, Tasko SM, Bless D, Heisey D, Ford CN (1997b) Psychological correlates of functional dysphonia: an investigation using the Minnesota Multiphasic Personality Inventory. Journal of Voice 11: 443–51.

Rugg T, Saunders MI, Dische S (1990) Smoking and mucosal reactions to radiotherapy. British Journal of Radiology 63: 554–6.

Russell J (1864) A case of hysterical aphonia. British Medical Journal 8: 619–21.

Russell A, Penny L, Pemberton C (1993) Speaking fundamental frequency changes over time in women: a longitudinal study. Journal of Speech and Hearing Research 38: 101–9.

Sabol JW, Lee L, Stemple J (1993) The value of vocal function exercises in the practice regimen of singers. Journal of Voice 9: 27–36.

Salassa JR, De Santo LW, Aronson AE (1982) Respiratory distress after recurrent laryngeal nerve sectioning for adductor spastic dysphonia. Laryngoscope 92: 240–5.

Sampaio C, Ferreira J, Simoes F, Rosas M, Magalhaes M, Correira A, Bastos-Lima A, Martins R, Castro-Caldas A (1997) DYSBOT: a single-blind, randomized parallel study to determine whether any differences can be detected in the efficacy and tolerability of two formulations of botulinum toxin type A Dysport and Botox – assuming a ratio of 4–1. Movement Disorders 12 : 1013–18.

Sapienza CM (1997) Aerodynamic and acoustic characteristics of the adult African American voice. Journal of Voice 11: 410–16.

Sapienza C, Stathopoulos ET (1994) Respiratory and laryngeal measures of children and women with bilateral vocal fold nodules. Journal of Speech and Hearing Research 37: 1229–43.

Sapir S, Atlas J, Shahar A (1990) Symptoms of vocal attrition in women army instructors and new recruits: results from a survey. Laryngoscope 100: 991–4.

Sapir S, Keidar A, Mathers-Schmidt B (1993) Vocal attrition in teachers: survey findings. European Journal of Disorders of Communication 28: 177–85.

Sasaki CT, Leder SB, Petcu L, Friedman CD (1990) Longitudinal voice quality changes following Isshiki thyroplasty type 1: the Yale experience. Laryngoscope 100: 849–52.

Sataloff RT (1987a) Clinical evaluation of the professional singer. Ear, Nose and Throat Journal 66: 267–77.

Sataloff RT (1987b) The professional voice Part II: Physical examination. Journal of Voice 1: 191–201.

Sataloff RT (1987c) The professional voice: Part III. Common diagnoses and treatments. Journal of Voice, 1: 283–92.

Sataloff RT (1991) Professional Voice: The Science and Art of Clinical Care. New York: Raven.

Sataloff RT (1995) Genetics of the voice. Journal of Voice 9(1): 16–19.

Sataloff RT (ed.) (1997) Professional Voice Care: The Science and Art of Voice Care. San Diego, CA: Singular Publishing Group.

Sataloff RT, Emerich K, Hoover CA (1997a) Endocrine dysfunction. In Sataloff RT (ed.) Professional Voice: The Science and Art of Clinical Care. San Diego, CA: Singular Publishing Inc.

Sataloff RT, Rosen DC, Hawkshaw M, Spiegel JR (1997b) The three ages of man: the aging adult voice. Journal of Voice 11(2): 156–60.

Saxman JH, Burk KW (1967) Speaking fundamental frequency characteristics of middle aged females. Folia Phoniatrica 19: 167–72.

Schaefer SD (1983) Neuropathology of spasmodic dysphonia. Laryngoscope 93: 1183–1204.

Schaefer SD, Finitzo-Hieber T, Gerling J, Freeman FJ (1983) Brainstem conduction abnormalities in spasmodic dysphonia. Annals of Otology, Rhinology and Laryngology 92: 59–64.

Schalen S, Anderrson K, Eliasson I (1992) Diagnosis of Psychogenic Dysphonia. Acta Otolaryngologica (Stockholm) Supplement 492: 110–12.

Scherer KR (1995) Expression of emotion in voice and music. Journal of Voice 9: 235–48.

Scherer RC, Titze IR, Raphael BN, Wood WP, Ramig LA, Blager RF (1991) Vocal fatigue in a trained and an untrained voice user. In Baer T, Sasaki C, Harris K (eds) Laryngeal function in phonation and respiration. Waltham, MA: College Hill Press.

Scherer RC, Alipour F, Finnegan E (1997) The membranous contact quotient: a new phonatory measure of glottal competence. Journal of Voice 11(2) 187–94.

Schutte H, Miller DG (1993) Belting and pop, nonclassical approaches to the female middle voice: some preliminary considerations. Journal of Voice 7: 142–50.

Scott A (1981) Botulinum toxin injection of eye muscles to correct strabismus. Trans Am Ophthalmol Soc. 79: 734–70.

Scott S, Caird FL (1983) Speech therapy for Parkinson's disease. Journal of Neurology, Neurosurgery and Psychiatry 46: 140–4.

Seaver EG, Andrews JR, Granata JJ (1980) A radiographic investigation of velar positions in hearing impaired young adults. Journal of Communication Disorders 13: 239–47.

Sederholm E (1995) Prevalence of hoarseness in ten-year-old children. Scandinavian Journal of Logopedics and Phoniatrics 20: 165–73.

Sederholm E (1998) Perception of gender in ten-year-old children's voices. Logopedics, Phoniatrics, Vocology 23: 65–8.

Segre R (1951) Spasmodic Aphonia. Folia Phoniatrica 3: 150–7.

Seligman MEP (1975) Helplessness. San Francisco, CA: Freeman.

Selye H (1956) The Stress of Life. New York. McGraw Hill.

Seth G, Guthrie D (1935) Speech in Childhood. Oxford: Oxford University Press.

Shapsey SM, Hybels RL (1985) Treatment of cancer of the larynx: analysis of success and failure. Otolaryngologic Clinics of North America 18(3): 461–8.

Shaw GY, Searl JP, Young, JL, Miner PB (1996) Subjective, laryngoscopic, and acoustic measurements of laryngeal reflux before and after treatment with Omeprazole. Journal of Voice 10: 410–18.

Shaw GY, Szewczyk MA, Searl J, Woodroof J (1997) Autologus fat injection into the vocal folds: technical considerations and long-term follow-up. Laryngoscope 107: 177–86.

Sherrod LR (1981) Issues in cognitive-perceptual development: the special case of social stimuli. In Lamb ME, Sherrod LR (eds) Infant Social Cognition: Empirical and Theoretical Considerations. Hillsdale, NJ: Erlbaum.

Shoulson I, Fahn S (1989) Parkinson study group: effect of deprenyl on the progression of disability in early Parkinson's disease. New England Journal of Medicine 321: 1364–71.

Sikora K, Halnan KE (eds) (1990) Treatment of Cancer 2nd edn. London: Chapman & Hall Medical.

Silverman EM, Zimmer CH (1975) Incidence of chronic hoarseness among school age children. Journal of Speech and Hearing Disorders 40(2): 211–15.

Simpson IC (1971) Dysphonia: the organisation and working of a dysphonia clinic. British Journal of Disorders in Communication 6: 70.

Simpson L (1981) The origin, structure and pharmacological activity in botulinum toxin. Pharmacological Review. The American Society for Pharmacology and Experimental Therapeutics.

Slavit DH, Maragos NE (1994) Arytenoid adduction and Type I thyroplasty in the treatment of aphonia. Journal of Voice 8: 84–91.

Smith S (1954) Remarks on the physiology of the vibrations of the vocal cords. Folia Phoniatrica 6: 166–78.

Smith S (1957) Chest register versus head register in the membrane-cushion model of the vocal cords. Folia Phoniatrica 9: 32–6.

Smith ME, Ramig LO (1995) Neurological disorders and the voice. In Rubin JS, Sataloff RT, Korovin GS, Gould WJ (eds) Diagnosis and Treatment of Voice Disorders: 203–24. New York: Igaku-Shoin.

Smith S, Thyme K (1978) Accent Metoden. Herning: Special Paedagogisk Forlag.

Smith E, Verdolini K, Gray S, Nichols S, Lemke J, Barkmeier J, Dove H, Hoffman H (1996) Effect of Voice Disorders on Quality of Life. Journal of Medical Speech-Language Pathology 4: 223–44.

Smith E, Gray SD, Dove H, Kirchner L, Heras H (1997) Frequency and affects of teachers' voice problems. Journal of Voice 11(1): 81–7.

Smith E, Kirchner HL, Taylor M, Hoffman H, Lemke JH (1998) Voice problems among teachers: differences by gender and teaching characteristics. Journal of Voice 12: 328–34.

Smith E, Lemke J, Taylor M, Kirchner HL, Hoffman H (1998a) Frequency of voice problems among teachers and other occupations. Journal of Voice 12: 480–8.

Smith E, Taylor M, Mendoza M, Barkmeier J, Lemke J, Hoffman H (1998b) Spasmodic dysphonia and vocal fold paralysis: outcomes of voice problems on work-related functioning. J Voice 12: 223–32.

Sobin LH , Wittekind C (eds) (1997) TNM – Classification of Malignant Tumours, UICC International Union against Cancer. New York: Wiley.

Sodersten M, Lindestadt PA (1987) Vocal fold closure in young adult normal-speaking females. Phoniatric and Logopedic Progess Report. Sweden: Karolinska Institute. 5: 12–19.

Sodersten M, Lindestadt PA (1992) Comparison of vocal fold closure in rigid telescopic and flexible fibreoptic laryngostroboscopy. Acta Otolaryngologica 112: 144–50.

Sorenson D, Horii Y, Leonard R (1980) Effects of topical anaesthesia on voice fundamental frequency perturbation. Journal of Speech and Hearing Research 23: 274–83.

Spiegel JR, Sataloff RT, Emerich KA (1997) The young adult voice. Journal of Voice 11: 138-43.

Stager S, Ludlow C (1994) Responses of stutters and vocal tremor patients to treatment with botulinum toxin. In Jankovic J, Hallet M (eds) Therapy with Botulinum Toxin (pp. 481–90). New York: Dekker.

Stanton AL (1987) Determinants of adherence to medical regimens by hypertensive patients. Journal of Behavioural Medicine 10: 377–94.

Stark R (1972) Some features of the vocalizations of young deaf children. In Jones F, Bosma JF (eds) Third Symposium on Oral Sensation and Perception. Springfield, IL: Charles C. Thomas.

Stell PM, Morrison MD (1973) Radiation necrosis of the larynx. Archives of Otolaryngology 98: 111–13.

Stemple JC (1984) Clinical Voice Pathology. Columbus, OH: Merrill.

Stemple JC (1993) Voice Therapy: Clinical Studies. St Louis, Baltimore, MD: Mosby Year Book.

Stemple JC, Weiler E, Whitehead W, Komray R (1980) Electromyographic biofeedback training with patients exhibiting a hyperfunctional voice disorder. Laryngoscope 90: 471–6.

Stemple JC, Lee L, D'Amico B, Pickup B (1994) Efficacy of vocal function exercises as a method of improving voice production. Journal of Voice 8: 271–8.

Stemple JC, Glaze LE, Gerdeman BK (1995a) Clinical voice pathology: theory and management 2nd edn. San Diego, CA: Singular Publishing Group.

Stemple JC, Stanley J, Lee L (1995b) Objective measures of voice production in normal subjects following prolonged voice use. Journal of Voice 9: 127–33.

Stevens KN (1977) Physics of laryngeal behaviour and larynx. Modes-Phonetica 34: 264–79.

Stevens KN (1988) Modes of vocal fold vibration based on a two section model. In Fujimura O (ed.) Vocal Fold Physiology, vol. 2. New York: Raven Press.

Stewart CF, Allen EL, Tureen P, Diamond BE, Blitzer A, Brin MF (1997) Adductor spasmodic dysphonia: standard evaluation of symptoms and severity. Journal of Voice 11(1): 95–103.

Stoicheff M (1975) Voice following radiotherapy. Laryngoscope 85(I): 608–17.

Stoicheff M (1991) Adductor spastic dysphonia: diagnosis and management. Ch. 13 in Fawcus M (ed.) Voice Disorders and their Management 2nd edn. London: Croom Helm.

Stoicheff M, Ciampi A, Passi JE, Fredrickson JM (1983) The irradiated larynx and voice: a perceptual study. Journal of Speech and Hearing Research 26: 482–5.

Stoker RG, Lape WN (1980) Analysis of some non-articulatory aspects of the speech and hearing children. Volta Review 82: 137–48.

Stone RE (1983) Issues in clinical assessment of laryngeal function: contraindications for subscribing to maximum phonation time and optimum fundamental frequency. In Bless DM, Abbs JH (eds) Vocal Fold Physiology: Contemporary research and clinical issues. San Diego, CA: College-Hill Press.

Stone RE Jnr., Sharf DJ (1973) Vocal pitch associated with the use of atypical pitch and intensity levels. Folia Phoniatrica 25: 91–103.

Strong MS (1975) Laser excision of carcinoma of the larynx. Laryngoscope 85: 1286–9.

Studdert-Kennedy M (1991) Language development from an evolutionary perspective. In Perkell JS, Klatt D (eds) Invariance and Variability in Speech Processes. Hillsdale, N.J: Erlbaum.

Subtelny J (1975) Speech assessment of the deaf adult. J Acad Rehabil Audiol 8: 110–18.

Sulter AM, Schutte HK, Miller DG (1996) Standardised laryngeal videostroboscopic rating: differences between untrained and trained male and female subjects, and effects of varying sound intensity, fundamental frequency and age. Journal of Voice 10(2): 175–89.

Sundberg J (1987) The Science of the Singing Voice. Illinois: Northern Illinois University Press.

Svec JG, Schutte HK (1996) Videokymography: high-speed line scanning of vocal fold vibration. Journal of Voice 10(2): 201–5.

Swain J, Finkelstein V, French S, Oliver M (1994) Disabling Barriers: Enabling Environments. London: Sage.

Syder D (1998) Some counselling issues in speech and language therapy. In Syder D (ed.) Wanting to talk: counselling case studies in communication disorders. London: Whurr.

Takahashi H, Koike Y (1975) Some perceptual dimensions and acoustic correlates of pathologic voices. Acta Otolaryngologica (Stockholm) 338: 1–24.

Tandan R, Bradley WG (1985) Amyotrophic lateral sclerosis: Part I. Clinical features, pathology, and ethical issues in management. Annals of Neurology 18: 271–80.

Teacher Training Agency (1997) Training Curriculum and Standards for New Teachers. London.

Terris DJ, Arnstein DP, Nguyen HH (1992) Contemporary evaluation of unilateral vocal cord paralysis. Otolaryngology Head and Neck Surgery 107: 84–90.

Thiery M, Yo Le Sian A, Vrijens M, Janssens D (1973) Vagitis Uterinus. Journal of Obstetrics, Gynaecology British Commonwealth 80: 183–5.

Thomas, DV (1993) Hoarseness and sore throat after tracheal intubation. Anesthesia 48(4): 355–6.

Thurman WL (1977) Restructuring voice concepts and production. In Cooper M, Cooper MH (eds) Approaches to Vocal Rehabilitation. Springfield, IL: CC Thomas.

Titze I (1981) Biomechanics and distributed mass models of vocal fold vibration. In Stevens KN, Hirano M (eds) Vocal Fold Physiology. Tokyo: University of Tokyo Press.

Titze IR, (1988) The physics of small-amplitude oscillation of the vocal folds. J. Acoust Soc Am 83(4): 1536–52

Titze IR (1990) Interpretation of the electroglottographic signal. Journal of Voice 4: 1–9.

Titze IR (1994) Principles of Voice Production. Englewood Cliffs, NJ: Prentice-Hall.

Traube L (1871) Spastiche form der nervosen heiserkeit. In: Traube L (ed.) Gesammelte Beitraege zur pathologie und phsyiologie 2 (pp. 674–8). Berlin: Hirschwald.

Troung D, Rantal M, Rolnick M, Aronson A, Mistura K (1991) A double blind controlled study of botulinum toxin in adductor spasmodic dysphonia. Laryngoscope 101: 630–4.

Trudgeon AM, Knight C, Hardcastle W et al. (1988) A multi-channel physiological data acquisition system based on an IBM PC and its application to speech therapy. Proceedings of the 7th FASE Symposium: Speech 88, Edinburgh, 3, 1093.

Tsunoda K, Takanozawa M, Choh K (1998) Sudden onset aphonia caused by a Japanese-style bath. Journal of Laryngology and Otology 112: 480–1.

Tucker HM (1978) Human laryngeal reinnervation: long-term experience with the nerve-muscle pedicle technique. Laryngoscope 88: 598–604.

Tucker HM (1993) The Larynx 2nd edn. New York: Thieme Medical.

Tulkin SR (1973) Social class differences in infants' reactions to mother's and stranger's voices. Developmental Psychology 8: 137.

Van den Berg JW (1958) Myoelastic-aerodynamic theory of voice production. Journal of Speech and Hearing Research 1: 227–34.

Van den Berg JW, Vennard W, Berger D, Shervanian C (1960) The Vibrating Larynx. Utrecht: Stichting Film en Watenshap.

Van Den Broek P (1987) Acute and chronic laryngitis. In Stell J (ed.) Oto-laryngology vol.5. London: Butterworths.

Van Lawrence M (1979) Laryngological observations on belting. Journal of Research in Singing 2: 26–8.

Van Lawrence M (1987) Common medications with laryngeal effects. Ear, Nose and Throat Journal 66: 318–22.

Van Riper C, Irwin JV (1958) Voice and Articulation. Englewood Cliffs, NJ: Prentice Hall.

Van Thal JH (1961) Dysphonia. Speech Pathology and Therapy 4: 1-21.

Verdolini K (1994) Voice disorders. In Tomblin JB, Morris HL, Spriesterbach DC (eds) Diagnosis in Speech-Language Pathology. San Diego, CA: Singular Publishing Group.

Verdolini-Marston K, Sandage M, Titze IR (1994) Effect of hydration treatments on laryngeal nodules and polyps and related voice measures. Journal of Voice 8:1 30–47.

Verdolini-Marston K, Burke MK, Lessac A, Glaze L, Caldwell E (1995) Preliminary study of two methods of treatment for vocal nodules. Journal of Voice 9: 74–85.

Verdolini K, Ramig L, Jacobsen B (1998) Outcomes Measurement in Voice Disorders. In Frattali CM (ed.) Measuring Outcomes in Speech-Language Pathology. New York: Thieme.

Verdonck-de Leeuw I (1998) Voice characteristics following radiotherapy; the development of a protocol. Studies in Language and Language Use. Amsterdam: Uitgave IFOTT.

Vilkman E, Alku P, Laukkanen AM (1995) Vocal-fold collision mass as a differentiator between registers in the low-pitch range. Journal of Voice 9(1): 66–73.

Vitek J, Zhang J, Evatt K, DeLong M, Hashimoto T, Triche S, Bakery R (1998). GPI Pallidotomy for Dystonia: clinical outcome and neuronal activity. Dystonia 3: Advances in Neurology, Vol. 78. Philadelphia, PA: Lippincott-Raven.

Voelker CH (1935) A preliminary stroboscopic study of the speech of the deaf. Am Ann Deaf 80: 243–59.

Wallston KA, Wallston BS (1982) Who is responsible for your health? The construct of health locus of control. In Sanders GS, Suls J (eds) Social Psychology of Health and Illness. Hillsdale NJ: Lawrence Erlbaum Associates.

Walton J (1977) Muscular dystrophy: some recent developments in research. Israel Journal of Medical Sciences 13(2): 152–8.

Wang CC (1974) Treatment of glottic carcinoma by megavoltage radiation therapy results. American Journal of Roentgenology 120: 157–63.

Ward PH, Hanson D, Berci G (1981) Photographic studies of the larynx in central laryngeal paresis and paralysis. Acta Otolaryngologica 91: 353–67.

Watkin KL, Ewanowski SJ (1985) Effects of aerosol corticosteroids on the voice: Triamcinolone Acetonide and Beclomethasone Dipropionate. Journal of Speech and Hearing Research 28: 301–4.

Watson PJ, Hixon TJ, Stathopoulos E, Sullivan D (1990) Respiratory kinematics in female classical singers. Journal of Voice 4: 120–8.

Weiner W, Lang A (eds) (1995) Behavioral Neurology of Movement Disorders: Advances in Neurology, 65. Philadelphia, PA: Lippincott-Raven.

Wendahl RW (1963) Laryngeal analog synthesis of harsh voice quality. Folia Phoniatrica 15: 241–50.

Werner-Kukuk E, Von Leden H, Yanagihara N (1968) The effects of radiation therapy on laryngeal function. Journal of Laryngology and Otology.

West R, Ansberry M, Carr A (1957) The Rehabilitation of Speech. New York: Harper.

Wexler DB, Jiang JJ, Gray SD, Titze IR (1989) Phonosurgical studies: fat-graft reconstruction of injured canine vocal cords. Annals of Otology, Rhinology and Laryngology 98: 668–73.

White PD, Moorey S (1997) Psychosomatic illnesses are not 'all in the mind'. Journal of Psychosomatic Research 42: 329–32.

White A, Deary IJ, Wilson JA (1997) Psychiatric disturbance and personality traits in dysphonic patients. European Journal of Disorders of Communication 32: 307–14.

Whittet HB, Lund VJ, Brockbank M, Feyerabend C (1991) Serum cotinin as an objective marker for smoking habit in head and neck malignancy. Journal of Laryngology and Otology 105(12): 1036–9.

Whurr R, Moore PA (1994) Assessment and diagnosis of spasmodic dysphonia. In Moore PA (ed.) Handbook of Botulinum Toxin. Oxford: Blackwell.

Whurr R, Lorch M, Fontana H, Brookes G, Lees A, Marsden CD (1993) The use of botulinum toxin in the treatment of adductor spasmodic dysphonia. Journal of Neurology, Neurosurgery and Psychiatry: 526–30.

Whurr R, Lorch M, Nye C (1997) The treatment of spasmodic dysphonia with botulinum toxin injection. Neurology Reviews International 1(2): 11–15.

Whurr R, Lorch M, Lindsay M, Brookes G, Marsden CD, Jahanshahi M (1998) Psychological function in spasmodic dysphonia before and after treatment with botulinum toxin. Journal of Medical Speech-Language Pathology 6(2): 81–91.

Widdicombe J, Davies A (1983) Respiratory Physiology. London: Arnold.

Wiedenfeld SA, O'Leary A, Bandura A, Brown S, Levine S, Raska K (1990) Impact of perceived self-efficacy in coping with stressors on immune function. Journal of Personality and Social psychology 59: 1082–94.

Wilder CN (1983) Chest wall preparation for phonation in female speakers. In Bless DM, Abbs JH (eds) Vocal Fold Physiology. San Diego, CA: College Hill Press.

Williams AJ, Hanson D, Calne DB (1979) Vocal cord paralysis in the Shy Drager syndrome. Journal of Neurology, Neurosurgery and Psychiatry 42: 151–3.

Williamson IJ, Matusiewicz SP, Brown PH, Greening A, Crompton GK (1995) Frequency of voice problems and cough in patients using pressurized aerosol inhaled steroid preparations. European Respiratory Journal 8: 590–2.

Wilson DK (1979) Voice Problems of Children. London: Williams & Wilkins.

Wilson DK (1987) Voice Problems of Children 2nd edn. Baltimore, MD: Williams & Wilkins.

Wilson JA, Deary IJ, Scott S, MacKenzie K (1995) Functional dysphonia. British Medical Journal. 311: 1039–40.

Winkworth AL, Davis PJ (1997) Speech breathing and the Lombard Effect. Journal of Speech, Language and Hearing Research 40: 159–69.

Wippold FJ (1998) Diagnostic imaging of the larynx. In Cummings CW et al. (eds) Otolaryngology Head and Neck Surgery 3rd edn. New York: Mosby.

Wirz S (1986) The voice of the deaf. In Fawcus M (ed.) Voice Disorders and their Management. London: Croom Helm.

Wirz S (1987) Unpublished PhD thesis. Edinburgh: University of Edinburgh.

Wirz SL (1995) Assessing communication skills in diverse clients groups. In Wirz S (ed.) Perceptual Approaches to Communication Disorders. London: Whurr.

Wirz SL (1996) Opportunities and responsibilities towards people with communication disorders in less developed countries. In Caring to Communicate, Proceedings of the RCSLT Conference, York, Oct 1995.

Wirz S, Subtelny J, Whitehead R (1980) A perceptual and spectrographic study of vocal tension in deaf and hearing speakers. Folia Phoniatrica 33: 23–36.

Wolfe VI, Garvin JS, Bacon M, Waldrop W (1975) Speech changes in Parkinson's disease during treatment with l-dopa. Journal of Communication Disorders 8: 271–9.

Wolfe VI, Ratusnik DL, Smith FH, Northrop G (1990) Intonation and fundamental frequency in male to female transsexuals. Journal of Speech and Hearing Disorders 55: 43–50.

Wolff C. (1977) Bisexuality: A Study. London: Quartet Books.

Wolski W (1967) Hypernasality as the presenting system of myasthenia gravis. Journal of Speech and Hearing Disorders 32(1): 36–8.

Woo P (1998) Laryngeal Electromyography is a cost-effective clinically useful tool in the evaluation of vocal fold function. Archives of Otolaryngology Head and Neck Surgery 124: 472–5.

Woo P, Colton RH, Brewer DW, Casper JK (1991) Functional staging for vocal fold paralysis. Otolaryngology Head and Neck Surgery 105: 440–8.

Woo P, Casper J, Colton R, Brewer D (1992) Dysphonia in the aging: physiology versus disease. Laryngoscope 102(2): 139–44.

Woodson GE (1998) Clinical value of laryngeal EMG is dependent on experience of the clinician. Archives of Otolaryngology Head and Neck Surgery 124: 476.

Woodson G, Murry T, Zwirner P, Swenson M (1991) Acoustic, aerodynamic and videoendoscopic assessment of unilateral thyroartenoid muscle injection with spasmodic dysphonia. Journal of Voice 5: 24–31.

World Health Organization (WHO) (1980) The International Classification of Impairments, Disabilities and Handicaps. Geneva: WHO.

Wu YR, Chen CM, Ro LS, Chen ST, Tang LM (1996) Vocal cord paralysis as an initial sign of multiple system atrophy in the central nervous system. J Formosan Med Assoc 95: 804–6.

Wyatt GI (1941) Voice disorders and personality conflicts. Mental Hygiene XXV: 237–50.

Wyke BD (1983a) Neuromuscular Control Systems in Voice Production. In Bless DM, Abbs JH (eds) Vocal Fold Physiology. San Diego, CA: College Hill Press.

Wyke BD (1983b) Reflexogenic contributions to vocal fold control systems. In Titze IR, Scherer RC (eds) Vocal Fold Physiology. Denver: Denver Center for the Performing Arts.

Wynter H (1974) An investigation into the analysis and terminology of voice quality and its correlation with the assessment reliability of speech therapists. British Journal of Disorders of Communication 9.

Yahr M, Bergmann K (1986) Parkinson's Disease: Advances in Neurology. Vol. 45. Philadelphia, PA: Lippincott-Raven.

Yanagisawa E, Estill J, Kmucha ST, Leder SB (1989) The contribution of aryepiglottic constriction to 'ringing' voice quality – a videolaryngoscopic study with acoustic analysis. Journal of Voice 3: 342–50.

Yano J et al. (1982) Personality factors in pathogenesis of polyps and nodules of the vocal chords. Auris Nasus Larynx 9: 105–10.

Yiu E, Ho P (1991) Voice problems in Hong Kong: a preliminary report. Australian Journal of Human Communication Disorders 19: 45–58.

Yorkston K, Beukelman D, Bell K (1988) Clinical management of dysarthric speakers. Boston, MA: College-Hill Press.

Young JL Jr, Perce CL, Asire AJ (eds) (1981) Surveillance, Epidemiology and End results: Incidence and Mortality Data 1973–77. NCI Monograph 57 NIH, PHS, DHEW Publication No (NIH) 81–2330.

Yumoto E, Gould WJ, Baer T (1982) Harmonics-to-noise as an index of hoarseness. Journal of the Acoustical Society of America 71: 1544–50.

Yumoto E, Sasaki Y, Okamura H (1984) Harmonics-to-noise ratio and psychological measurement of the degree of hoarseness. Journal of Speech and Hearing Research 27: 1–6.

Zealear DL, Rainey CL, Herzon GD, Netterville JL, Ossoff RH (1996) Electrical pacing of the paralyzed human larynx. Annals of Otology, Rhinology and Laryngology 105: 689–93.

Zeitels SM, Hochman I, Hillman RE (1998) Adduction arytenopexy: a new procedure for paralytic dysphonia with implications for implant medialization. Annals of Otology, Rhinology and Laryngology, Supplement 173: 2–24.

Zemlin WR (1968) Speech and Hearing Science. Englewood Cliffs, NJ: Prentice Hall.

Zwirner P, Murry T, Swenson M, Woodson G (1991) Acoustic changes in spasmodic dysphonia after Botulinum Toxin injection. Journal of Voice 5(1): 78–84.

Zwirner P, Murry T, Swenson M, Woodson G (1992) Effects of Botulinum Toxin therapy in patients with adductor spasmodic dysphonia: acoustic, aerodynamic and videopendoscopic findings. Laryngoscope 102(4): 400–6.

Zyski BJ, Bull GL, McDonald WE, Johns ME (1984) Perturbation analysis of normal and pathologic larynges. Folia Phoniatrica. 36(4):190–8.

Index

abductor paralysis 37
  bilateral 38, 41
  unilateral 38
abductor spasmodic dysphonia 164, 197
  botulinum toxin treatment 211–12
accent method 131–2, 154–5
acetazolamide 167
acid reflux, as laryngeal irritant 35
acoustic voice quality measurements,
    after radiotherapy 277–9
acoustics, effect on professional voice
    users 294, 296
actors
  and ageing 29, 294
  dehydration 297
  laryngeal manipulation 324
  vocal usage level 283
  see also professional voice users
Adam's apple 24
adduction arytenopexy 188–9
adductor laryngospasms 198
adductor paralysis 37
  bilateral 38
  pseudo bilateral 39
  unilateral 38, 45
adductor spasmodic dysphonia 164,
    194, 195, 196–7
  botulinum toxin treatment 208–9,
    211–12
  physiological behaviour 196–7
adenoids, during puberty 24
adherence 297–8
adolescents 25–6, 67
  female 242–3

adults 26–7
  male-female difference in voice and
    speech 26–7
aerobic instructors, vocal attrition 284–5
aerodynamic voice measurements 80–1
  after radiotherapy 277–9
African languages 5
ageing
  biological vs. chronological 29
  and deaf speakers 232
  and fundamental frequency 29, 234,
    243
  laryngeal disorders 40, 67–8
  professional voice users 294
  voice changes in 28–31
  voice disorder prevalence 50
air flow
  equipment for measuring 331
  patient assessment 80–1
  after radiotherapy 277–8
  in vocal fold paralysis 180, 185
air pollutants, as laryngeal irritants 116
air pressure, in vocal fold paralysis 185
  studies 180
air traffic controllers, vocal attrition
    285
airport announcers, vocal attrition 285
airway, artificial 41
airway maintenance
  in children 42
  surgery for 41–2
alaryngeal dysphonia 63
Albany Trust 257
alcohol

and laryngeal cancer 270, 274
    as laryngeal irritant 35, 116
Alexander Technique 298
allergic laryngitis 67
allergic rhinitis 67
allergies 67, 145
    as cause of aphonia 153
alprazolam 167
ALS, see amyotrophic lateral sclerosis
amplitude perturbation (shimmer) 82,
        84, 278
amplitude perturbation quotient 84
amplitude variability index 84
amyotrophic lateral sclerosis (ALS) 160,
        199
    incidence 161
    symptoms and signs 162
    and vocal fold movement 175
    voice characteristics, endoscopic
        findings 165
    voice characteristics, perceptual
        findings 164
androgens 28, 39, 60
animals, communication patterns 5
ansa hypoglossi 45
antibiotics 145
anticholinergics 207
    as laryngeal irritants 116
antidepressants, as laryngeal irritants
        116
antidopaminergic agents 167
antihistamines, as laryngeal irritants 116
antihypertensive drugs, as laryngeal
        irritants 116
antipsychotic agents, as laryngeal
        irritants 116
antiseizure medications 167
anxiety, professional voice users 289
anxiety state 62
aphonia 152–4
    causes 153
    conversion aphonia 66
    as a conversion disorder 139, 152
    functional 143–4
    hysterical 59
    intermittent 153–4
    psychogenic 143–4
    symptoms and signs 153

    therapy techniques 153
    whispering aphonia 143
apraxia 62
army instructors, see military training
        instructors
arthritis, see cricoarytenoid arthritis;
        rheumatoid arthritis
articulation 1
articulation techniques, transsexuals 264
artificial airway 41
aryepiglottic narrowing 130
arytenoid adduction 188
arytenoid granulomata, laryngeal manip-
        ulation in 324
arytenoidectomy 41–2, 190
Asian languages 5
aspirate initiation of voicing 129–30
aspiration, in vocal fold paralysis 182,
        183, 190
assessment, see patient assessment
asthma 67, 145
    vocal hyperfunction and 115, 116
ataxia, cerebellar 62
ataxic voice disorders 159
    intensive voice treatment 170
    voice characteristics, perceptual
        findings 163
athetosis 62
atresia, of larynx 35
attrition, see vocal attrition
audio-recording 330
audit, multidisciplinary voice clinics
        336–7
auditory voice quality ratings 73–5
    difficulty of judging 73–4
    rating scales 73–4
augmentative communication, neurolog-
        ical voice disorders 170
autologous fat 45, 187
axonal sprouting, botulinum toxin treat-
        ment and 212, 217

babbling 21–2
baclofen 207
Beaumont Society 257
Beck Depression Inventory (BDI) 205
behaviour modification programmes
        123–6

behavioural descriptions of voice disor-
    ders 140–1
behavioural differences, male/female
    265
behavioural treatment, neurological
    voice disorders 167
behavioural voice disorders 62
belting 113, 125
benzhexol 207
benzodiazepines 167, 207
Bernoulli effect 6
birds, communication patterns 5
birth cry 18, 20
body alignment, patient's 76–7
body language, gender differences 265
Bogart–Bacall syndrome 119
bone growth, during puberty 24–5
Botox 166, 167
    see also botulinum toxin
botulinum toxin 217–18
    Botox vs. Dysport 218
    potency 208, 218
    preparation and dosage 218
botulinum toxin treatment
    abductor spasmodic dysphonia
        211–12
    adductor spasmodic dysphonia
        208–9, 211–12
    axonal sprouting and 212, 217
    evaluation methods 208–9
    injection technique 209
    laryngeal dystonia 166
    long-term effects 212
    overview 211–12
    psychosocial aspects 210–11
    results of 209–11
    side effects 209
    in spasmodic dysphonia 45–6, 207–8
    vocal change after injection 210
bowing of vocal folds 30
    classification 65
    distribution by age and gender 52
    prevalence 51
breath control, deaf speakers 222–3
breathiness 74
    see also 'breathy'; breathy (confiden-
        tial) voice
breathing, for transsexuals 262–3

breathing exercises, professional voice
    users 299
'breathy' 56–7
    benign vs. cancerous lesions 275
    after radiotherapy 276
    see also breathiness
breathy (confidential) voice 56, 57, 129
bromocriptine 166
Buffalo III Voice Profile 74
bulbar palsy 62
bulimia 67
business people, vocal usage level 283

caffeine, as laryngeal irritant 116, 122
call signs, infants' 21
cameras 329
cancer 65
    control rates 272
    distribution by age and gender 50, 52
    fear of 33
    prevalence 50, 51
    see also carcinoma; glottal cancer;
        laryngeal cancer; laryngeal carci-
        noma; lung cancer
Cantonese 5
capillary telangiectases, phonosurgery
    305–6
    indications 305–6
    the operation 306
    postoperative follow-up and results
        306
carbamazepine 207
carbon dioxide (CO_2) lasers 42, 43, 44,
    303
carcinoma
    glottic 270
    TNM staging 269
    see also laryngeal carcinoma
case discussion 152
case history interviews 70–3, 149–50,
    213–14
    basic questions 85
    history of voice problem 70–1, 85
    medical history 71–2, 85
    occupational factors 72–3, 85
    open-ended questions 70
    patient questionnaires 70, 72, 76,
        86–8, 335

personality factors 72
professional voice users 289–90
psychological considerations 72, 85
questioning technique 70
social factors 72–3, 85
standard formats 70
cerebellar ataxia 62
cervicomedullary compression 179
chanting 133
CHART (continuous, hyperfractionated, accelerated radiotherapy) 272, 273
chemical fumes, as laryngeal irritants 116
chest growth, during puberty 25
chest register 237
chest resonance, in transsexuals 260, 264
chest X-ray, vocal fold paralysis 178
chewing technique 132
children
    airway maintenance 42
    breathing and vocalization studies 242
    chewing technique 132
    deaf speakers 221, 223, 225
    dysphonia 67
    early school years to puberty 23
    fundamental frequency 224, 241–2
    gender differences in voice and speech 23
    hoarseness 23
    hyperfunctional behaviour 92, 123
    hypertonicity 92
    hypofunctional behaviour 92
    hypotonicity 92
    incidence of voice disorders 89
    intonation patterns 23
    knowledge base 90
    learning from parents 22–3
    psychosocial behaviours 96
    puberty 24–6
    resonance 92, 100
    respiration 95–6
    speaking fundamental frequency (SFF) 23
    stenosis 42
    vocal fold paralysis 42, 94
    vocal frequency range in 23

voice conveying feeling 90–1
voice therapy, see children, treatment of voice problems
see also adolescents; infants; neonates
children, treatment of voice problems 89–109
    adequate hydration 94
    aetiology 93–4
    assessing vocal capabilities 94–6, 103–5
    case example 93–109
    general awareness phase of treatment 96, 97–8
    general principles 90–2
    individualized treatment plan 102
    microsurgery 316–17
    motivation 92
    multidisciplinary approach 91
    parental involvement and education 91
    pre-test/post-test items 103–5
    production phase of treatment 99–100
    response to voice therapy 89
    specific awareness phase of treatment 96–7, 98–9
    stories 92, 100
    substituting appropriate vocal options 100–2
    tracheotomy 42
    treatment programmes 96–100
chorea 62
chronic obstructive airways disease, vocal hyperfunction 115
cleft palate 62
clergy
    ageing 294
    vocal attrition 285
    vocal usage level 283
    see also professional voice users
clerks, vocal usage level 283
clients, see patients
clinical supervision 152
clinics, see multidisciplinary voice clinics
clonazepam 207
Co-phenylcaine forte spray 329
cocaine, as laryngeal irritant 116, 122

cochlear implants 221
collagen 12, 45, 187, 314
comfort sounds 21
communication, gender differences 265
communication skills, transsexuals 256
    non-verbal 265
compliance 297
Compulsory Figures for Voice 125
computed tomography (CT) scan, vocal
    fold paralysis 178
Computer Speech Lab voice analysis
    system 78
confidential voice, *see* breathy (confi-
    dential) voice
conflict over speaking out (CSO) 143
congenital laryngeal disorders 35–6
contact ulcers
    classification 62, 63, 65
    distribution by age and gender 52
    prevalence 51
continuous, hyperfractionated, acceler-
    ated radiotherapy (CHART) 272,
    273
contraception, oral 28
control rates, cancer 272
conversion aphonia 66
conversion disorder 148
    aphonia as 139, 152
    spasmodic dysphonia as 193
conversion dysphonia 66
conversion symptoms 62
coping styles and strategies 147–8
cordectomy 41–2
cordotomy 44, 310
    laser 190
corticosteroids, as laryngeal irritants 116
cough suppressants, as laryngeal
    irritants 116
coughing 113, 115
    see also hyperfunction
counselling
    laryngeal dystonia 211
    transsexuals 257
counsellors, in multidisciplinary voice
    clinics 326–7
creak (glottal fry) 8, 112, 134, 135,
    238–9
cricoarytenoid arthritis

classification 62
distribution by age and gender 53
prevalence 51
cricoarytenoid muscles
    lateral 13
    posterior 13, 174
cricopharyngeal myotomy 46
cricothyroid muscle 13
    role in falsetto 237
cricothyroid visor 339
Crown and Crisp Experiential Index
    (CCEI) 205
crying 113
CT, *see* computed tomography
cysts
    classification 62, 65
    distribution by age and gender 52
    prevalence 51
    see also epidermoid cysts; mucus
        retention cysts

dance teachers, vocal attrition 284–5
deaf speakers 219–33
    ageing and 232
    breath control 222–3
    children 221, 223, 225
    education choice 221
    falsetto voice 231, 236
    fundamental frequency 224
    vs. hearing groups 227–31
    vs. hearing impaired speakers 220
    high pitch 223–4
    laryngeal features 222–4
    literature review 222–5
    loudness 230
    miscellaneous factors affecting voice
        231–3
    nasal voice quality 224
    non-neutral supralaryngeal, laryngeal
        and prosodic features 229
    personality affecting voice disorder
        232
    pitch 223–4, 230
    prosodic aspects, miscellaneous
        224–5
    range of articulatory movements
        228–30
    secondary voice disorder 231–2

tense/harsh voice 223
tension 230
time of onset of hearing loss 220
velopharyngeal features 224
voice quality in 222–3
voices different from those of hearing
    speakers 220, 221–2
decongestants, as laryngeal irritants 116
deglutition, see swallowing
dehydration
    and professional voice users 297
    see also hydration
dentures, effect on articulation 30
Deprenyl 166
diabetes, and vocal fold movement 175
diadochokinetic rates, laryngeal 77
diagnosis 149–52
    interview 149–50
    and musculoskeletal tension 150–1
    personal factors in 151
    psychosocial factors in 151
    reflection and supervision 152
    sifting the information 151–2
    stress and 150
diaphragmatic-abdominal breathing 128,
    131–2
directional perturbation factor 83, 84
disability, WHO definition 287
discomfort, to the patient 55
discomfort sounds 21
distress 288
dopamine precursors/agonists 166
drug therapy, adverse 62
drugs
    as laryngeal irritants 116, 122
    see also individual drugs and drug
        types
dust, as laryngeal irritant 35, 116
dysarthria
    background 156–7
    classification 156
    developments in diagnosis and treat-
        ment 157–8
    treatment options 165–70
    see also neurological voice disorders
dysarthric dysphonia 63
dysarthrophonias 156
dysarthrophonic syndrome 48

dysphagia 273
dysphonia
    childhood 67
    classification 63
    conversion dysphonia 66
    functional, see functional dysphonia
    habitual 139–40
    hyperfunctional 71
    hysterical 48
    intermittent 71, 143–4, 153–4
    with no apparent pathology (normal
        on exam) 50, 51, 52
    physiological studies in management
        of 15–17
    psychogenic, see psychogenic
        dysphonia
    psychosocial consequences 72–3
    significance of 55
    spasmodic, see spasmodic dysphonia
    spastic, see spasmodic dysphonia
    studies 143–4
    whispering dysphonia 144
    see also voice disorders
dysplastic dysphonia 63
Dysport, see botulinum toxin
dystonia 160
    mechanism 195
    prevalence 161
Dystonia Society, UK 211, 215

Ear, Nose and Throat (ENT) depart-
    ments 32
education, deaf children 221
elastin 12–13
electroglottograph 154, 330–1
    see also laryngography
electrolaryngograph 330–1
electrolaryngography (ELG) 281
    see also laryngography
electromyography (EMG)
    laryngeal (LEMG) 179
    in spasmodic dysphonia 196–7
electronic keyboards 238
emotions, and physiology 17
endocrine disorders 39–40, 61, 62
endocrine dysphonia 63
endoscopes 328–9
    rhinolaryngeal video endoscopes 328

endoscopy
    laryngeal 178
    rigid 75
    see also nasendoscopy
endotracheal intubation 39, 41
environmental factors, professional
    voice users 286, 293–4, 296–7
epidermoid cysts, phonosurgery 309–11
    indications 310
    the operation 310–11
    postoperative follow-up and results
    311
epiglottis, during puberty 24
epiglottopexy 38
equipment, in multidisciplinary voice
    clinics 327–32
essential tremor
    causes 159
    neuropharmacological treatment 167
    prevalence 161
    signs 162
    voice characteristics, perceptual
    findings 164
exercises
    professional voice users 298–9
    vocal function 134
expiration, prephonatory phase 7
extrapyramidal disease 66

facial buzz 92, 100, 102
facial language 265
falsetto 8, 234, 236–7
    auditory factors 236
    deaf speakers 231, 236
    mutational 66, 235
    singers 236–7
    see also loft register
feeding difficulties, in neonates 36
feeling, and physiology 17
fibreoptic laryngoscopy 32, 75
fibreoptic nasendoscopy 75, 328
fibreoptic nasolaryngoscopy 199
fibreoptic nasopharyngoscopes 329
fibroblasts 12
fight and flight response 146, 147
flaccid voice disorders 158
flexible fibreoptic laryngoscopy 32, 75
flexible fibreoptic nasendoscopy 75

frequency, *see* fundamental frequency;
    speaking fundamental frequency
frequency control 7–8
frequency perturbation (jitter) 82, 83,
    278
frequency perturbation quotient 84
Friedreich's ataxia
    prevalence 160
    symptoms 161
    voice characteristics, perceptual
    findings 163
'front of mouth' voice 100
'functional'
    functional-organic dichotomy 58–61,
    139, 142
    meaning 59, 137–8, 139
    vs. 'psychogenic' 141
functional aphonia, studies 143–4
functional dysphonia 48
    distribution by age and gender 52
    prevalence 51
functional voice disorders 137, 140, 142
    in deaf speakers 231, 232
    physical vs. psychological factors 140
fundamental frequency 255
    adolescents, female 242–3
    ageing and 234, 243
    children 224, 241–2
    deaf speakers 224
    gender differences 80, 234, 243–4,
    255
    harsh voices 57
    in puberty 24, 234
    after radiotherapy 278–9, 281–2
    in voice measurement 80
    women 234, 242–3
    see also speaking fundamental
    frequency
funding, multidisciplinary voice clinics
    323
fungal infection 62

gastro-oesophageal reflux 67
GAX collagen 314
gelfoam 45, 187
gender differences
    adults 26–7
    behavioural differences 265

body language 265
children 23
communication 265
distribution of laryngeal pathologies
    52–3
facial language 265
functional voice disorders 145
fundamental frequency 80, 234,
    243–4, 255
  in puberty 24, 234
  speaking fundamental frequency
    (SFF) 26, 29, 80
hyaluronic acid 13
in neurological voice disorders 160–1
psychogenic voice disorders 54
in puberty 24, 25, 234
pulse register 8
register transition 9
respiration 3
speaking fundamental frequency
    (SFF) 26, 29, 80
speech habits 265
speech indicators 255
vocal tract changes in puberty 24
voice quality 26
gender reassignment
  preconditions for 247
  see also sex-change operations; trans-
    sexualism; transsexuals
General Adaptation Syndrome 146
General Health Questionnaire GHQ-60
    72
giggle posture 130
giggling 9, 236
globus, laryngeal manipulation in 324
glottal cancer
  control rates 272
  TNM staging 269
glottal fry (creak) 8, 112, 134, 135,
    238–9
glottal gap 26
glottal incompetence, due to vocal fold
    paralysis 187–8, 188
glottal vibration 6
glottis, posterior 65
glycosaminoglycans (GAGs) 12, 13
Gore-Tex 187
granuloma 62

distribution by age and gender 52
  prevalence 51
GRBAS scale 74, 275
group work, professional voice users
    299
growth, during puberty 24–5
Guillaine–Barré syndrome, and vocal
    fold movement 175
Gutzmann's pressure test 237

H2-receptor agonists 122
habitual dysphonia 63, 139–40
haemangioma, subglottic 42
Haemophilus influenzae 41
handicap, WHO definition 287
harsh voice 57
  in deaf speakers 223
  mean fundamental frequency 57
head, neck and shoulder girdle dysfunc-
    tion and dysphonia, research
    337–9
health, beliefs and cognitions about 148
health psychology 146–8
hearing groups, non-neutral supralaryn-
    geal, laryngeal and prosodic
    features 229
hearing impaired speakers, see deaf
    speakers
hearing loss 49
  effect on voice and speech 29
height, as index of vocal maturity 25
high pitch
  as compensatory behaviour in vocal
    fold paralysis 185
  in deaf speakers 223–4
  higher-pitched voices and vocal
    hyperfunction 111
  see also falsetto; loft register; pitch
high-quiet singing 77
history taking
  in multidisciplinary voice clinics 335
  see also case history interviews
hoarseness 32, 57
  children 23
  definition 57
  outcome measurement 337
  priority in assessment 334
  after radiotherapy 272, 277, 280

as symptom of laryngeal cancer 37,
     268, 279
homemakers 54
homosexuality 248, 250
hormonal voice disorders
     distribution by age and gender 53
     prevalence 51
hormone therapy, transsexuals 245, 247,
     249
hormones, sex hormones 39–40
     female 27–8
humming 132
Huntington's disease 159
     medical treatment 167
     prevalence 160–1
     symptoms and signs 161
     voice characteristics, endoscopic
          findings 165
     voice characteristics, perceptual
          findings 164
husky voice 57
hyaluronic acid 12–13
     gender differences 13
hydration 122, 130
     children, treatment of voice problems
          94
     see also dehydration
hyperadduction 165
     treatment 168–9
hyperfunction (vocal) 57
     adducted 120
     assessment 121
     asthma and 115, 116
     behaviour modification programmes
          123–6
     behaviours associated with 112–13
     children 92
     chronic obstructive airways disease
          and 115
     classification and measurement
          117–21
     compensatory mechanism 116
     compensatory strategies 124
     damage to vocal folds 111
     experimental studies 111–12
     from faulty learning mechanisms 122
     general use of term 110
     genetic predisposition 113

'inappropriate vocal components'
     118
indicators of 120–1
laryngeal irritants 35, 116, 122
and laryngopharyngeal reflux 114,
     115, 122
learning factors 115
lung cancer 115
management of voice disorders
     associated with 121
measurement 117–21
medical factors 115–16
minimization of effects of underlying
     causes of 121–3
modification of vocal technique
     126–7
nature of 112–13
non-adducted 120, 130
pitch, direct modification of 134, 135
posture 114
predisposition to 113
psychogenic factors 117, 122–3
reasons for 114–17
recuperation time 124
respiration 114
respiratory dysfunction 127–8
signs 110, 113
sinusitis and 115
situational factors 114–15
therapy, see hyperfunction (vocal),
     therapy techniques
voice disorders associated with
     110–36
whooping cough and 115
see also coughing; screaming;
     shouting; throat clearing; vocal
     abuse; vocal misuse; yelling
hyperfunction (vocal), therapy
     techniques
accent method 131–2
categories of 127
chewing technique 132
diaphragmatic-abdominal breathing
     128, 131–2
exercises, see exercises
focusing on support functions 127–9
giggle/laughing posture 130
holistic therapy 131–4

modification of pitch, loudness and
    glottal fry 134–5
postural education 127, 128
to reduce muscle tension and
    constriction 129–35
resonant voice therapy 132–4
hyperfunctional behaviours 112–13
    children 92
hyperfunctional dysphonia 71
hyperfunctional voice 61
hyperfunctional voice disorders
    spasmodic dysphonia (SD) associated
        with 200–1
    see also hyperfunction
hyperkeratosis 35, 62
    distribution by age and gender 52
    prevalence 51
'hyperkinetic' 61
hyperkinetic phonation, see hyperfunc-
    tion
hyperkinetic voice disorders 159–60
hypertonicity, children 92
hypervalvular phonation 57, 61
hypoadduction, treatment 167–8
hypofunctional behaviour, children 92
hypofunctional voice 57, 61
'hypokinetic' 61
hypokinetic voice disorders 159
hypothyroidism 60, 94
hypotonicity, children 92
hypovalvular phonation 61
hysterical aphonia 59
hysterical dysphonia 48

iatrogenic scars 315–16
IBM Phonetic Workstation 16
illness, beliefs and cognitions about 148
imagery 133
impairment, WHO definition 287
implants
    cochlea implants 221
    implantable electrodes in laryngeal
        pacing 189
'inappropriate vocal components' 118
Indo-European languages 5
infants 20
    babbling 21–2

call signs 21
comfort/discomfort sounds 21
from vocalizations to spoken
    language 21–3
see also children; neonates
INSET training days, teachers 291
inspiration, prephonatory phase 6–7
inspiratory speech 193
instability, phonatory 169–70
instrumental voice measurements, see
    voice measurements, instrumental
interarytenoid muscle 13
intercostals 2, 5
intermittent aphonia 153–4
intermittent dysphonia 71, 143–4, 153–4
interviewing, professional voice users
    289
intonation 5
    in transsexuals 264
intonation patterns
    adults 26
    children 23
intubation, endotracheal 39, 41
intubation trauma 94

jaw exercises, professional voice users
    299
jitter (frequency perturbation) 82, 83,
    278
jitter factor 83
jitter ratio 84
juvenile papillomatosis 44

keratin 35
keratosis leukoplakia 65
keyboards, electronic 238
'kinesiologic' 62
knowledge base, children's 90

L-dopa (levodopa) 162, 207
labourers, vocal usage level 283
lamina propria 12–13, 28, 111
language groups and patterns 5
laryngeal cancer
    hoarseness as symptom of 37, 268,
        279
    and radiotherapy 43, 268

surgery 42–4, 268, 270
treatment aims 269
see also radiotherapy
laryngeal carcinoma 36–7
and alcohol 270, 274
hoarseness as symptom of 37
incidence 270
risk factors 270
and smoking 37, 270, 273–4
squamous cell carcinoma 36–7, 270
treatment for early tumours 270–2
see also radiotherapy
laryngeal diadochokinetic rates 77
laryngeal disorders
ageing 40, 67–8
benign swellings 43–4
classification 61, 62
combined treatments 33
congenital 35–6
differential diagnosis 32–3
inflammatory conditions 40
malignancies 36–7, 42–4
pathology of primary organic origin
35–40
pathology secondary to functional
disorder 34–5
primary non-organic or functional
(psychogenic) disorders 33–4
surgery for airway maintenance 41–2
surgery for diagnosis 40
surgical management 32–46
see also laryngitis; *and other
individual disorders*
laryngeal dystonia, *see* spasmodic
dysphonia
laryngeal electromyography (LEMG),
vocal fold paralysis 179
laryngeal endoscopy, vocal fold paralysis
178
laryngeal inlet 36
laryngeal irritants 35, 116, 122
laryngeal manipulation 324–5
laryngeal mucosa 62
laryngeal muscles
innervation 173–4
techniques to reduce tension 129–35
laryngeal nerve paralysis 62

unilateral recurrent laryngeal nerve
paralysis, phonosurgery 314–15
indications 314
the operation 314–15
postoperative follow-up and results
315
laryngeal nerves 173–4
superior laryngeal nerve injury 39
unilateral recurrent laryngeal nerve
resection 206
laryngeal pacing, electrical 189
laryngeal vibration 16
laryngeal webs 36, 62
children 42
laryngectomy
total 38, 43, 190
voice rehabilitation after 46
laryngitis 35, 40
allergic 67
classification 62, 65
distribution by age and gender 52
non-specific, causes of 30
prevalence 51
Laryngograph 16, 78, 298
in puberphonia 238
see also electrolaryngograph
laryngography 78–9
Lx waveform 78–9
see also electrolaryngography and
electroglottograph
laryngologists, in multidisciplinary voice
clinics 323
laryngomalacia 36
laryngopharyngeal reflux
control of 122
and vocal hyperfunction 114, 115
laryngoscopy 32, 40
direct 76
fibreoptic 32, 75
indirect 32, 75
rigid 75
see also microlaryngoscopy
laryngostroboscopes 17
laryngotracheoplasty 42
larynx
ageing 40, 67–8
atresia 35
benign swellings 43–4

control mechanisms 10
female hormone loss affecting 28
function test categories 202
functions of 4, 37, 112
in humans 5
neuromuscular activity 13–14
physical stress and 48
physiology 4–5
posterior clefts 36
reflex mechanisms 4, 11
reinnervation techniques 45
susceptibility to vocal hyperfunction
  112
transplant 46
trauma 44
 distribution by age and gender 52
 prevalence 51
vegetative function 4–5, 6
see also laryngeal *entries*
lasers
carbon dioxide (CO2) lasers 42, 43,
  44, 303
laser cordotomy 190
laser excision, for early laryngeal
  tumours 271
lateral cricoarytenoid muscle 13
laughing 9, 113, 236
laughing posture 130
lawyers
vocal usage level 283
see also professional voice users
La-zarus Training 256
learning, topographical learning 22
learning factors, vocal hyperfunction 115
learning mechanisms, faulty, resulting in
  vocal hyperfunction 122
learning styles, patients' 154–5
lecturers
vocal usage level 283
see also professional voice users
Lee Silverman Voice Treatment
  (LSVT(CM)) 158, 166, 170
LEMG, *see* laryngeal electromyography
lesions
classification 65
multiple 62
leukoplakia
distribution by age and gender 52

keratosis leukoplakia 65
prevalence 51
levodopa (L-dopa) 162, 207
life events theory of stress 146
lilt, in transsexuals 264–5
limb tremor 166
listening skills, in diagnostic interview
  149
locus of control 148, 149–50, 150
loft register 8–11, 234
mean air flow 9
see also falsetto
loudness 134–5
deaf vs. hearing speakers 230
LSVT(CM) (Lee Silverman Voice
  Treatment) 158, 166, 170
lung cancer, and vocal hyperfunction
  115
lung size, during puberty 25

magnetic resonance imaging (MRI) 17
vocal fold paralysis 178
male-female differences, *see* gender
  differences
manual circumlaryngeal therapy 131
manual laryngeal musculoskeletal
  tension reduction 131
marijuana, as laryngeal irritant 116, 122
Maximum Phonation Time (MPT) 77, 95
mechanical stress, *see* hyperfunction
mechanical voice disorders, *see* hyperfunction
medications
as laryngeal irritants 116
*see also individual drugs and drug
  types*
Meige's syndrome 193
membrane-cushion (mucosamuscle)
  theory of vocal fold function 14
meningitis, transient vocal fold paralysis
  in 176
menopause 28, 234
menstruation 25, 27
Mestinon 166
metaplasia 35
microlaryngoscopy 43, 44
suspension microlaryngoscopy 301,
  302

microsurgery
    in children 316–17
    for singers 317–18
'middlescents' 54, 67
military training instructors
    falsetto voice 8–9, 236
    vocal attrition 285
modal register 6–8
    mean air flow 8
Mood Adjective Check List (MACL) 205
motor neuron disease 62
movement disorders, organic 66
MRI, *see* magnetic resonance imaging
MS, *see* multiple sclerosis
mucosa
    fusiform thickening 304
    see also nodules
mucosal bridge, phonosurgery 313–14
mucosal wave 75–6
mucosamuscle (membrane-cushion)
        theory of vocal fold function 14
mucositis 274
mucus retention cysts, phonosurgery
        308–9
    indications 308–9
    the operation 309
    postoperative follow-up and results
        309
multidisciplinary teams
    children's voice therapy 91
    in spasmodic dysphonia diagnosis
        205
multidisciplinary voice clinics 319–39
    acoustics department 327
    administration 334–9
    advantages 319–22
    assessment 332–4
    audit 336–7
    clinical records 335
    continuity of care 320
    contributory medical factors 321
    cost-effectiveness 319
    counsellors in 326–7
    disadvantages 322–3
    equipment 327–32
    explanations to patients 335–6
    funding 323
    head, neck and shoulder girdle

dysfunction research 337–9
    history taking 335
    laryngologists in 323
    osteopaths in 324–5
    outcome and audit 336–7
    patient numbers 335
    patient satisfaction questionnaires
        337
    personnel 323–7
    phoneticians in 327
    physiotherapists in 324–5
    psychologists in 326–7
    psychotherapists 326–7
    referrals, inappropriate 321–2
    singing coaches in 325–6
    speech and language therapists in
        323–4
    support staff 336
    team decisions 320–1
    see also voice clinics
multiple sclerosis (MS)
    classification 62
    intensive voice treatment 170
    prevalence 161
    symptoms and signs 162
    and vocal fold movement 175
multiple system atrophy, vocal cord
        adduction and abduction 200
muscle tension, vs. stiffness 8
muscle tension dysphonias (MTDs)
    anteroposterior supraglottic contrac-
        tion (Type 3) 118, 119, 130
    laryngeal isometric pattern (Type 1)
        118
    lateral contraction (Type 2) 118, 119
    types of 118–19
    see also hyperfunction
muscles
    functions of, in vocal fold adjust-
        ments 13
    growth during puberty 24–5
    see also laryngeal muscles
muscular tension
    classification 62, 66
    stressors, exogenous and endoge-
        nous 140
muscular tension dysphonias, *see* hyper-
        function

musculoskeletal tension 150–1
    see also hyperfunction; stress
mutational falsetto 66
mutational retardation, male sexual 62
mutational voice disorders 234–44
    see also fundamental frequency;
        puberphonia
myasthenia gravis 39, 158
    classification 66
    pharmacological treatment 166
    prevalence 160
    surgical treatment 166
    symptoms 161
    transient vocal fold paralysis in 176
    voice characteristics, endoscopic
        findings 164–5
    voice characteristics, perceptual
        findings 163
myoelastic-aerodynamic theory of vocal
    fold function 14
myopathic dysphonia 63
myotomy, cricopharyngeal 46
myotonic muscular dystrophy 158
    prevalence 160
    symptoms 161
    voice characteristics, endoscopic
        findings 164–5
    voice characteristics, perceptual
        findings 163
myxoedema 62

nasal consonants 132, 133
nasal obstruction 62
nasal voice, in deaf speakers 224
nasendoscopy
    advantages 328–9
    disadvantage 329
    fibreoptic 75, 328
nasolaryngoscopy, fibreoptic 199
nasopharyngoscopes, fibreoptic 329
National Technical Institute for the Deaf
    (NTID) 223
neonates 19–20
    feeding difficulties 36
    subglottic stenosis 35–6
    see also infants
nerve-muscle junction dysfunctions 66

nerves
    vagus nerve 173, 179
    see also laryngeal nerves
neurochronaxic theory of vocal fold
    function 14
neurogenic voice disorders
    distribution by age and gender 52
    prevalence 51
neurolaryngology 173–4, 189
neurological voice disorders
    aetiology 158–60
    ataxic voice disorders 159, 170
    augmentative communication 170
    behavioural treatment 167
    classification 61, 62, 156–8
    definition 156
    demographic information 160–1
    diagnosis and findings 161–2
    flaccid voice disorders 158
    hyperadduction treatment 168–9
    hyperkinetic voice disorders 159–60
    hypoadduction treatment 167–8
    hypokinetic voice disorders 159
    incidence 160–1
    mixed voice disorders 160
    pathogenesis 158–60
    pharmacological treatments 166–7
    phonatory instability treatment
        169–70
    prevalence 160–1
    prognosis 170
    spastic (pseudobulbar) voice disor-
        ders 159, 163, 165
    speech pathology 167–70
    surgical treatment 166
    swallowing 162
    treatment options and outcomes
        165–70
    voice characteristics
        endoscopic findings 164–5
        perceptual findings 163–4
    voice evaluation 162
neurosis 62
nodules 34
    classification 62, 63, 65
    development of 58–9
    distribution by age and gender 50, 52

and hyperfunction 111
  phonosurgery 303–5
    indications 304–5
    the operation 304–5
    postoperative follow-up and results
      305
    preoperative speech therapy 304
    prevalence 50, 51
noise, in speech signal 83
'non-organic', meaning 137
non-organic voice disorders 137, 138,
    141
  classification 66
  in deaf speakers 231
non-verbal communication, transsexuals
    265
nucleus ambiguus 7

occupational factors, in patient assess-
    ment 72–3, 85
occupations requiring use of voice
    284–5
  see also professional voice users
oedema
  classification 62
  distribution by age and gender 50, 52
  and pitch range 67
  prevalence 50, 51
  after radiotherapy 272–3, 279
  vocal folds 34, 44
  see also Reinke's oedema
oesophagoscopy 40
oestradiol 28
oestrogen 28
omeprazole 122
opera singers
  vocal usage level 283
  see also professional voice users;
    singers
'organic'
  functional-organic dichotomy 58–61,
    139, 142
  meaning 137
organic movement disorders 66
organic voice disorders
  classification 62, 64
  in deaf speakers 231, 232

definition 58
osteopaths, in multidisciplinary voice
    clinics 324–5
over fortis 222, 225

Paedpharma 329
pallidotomy 166
palpation 325, 333, 339
palsy
  bulbar 62
  pseudobulbar 62
papilloma 65
  distribution by age and gender 52
  prevalence 51
papillomatosis 62
  juvenile 44
paralysis
  peripheral and central 66
  see also abductor paralysis; adductor
    paralysis; laryngeal nerve paralysis;
    vocal fold paralysis
paralytic dysphonia 63
paresis, see vocal fold paresis
parkinsonism 62, 159
Parkinson's disease
  classification 66
  hypokinetic voice disorders and 159
  idiopathic 160, 166
  neuropharmacological treatment
    166–7
  prevalence 160
  prognosis 170
  surgical treatment 166
  symptoms and signs 161, 162
  vocal cord adduction and abduction
    199–200
  and vocal fold movement 175
  voice characteristics, endoscopic
    findings 165
  voice characteristics, perceptual
    findings 163
patient assessment 69–88
  case history interviews, see case
    history interviews
  instrumental voice measurements, see
    voice measurements, instrumental
  multi-dimensional approach 69

in multidisciplinary voice clinics
    332–4
perceptual judgements, *see* percep-
    tual judgements in patient assess-
    ment
before phonosurgery 302
professional voice users 289–93
psychosocial 205
reasons for 69
of spasmodic dysphonia (SD)
    199–202, 215
transsexuals, male to female 259–61
of vocal hyperfunction 121
Patient Questionnaire of Vocal
    Performance 76, 86–8
patient satisfaction questionnaires 337
patients
    degree of effort 55
    discomfort to 55
    learning styles 154–5
    with ongoing problems 155
    psychological/psychosocial character-
        istics 143–5
    unable to respond to voice therapy
        154–5
PCLX voice analysis system 78
peaking, in transsexuals 264
perceptual judgements in patient assess-
    ment 73–7
    auditory voice quality ratings 73–5
    patient's opinion 76
    performance measures 77
    posture and body alignment 76–7
    visual laryngoscopic judgements 75–6
perceptual voice quality, after radio-
    therapy 275–7, 280
pergolide mesylate 166
period variability index 84
personal factors, in diagnosis and
    therapy 151
personality
    affecting voice disorder in deaf
        speakers 232
    and coping styles 147
    personality factors in patient assess-
        ment and management 72
    personality projection, transsexuals
        265

perturbation
    amplitude, *see* amplitude perturba-
        tion
    frequency, *see* frequency perturbation
    after radiotherapy 278
pharyngeal constriction, deaf vs. hearing
    speakers 230
pharyngitis 30
phenobarbital 167
phenothiazines 167
phonaesthesia 153, 154
Phonagel 314
phonation
    and articulation 1
    changes over time 234
    children 96
    hypervalvular 57, 61
    hypovalvular 61
    instability 169–70
    mode shift difficulties 236
    physiology of 1–17
    see also ventricular phonation
phonatory registers 6–11
    loft register 8–11
    modal register 6–8, 8
    pulse register 8
    register transitions 9
phoneticians, in multidisciplinary voice
    clinics 327
Phonetograms 81–2, 331–2
phoniatrists 63
phonosurgery 44–6, 301–18
    acquired benign lesions 303–9
    capillary telangiectases 305–6
    in children 316–17
    congenital lesions 309–15
    description 301
    epidermoid cysts 309–11
    equipment 302–3
    iatrogenic scars 315–16
    mucosal bridge 313–14
    mucus retention cysts 308–9
    nodules 303–5
    the operation 302–3
    polyps 306–7
    postoperative follow-up 303
    preoperative assessment 302
    Reinke's oedema 307–8

sulci 311–13
unilateral recurrent laryngeal nerve
    paralysis 314–15
videolaryngostroboscopy recording in
    assessment of 302
vocal assessment 302
vocal fold paralysis 186–9
  future direction 189
  intrafold injection procedures 186–8
  laryngeal framework surgery 188–9
  reinnervation techniques 189
  see also microsurgery
phonotrauma, *see* hyperfunction
physicians, vocal usage level 283
physiotherapists, in multidisciplinary
    voice clinics 324–5
pitch
  alteration of 45
  deaf speakers 223–4, 230
  direct modification of, in vocal hyper-
    function 134, 135
  establishment of, in transsexuals 263
  voice breaks 25
  see also high pitch
polyps
  classification 62, 63, 65
  distribution by age and gender 50, 52
  and hyperfunction 111
  phonosurgery 306–7
    indications 306
    the operation 307
    postoperative follow-up and results
      307
  prevalence 50, 51
posterior cricoarytenoid (PCA) muscle
    13, 174
posture
  patient's 76–7
  postural education 127, 128
  professional voice users 293, 297, 298
  vocal hyperfunction 114
pregnancy 28
presbylaryngis 30, 68
primidone 167
professional voice users 50–4, 283–300
  achieving change 294–6
  acoustics, effect of 294, 296
  and ageing 294

anxiety 289
breathing exercises 299
case history information 289–90
environmental factors 286, 293–4,
    296–7
exercises 298–9
factors in poor vocal practice 297–8
group voice work 300
intervention and management
    288–93, 299–300
interviewing 289
jaw exercises 299
levels of vocal usage 283
occupational demands on the voice
    293–4
patient's perspective 290–2
posture 293, 297, 298
stress and 292
treatment regimes 298–9
vocal abuse and misuse 287
vocal attrition incidence 284–5
vocal problems 299
voice care and development 285–6
voice care training 283–4, 285–6, 291,
    294–5
voice loss 287–8
voice production 286
voice use 286
see also occupations requiring use of
    voice; singers; teachers
progesterone 28
propranolol 167
prostaglandins 116
proteoglycans 12
pseudo-cysts 304
'pseudoauthoritative' voice 135
pseudobulbar palsy 62, 163
pseudobulbar voice disorders, *see*
    spastic (pseudobulbar) voice disor-
    ders
psychodynamic theory 139–40
'psychogenic'
  vs. 'functional' 141
  meaning 137–8, 141–2
psychogenic aphonia, studies 143–4
psychogenic dysphonia 48, 63
  distribution by age and gender 52
  examination for 200

prevalence 51
vs. spasmodic dysphonia 200
psychogenic voice disorders 59, 141–2
classification 60–2, 64
and gender 54
psychological characteristics, patients'
143–5
psychological considerations, in patient
assessment 72, 85
psychologists, in multidisciplinary voice
clinics 326–7
psychology, see health psychology
psychosocial consequences, of voice
disorders 72, 288
psychosocial factors
in diagnosis and therapy 151
patients' characteristics 143–5
in voice change 142–3
psychosocial issues 145
psychosocial problems, children 96
psychotherapists, in multidisciplinary
voice clinics 326–7
puberphonia
case histories 240–1
causes 234–7
classification 62
establishing the new voice 239–41
laryngography 238
rejection of new voice 239–40
tests 237–9
treatment 237–9
puberty 24–6
and climate 24
growth during 24–5
vocal tract changes 24
voice changes 25
pulmonary malignancy, as cause of vocal
fold paralysis 175
pulse register 8
see also glottal fry
pyridostigmine 166

quality of life 144–5
questioning techniques 70
questionnaires
in history taking 70, 72
Patient Questionnaire of Vocal
Performance 76, 86–8

patient satisfaction questionnaires
337

radiotherapy
aerodynamic/acoustic voice measurements 277–9
CHART (continuous, hyperfractionated, accelerated radiotherapy)
272, 273
complications 273
for early laryngeal tumours 270, 271
field sizes 273
fractionation schedules 272
for laryngeal cancer 43, 268
laryngeal tissues 272–4
oedema after 272–3, 279
time for voice to recover after 274
and vocal fold vibration, see vocal fold
vibration
voice quality after 268–82
voice therapy in patient rehabilitation
279–82
receptionists, vocal usage level 283
records, clinical records in multidisciplinary voice clinics 335
reflex mechanisms, larynx 4, 11
reflux oesophagitis 30
registers, see phonatory registers
Reinke's oedema 34, 40, 65
phonosurgery 307–8
indications 307
the operation 307–8
postoperative outcome and results
308
reinnervation 179, 180, 189
reinnervation techniques, larynx 45
relative average perturbation 83
relaxation 151, 298
for transsexuals 262
renal problems 94
repression, as coping mechanism 147–8
resonance
chest resonance in transsexuals 260,
264
children 92, 100
resonant voice therapy 132–4
respiration 1–4, 95–6
children 95–6

gender differences 3
pneumographic devices 4
vocal hyperfunction 114
respiratory dysfunction, in vocal hyper-
    function 127–8
respiratory tract, upper respiratory tract
    infections 67, 71, 324
respiratory volume, and ageing 30
rheumatoid arthritis 39, 179
rhinitis, allergic 67
role playing, transsexuals 265
rough voice
    benign vs. cancerous lesions 275
    after radiotherapy 276

s/z ratio 77
salespeople, *see* professional voice users
sarcoidosis 40
scars, iatrogenic 315–16
screamer's nodes 34
screaming 112, 113
    see also hyperfunction
secondary voice disorders 231–2
self-monitoring
    of loudness 134–5
    in resonant voice therapy 133
    of vocal performance 126–7
sex-change operations 246, 247, 249,
    252
sex chromosomes 248–9
sex hormones 39–40
    female 27–8
sexual mutational retardation, male 62
SFF, *see* speaking fundamental
    frequency
Sharma effect 298
shimmer (amplitude perturbation) 82,
    84, 278
shouting
    teaching less harmful methods of
    124–5
    see also hyperfunction
Shy Drager syndrome 189
    vocal cord adduction and abduction
    200
    and vocal fold movement 175
sigh 129–30
sighing 236

sign language 221
silicone 187
singers 128
    and ageing 29, 294
    castrati 236
    counter-tenors 236
    dehydration 297
    falsetto 236–7
    'grace days' 27
    hormonal changes 27
    laryngeal manipulation 324
    male altos 236, 238
    microsurgery 317–18
    oedema 67
    popular singers 236–7
    pre-menstrual phase 25
    training 125
    vocal usage level 283
    voice care training and development
    291
    voice disorders in 54
    see also professional voice users
singer's nodes 34
singing
    belting 113
    high-quiet singing 77
    hyperfunctional behaviours 112
singing coaches, in multidisciplinary
    voice clinics 325–6
sinusitis, and vocal hyperfunction 115
situational factors, vocal hyperfunction
    114–15
smoking
    ignoring medical advice 150
    and laryngeal carcinoma 37, 270
    as laryngeal irritant 35
    and radiotherapy 270, 273–4
    and vocal fold oedema 34
sneezing 113
social factors, in patient assessment
    72–3, 85
social issues 145
spasmodic (spastic) dysphonia (SD) 138,
    162, 192–218
    abductor spasmodic dysphonia, *see*
    abductor spasmodic dysphonia
    adductor spasmodic dysphonia, *see*
    adductor spasmodic dysphonia

assessment 199–202
by speech and language therapist
    201, 215
voice assessment protocol 201–2,
    214–15
asymptomatic vocal behaviour 194–5
background 193
case history format 201, 213–14
classification 66
compensatory modes of speaking
    197–8
as a conversion disorder 193
current thoughts 193
definition 193–4
degrees of severity 198
description 192–3
diagnosis and the multidisciplinary
    team 205, 215
differential diagnosis 199–202
distribution by age and gender 53
epidemiology 194–5
hyperfunctional voice disorders
    associated with 200–1
idiopathic 201
incidence 194
management 216
mechanism of 195
medical treatment 167
misdiagnosis 205
neurological examination 199–200
one disorder or many? 198–9
otolaryngological investigation 199
perceptual voice ratings 203–4
prevalence 51, 194
psychiatric assessment 200
vs. psychogenic dysphonia 200
psychosocial assessment 205
referral for neurological opinion 33–4
speech and language therapist's role
    201, 215–17
stigma, concept and management of
    211
symptomatology 194
symptoms 198
treatment 206–9, 216–17
with botulinum toxin, see botulinum
    toxin treatment

counselling 211
non-medical 206
pharmacological 207
previous methods 206
surgical 45–6, 206
voice therapy 206, 216–17
video recordings 202, 205
voice assessment methods 202–5
voice assessment protocol 201–2,
    214–15
voice characteristics 195–8
perceptual findings 164
as a voice sign 205
voice tests, classification 202
Spasmodic Dysphonia Society, USA 211
spastic aphonia 193
spastic dysphonia, see spasmodic
    dysphonia
spastic (pseudobulbar) voice disorders
    159
voice characteristics, endoscopic
    findings 165
voice characteristics, perceptual
    findings 163
speaking fundamental frequency (SFF)
    26, 80
and ageing 29
and children 23
gender differences 26, 29, 80
mean vs. modal 80
ranges 23, 26
reading vs. conversational 80
women 26–7, 29
see also fundamental frequency
spectrography 331
spectrographic analysis 202, 203
speech, gender indicators 255
speech and language therapists
in multidisciplinary voice clinics
    323–4
role in male to female transsexualism
    256–66
role in spasmodic dysphonia (SD)
    201, 215–17
speech habits, gender differences 265
speech markers 255
speech stereotypes 255

Speech Viewer 154
speech waveform, acoustic analysis 82–3
squamous cell carcinoma (SCC) 36–7,
    270
stability, vocal 74
stammering 239
stenosis
    children 42
    distribution by age and gender 53
    prevalence 51
    subglottic 35–6
steroids 60, 324
stiffness, vs. muscle tension 8
Stock Exchange dealers, vocal attrition
    285
strabismus 207
strain 74
stress 144, 146, 150
    coping with 147
    life events theory 146
    ongoing 143, 146
    phases of 146
    and professional voice users 292
    see also musculoskeletal tension
stress patterns in speech 5
stressors, exogenous and endogenous
    140
stretch marks 311–12, 312, 313
strident voice, see harsh voice
stridor 35, 36, 41, 176
stroboscopes 328
stroboscopic observations, after radio-
    therapy 274–5
stroboscopy 75–6, 327, 332–3
    differentiating between vocal fold
        paralysis and immobility 178
stroke
    incidence 160
    intensive voice treatment 170
structural abnormalities 61, 62
subglottic haemangioma 42
subglottic stenosis 35–6
sulci, phonosurgery 311–13
    indications 312
    the operation 312–13
    postoperative follow-up and results
        313

sulcus glottidis 311, 312
sulcus vocalis 65, 305
supervision, see clinical supervision
suppression, as coping mechanism
    147–8
supraglottitis 41
supranuclear palsies, vocal cord adduc-
    tion and abduction 200
surgery
    for airway maintenance 41–2
    for diagnosis of laryngeal disorders 40
    in disease cure or control 42–4
    laryngeal disorders 32–46
    laryngeal malignancies 42–4, 268, 270
    neurological voice disorders 166
    sex-change operations 246, 247, 249,
        252
    spasmodic dysphonia 45–6, 206
    vocal cord surgery for transsexuals
        266
    voice rehabilitation after laryngec-
        tomy 46
    see also microsurgery; phonosurgery
surgical trauma 176
suspension microlaryngoscopy 301, 302
swallowing (deglutition) 4, 100, 162
    in neonates 20
symptomatic voice therapy 141, 143
syphilis 40

teachers
    and ageing 294
    environmental factors 293–4, 296–7
    high risk of voice disorder 287–8
    INSET training days 291
    perceptual effects of teaching on the
        voice 292–3
    postural effects 293
    specific vocal problems 299
    vocal attrition 284, 285
    and vocal hyperfunction 111
    vocal usage level 283
    voice care training and development
        285–6, 287, 291
    voice disorders in 54
    see also professional voice users
Teflon 45, 186–7, 314, 315

telangiectases, *see* capillary telangiectases
telescopes 328–9
television monitors, high resolution
   329–30
Ten-step (10-step) Outline for Voice
   Abuse 123
tense voice
   in deaf speakers 223
   after radiotherapy 276
tensilon 166
tension, laryngeal, deaf vs. hearing
   speakers 230
thalamectomy 166
thalamotomy 166
therapy
   adverse drug therapy 62
   children, *see* children, treatment of
      voice problems
   hormone therapy for transsexuals
      245, 247, 249
   manual circumlaryngeal therapy 131
   personal factors in 151
   psychosocial factors in 151
   vocal fold paralysis
      bilateral 190
      unilateral 180–9
   see also radiotherapy; voice therapy;
      and under individual disorders
throat clearing 113, 115
   see also hyperfunction
thymectomy 166
thyroplasty 45, 166
   Isshiki Type 1 188
thyrotoxicosis 62
thyroxine 40
tissue changes, classification 65
tobacco, as laryngeal irritant 116, 122
tonal languages 5
tone focus alteration 132–3
tonsils, during puberty 24
topographical learning 22
total laryngectomy 38, 43, 190
tracheobroncoscopy 40
tracheotomy 41, 190
   in bilateral abductor paralysis 38
   in children 42
   in juvenile papillomatosis 44

training, in voice care, professional voice
   users 283–4, 285–6, 291, 294–5
transplants
   adrenal and fetal cells 166
   laryngeal 46
transsexualism 49, 245–50
   cause 248
   conflict 62
   hormone therapy 245, 247, 249
   vs. transvestism 250
transsexuals, male to female 245–67
   acoustic and linguistic considerations
      255
   'acting' 258–9
   articulation techniques 263, 264
   assessment for voice therapy 259–61
   breathing 262–3
   case histories 251–4
   chest resonance elimination 260, 264
   communication skills 256
      non-verbal 265
   counselling 257
   definition 248
   electrolysis 257
   group learning and support 246–7
   instrumentation in voice therapy 266
   intonation 264
   lilt 264–5
   linguistic considerations 255
   marriage 250
   name changing 256
   pattern of progress 250
   peaking 264
   personality projection 265
   pitch establishment 263
   preconditions for gender reassign-
      ment 247
   proof of ongoing medical treatment
      256–7
   referral to other agencies 256–7
   referral to speech and language thera-
      pist 247
   relaxation 262
   role playing 265
   sex-change operations 246, 247, 249,
      252
   speech and language therapist's
      responsibilities 256–66

summary 266–7
therapist's personal involvement 257
vocal cord surgery 266
vocal experimentation 262
voice modification 256, 257–9
transvestism 250
trauma
as cause of vocal fold paralysis 175,
176, 177, 189
classification 62, 65
intubation trauma 94
laryngeal 44
distribution by age and gender 52
prevalence 51
mechanical, vocal folds 111
surgical, transient vocal fold paralysis
in 176
traumatic dysphonia 63
travelling wave, *see* mucosal wave
treatment, *see* therapy
tremor 62, 161, 162
see also essential tremor; limb
tremor; vocal tremor
tuberculosis 40
tumours 62
TNM staging 269
TV monitors, high resolution 329–30
twang 125–6, 130

ulcers, *see* contact ulcers
'um-hum' procedure 132, 135
Unified Spasmodic Dysphonia Rating
Scale (USDRS) 204
upper respiratory tract infections 67, 71,
324

vagitis uterinus 20
vagus nerve 173–4, 179
vascular corditis 305
vasomotor monochorditis 63
vegetative function, larynx 4–5, 6
ventricular phonation 66, 185, 186
distribution by age and gender 52
prevalence 51
VHI (Vocal Handicap Index) 288
vibration
glottal 6
laryngeal 16

see also vocal fold vibration
video equipment 329–30
video recorders 329
video recording 202, 205
videoendoscopy, to assess vocal hyperfunction 119, 120
videokymography 333
videolaryngostroboscopy in assessment
for phonosurgery 302
videostrobolaryngoscopy, in voice clinics
322
videostroboscopy, in voice clinics 332
Vietnamese 6
virilization, female 60, 62
vision, and speaker–listener distances 29
Visipitch 154, 298
Visispeech 203, 266
vitamin C, as laryngeal irritant 116
vocal abuse 59
as cause of nodules 34
definition 117–18
industrial attempts to mitigate 285
as laryngeal irritant 35
professional role affecting 287
psycho-emotional causes 138
radiotherapy and 280
symptom-based therapy 140
vs. vocal misuse 118
see also hyperfunction
Vocal Abuse Reduction Program 123
vocal accommodation 22
vocal attrition 54
incidence in professional voice users
284–5
'vocal elite' 19
vocal fold function
membrane-cushion (mucosamuscle)
theory 14
myoelastic-aerodynamic theory 14
neurochronaxic theory 14
theories of 14–15
vocal fold paralysis 37–9, 172–3
abductor paralysis, *see* abductor
paralysis
adductor paralysis, *see* adductor
paralysis
aetiology 175–6, 177
airflow/air pressure studies 180, 185

aspiration 182, 183, 190
bilateral 189–90
  aetiology 177
  children 42
  congenital 176
  lesions involved 174
  tracheotomy 41, 42
chest X-ray 178–9
children 42, 94
compensatory behaviours 184–5, 186
congenital vs. acquired 176
diagnosis 176–80
diagnostic practices and cost effective-
    ness 180
diagnostic testing and evaluation
    177–80
distribution by age and gender 50, 52
imaging studies 178–9
incidence 174–5
laryngeal electromyography (LEMG)
    179
laryngeal endoscopy 178
phonosurgery 186–9
prevalence 50, 51, 174–5
pulmonary malignancy as cause of
    175
related conditions 39
superior laryngeal nerve injury 39
transient 176
trauma as cause of 175, 176, 177, 189
unilateral 174, 190–1
  glottal incompetence due to 187–8,
    188
  phonosurgery 186–9
  treatment 180–9
  voice therapy 183–6
vocal fold paresis 172–3
  distribution by age and gender 52
  prevalence 51
  unilateral 174
vocal fold vibration, effect of radio-
    therapy on 274–9
  acoustic voice quality measurements
    277–9
  aerodynamic voice quality measure-
    ments 277–9
  airflow measures 277–8
  fundamental frequency 278–9, 281–2

perceptual and self-rated voice quality
    275–7, 280
  perturbation measures 278
  stroboscopic observations 274–5
vocal folds
  atrophy after radiotherapy 275
  body-cover structure 14–15
  bowing, see bowing of vocal folds
  experimental inflammation 57
  function, see vocal fold function
  immobility 173, 179
  mechanical trauma 111
  medialization 45
  movements of 48
  muscle functions 13
  nodules, see nodules
  oedema 34, 44
  paralysis, see vocal fold paralysis
  paresis, see vocal fold paresis
  during puberty 24
  structure 11–13
  surgery, transsexuals 266
  vibration, see vocal fold vibration
vocal frequency, see fundamental
    frequency; speaking fundamental
    frequency; and frequency entries
vocal function exercises 134
vocal gymnastics 141
Vocal Handicap Index (VHI) 288
vocal hyperfunction, see hyperfunction
vocal instability, treatment 169–70
vocal maturity, height vs. age as influ-
    ence on 25
vocal misuse 59
  definition 117, 118
  industrial attempts to mitigate 285
  laryngeal structure changes associ-
    ated with 231
  professional role affecting 287
  psycho-emotional causes 138
  symptom-based therapy 140
  vs. vocal abuse 118
  see also hyperfunction
vocal performers, see professional voice
    users
Vocal Profile Analysis (VPA) 74, 74–5,
    225–7, 232–3
  neutral points 227

parameters included in 228
supralaryngeal, laryngeal and
    prosodic features 226–7, 228, 229
tension features 228, 229
vocal profiles, deaf vs. hearing groups
    227–31
vocal stability 74
vocal strain 139–40
vocal trauma, *see* hyperfunction
vocal tremor 159, 161
    endoscopic findings 165
    treatment 167
'vocal yokels' 19
vocalis muscle 13
voice, intelligibility vs. acceptability 221
voice analysis systems 78
voice assessment, *see* patient assessment
Voice Break Factor (VBF) 202
voice care training, professional voice
    users 283–4, 285–6, 291, 294–5
voice changes
    in later life 28–31
    psychosocial factors 142–3
    voice breaks during puberty 25
voice clinics 16, 32, 33
    see also multidisciplinary voice clinics
voice development 18–31
voice disorders
    behavioural descriptions 140–1
    behavioural vs. organic 61, 62
    causes 48–50
    continuum of 140
    children's, incidence 89
    classification 55–8, 62
    aetiological 63–6
    based on acoustic phenomena 56–8
    definitions 47, 49
    developmental perspective 67–8
    distribution by age and gender 52–3
    functional, *see* functional voice disor-
        ders
    functional vs. organic factors 58–61
    as interactive process 142–3
    neurological, *see* neurological voice
        disorders
    non-organic, *see* non-organic voice
        disorders
    organic, *see* organic voice disorders

prevalence 50–4
psychogenic, *see* psychogenic voice
    disorders
see also dysphonia
Voice Handicap Index 72, 76
voice history interviews, *see* case history
    interviews
voice loss, in professional voice users
    287–8
voice measurements, instrumental
    acoustic analysis of speech waveform
        82–3
    aerodynamic measurements 80–1
    after radiotherapy 277–9
    amplitude perturbation (shimmer)
        82, 84
    frequency perturbation (jitter) 82, 83
    fundamental frequency, *see* funda-
        mental frequency; speaking funda-
        mental frequency
    laryngography, *see* Laryngograph;
        electrolaryngography
    noise in speech signal 83
    vs. 'objective' 78
    Phonetograms 81–2, 331–2
voice measures, objective 78, 202–5
    perceptual voice ratings 203–4
    psychosocial assessment 205
    test classification 202
    video recording 205
voice modification, transsexuals 257–9
voice pictures 101
voice production
    listeners' judgements 49–50
    professional voice users 286
Voice Program for Children 123
voice quality
    definition 225
    gender differences 26
    in hearing impaired speakers 222–3
    parameters of 55–6
    after radiotherapy, *see* radiotherapy
    see also auditory voice quality ratings
voice rehabilitation after laryngectomy
    46
voice tests, classification 202
voice therapy
    patients unable to respond to 154–5

rehabilitation after radiotherapy
    279–82
resonant voice therapy 132–4
symptomatic 141, 143
transsexuals 256, 257–9
unilateral vocal fold paralysis 183–6
see also therapy
vowel play 131
VPA, *see* Vocal Profile Analysis

war cries 8–9, 236
wellness programmes 29
whispering aphonia 143
whispering dysphonia 144
whistle register 237
whooping cough, and vocal hyperfunc-
    tion 115
women
    fundamental frequency 234, 242–3
    speaking fundamental frequency
        26–7, 29

hormones 27–8
psychological difficulties 145
speaking fundamental frequency
    26–7, 29
and voice disorders 144, 145
see also gender differences
World Health Organization, classifica-
    tion of impairments, disabilities
    and handicaps 287

X-ray, chest, in vocal fold paralysis 178
Xylocaine 329

yawn-sigh 100, 129–30
yawning 100, 236
Ybuzz 133
yelling 112, 113
    'yell well' 125
    see also hyperfunction
yodelling 9, 236